The International Library of Psychology

THE LAW WITHIN

Founded by C. K. Ogden

The International Library of Psychology

GENERAL PSYCHOLOGY
In 38 Volumes

THE LAW WITHIN

SIR BAMPFYLDE FULLER

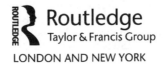

Routledge
Taylor & Francis Group

LONDON AND NEW YORK

First published in 1926 by
Kegan Paul, Trench, Trubner & Co., Ltd

2 Park Square, Milton Park, Abingdon, Oxfordshire OX14 4RN
711 Third Avenue, New York, NY 10017

First issued in paperback 2014

Routledge is an imprint of the Taylor and Francis Group, an informa business

British Library Cataloguing in Publication Data
A CIP catalogue record for this book
is available from the British Library

The Law Within
ISBN 978-0415-21021-8
General Psychology: 38 Volumes
ISBN 0415-21129-8
The International Library of Psychology: 204 Volumes
ISBN 0415-19132-7

ISBN 13: 978-1-138-87526-5 (pbk)
ISBN 13: 978-0-415-21021-8 (hbk)

CONTENTS

vii

CONTENTS

THE LAW WITHIN

INTRODUCTION

I wonder that you will still be talking, Signor Benedick: nobody marks you.

During the last fifteen years my thoughts have been occupied very closely with endeavours to discover the *laws* which underlie human nature—to bring within the domain of scientific generalization man's various activities—whether in industry, politics or war, in self-centred, social or religious life, in science or in art. I have written several books on the subject, which, it must be confessed, have met with very scant attention. For this they have in some measure themselves to blame. In exploring an uncharted country, I have at times been misled by what seemed to be landmarks, and have strayed into " dead ends ", the only escape from which is through a wilderness of words. But the general correctness of my alignment is proved by the fact that, in advancing along it, clues have continually presented themselves that guide one's steps over difficulties which seemed to be insurmountable, so that each excursion, while more successful than its predecessor, has, nevertheless, been a continuation of it. I now make a further attempt to attract attention to what is practically a new science. It is mainly concerned with the living energies of motive, emotion and thought which intervene between the *stimuli* to which we are subject and our behaviour in response to their stimulation. They may be compared to the electric current which passes between the transmitter and receiver of a telephonic circuit, or to the ethereal radiations that flash between a distributing station and the instruments that give voice to its messages. In both cases, an immaterial energy that is unperceivable by the senses, intervenes between stimuli and manifestations that are of material character or origin. But, whereas we can know nothing of electricity or radiation except by inference, we are, through consciousness, in direct touch with our motives, emotions and thoughts.   The information that we receive is cryptic and confusing.   But it may be possible to interpret it.

This science may not inappropriately be named *Biothymology*.[1] It differs radically from Psychology.   For this confesses in its very name that it is limited to one side only of our dual constitution— the animative—not realizing that the truth is undiscoverable if the contributing forces are considered apart.   Our motives are *blends* of the animative and the physical, or compulsive.   It is for this reason that psychology, promising so much, has accomplished so little.   What has it given us in the way of *laws*, the discovery of which distinguishes scientific knowledge from simple experience ?   Its vague generalities are no doubt pleasing to those who, while distrusting religious dogmas, wish to feel, nevertheless, that there is something of the supernatural within them.   And, since one may excel in badness as well as goodness, there is something attractive in the preposterous idea of the Freudian school that man's imaginative faculties are the fruits of sexual lust, or *libido*. Nor is the failure of psychology to be wondered at.   For it has closed its eyes to the avenues that lead to truth.   It has practically ignored the law of evolution, which, like the thread of Ariadne, can guide us through the obscurest problems.   If we accept this law, we must search for the germs of our faculties in the humblest animals.   They also must have souls, although in embryo.   It has, moreover, erred in taking too " objective " a view of life ; it has given too large a share of its attention to our *measurable* relations with the outside world through sensation and behaviour, whereas the causes, or motives, of our various activities are nervous conditions that are within us, and can only be detected by self-observation.   Our sensations, it may be urged, are *causes*.   But only so far that they " set off " internal forces as a match explodes gunpowder.   A stimulus has no effect upon us if we do not meet it with the explosive energy of a like or dislike.   Food does not tempt us if we have no appetite ; repose is not alluring if we are not fatigued. The causes of our behaviour are conditions—in consciousness " feelings "—that are within us and are discernible only by " subjective perception ", so to speak—by a laborious process of self-observation. The behaviour of other persons—and of animals generally—is of evidential use only as manifesting internal conditions which are similar or analogous to our own.

It is obvious that if we behave angrily it is because we feel angry.

[1] The meaning of θυμός is sufficiently broad to include all the vital forces of

Behaviour can no more be dissociated from the internal energies that actuate it than can the vibrations of a telephone from the electric current that is their cause. Yet there are psychologists who appear to regard feelings as merely *accompanying* actions and utterances—as a " descant " upon them, so to speak—so that one is afraid *because* he runs away, or sorrowful *because* he weeps. There is, no doubt, something in experience that supports this inversion of the real order of things. It is a fact that by deliberately smiling we can keep up our spirits, that anger grows if we express it violently, so that in a measure it is true that " manners makyth man ". But these are simply illustrations of auto-suggestive, or memorial, re-stimulation, and this commonly runs backwards. Apart from it, conduct and speech are the outcome of internal nervous conditions which urge external activity, and are relieved by it. Is there anyone who, under the influence of strong emotion, has not felt the relief that is given by doing or saying something ?

The sciences of Biology and Physiology have been similarly prejudiced by the idea that functional are wholly distinct from " motiving " activities, so that physical researches can logically stop short of investigating passions and thoughts—conditions which exist as actually as secretion or fatigue. Moreover, these sciences have closed their eyes to the duality which must exist in the constitution.of all living organisms—whether animals or plants—that are formed by the combination of two sexual elements. Consequently the mass of facts which they have accumulated tends to obscure truths of a general kind rather than to reveal them. The law of evolution was a great discovery. It is a fact that an individual comes to maturity by the growth of new points out of old ; and it seems clear that individuals have been diversified, and new species created, by a similar process of differentiating growth. But the cause of evolution, and the instruments by which it introduces its novelties, are still in dispute. Influenced by the utilitarian spirit of the age, biologists have clung to the belief that the changes which have come about in the forms and faculties of living things were always *purposeful*, in the sense that they were of service in enabling a plant or animal to struggle for its life or propagate its kind. They have, for instance, eagerly seized hold of any instances in which form or colour may have a protective use, and have ignored the multitude of cases in which they advertise an animal's existence to its enemies. If one butterfly is so coloured as to be inconspicuous, hundreds gaily flaunt themselves in bravado. How *dangerous*, from the utilitarian point of

pursuers.   A utility is found for it in attracting the female's admiration.   But the sparrow—with no song but a chirp—is by no means
an unsuccessful lover.   Evolution may be *expressive* as well as
useful.   Nature may be as magnificently purposeless as Art.

If we bring the working of evolution to the only test in our power—
the development of our own faculties—we find that each new attainment is the product of surplus nervous energy, and comes about
through the endowment of a consequence, or an instrument, with
activity.   Pleasure is surplus energy ; it becomes the cause of the
conditions of attractedness of which we are conscious as " likes ".
Success is the consequence of an effort ; an idea of it is the directive
force in willing, and in the various forms of ambition which play so
immensely important a part in human life.   Exhilaration is the
consequence of success ; it becomes admiration by stimulating a
like ; and admiration, with its fruit in respect, is the cause of the
loyalties which bind society together into an ordered whole.   Moreover, admiration stimulates the imaginative faculties ; an artist is
inspired by admiration of his subject.   Language and dress are
primitively *instruments ;* they become the subjects of cult in themselves, because they are admirable.   If faculties evolve in this way,
there is a *prima facie* case for holding that organs do so also, and
that evolution has advanced through the production and utilization
of surplus energy.   When none is generated, life stagnates.

The studies with which this book is occupied are, then, so far
biological that they proceed by the method of evolution.   They
bring living energies within the domain of law by tracing them back
to their simplest manifestations.   It will commonly be held that
there is no " success " in this achievement—that, in reducing human
nature to law, we are humiliating it by depriving it of all spontaneity
of action and nobility of descent.   This argument, however, would
rob the heavens of their majesty because their movements can be
calculated.   It would deny beauty to flowers because they spring
from insignificant seeds and are rooted in earth.   Human nature has
its flowers which we shall appreciate none the less because we know
their natural history.   And our knowledge will be of inestimable
practical value in teaching us how to cultivate them.

There are particular reasons why science has turned its eyes
away from the energies of human life, and has accepted them as
insolubly mysterious.   Their real character is obscured by the form
in which we are conscious of them ; they are confused with their
mental presentments as " feelings "—that is to say, with " the

but are inclined to regard them as merely incidental to action and speech—as conditions of mind as opposed to those of body. But, in fact, they exist quite apart from our consciousness of them. Certain primitive likes and dislikes, for instance, affect us during sleep, and we can, when asleep, make an effort in response to a disagreeable stimulus. The nerves are affected by the shock of an injury irrespective of any consciousness of pain, so that patients may suffer very greatly from the effects of surgical operations which they have not felt. It seems that we can even think in some fashion when asleep, for we not infrequently awake with the solution of a difficulty that had puzzled us over-night. Consciousness is a faculty which is as distinct from the internal energies of which it makes us aware as the sight of the moon is from the moon itself. A motive or emotion may present itself in a purely mental form as a *thought* or a *recollection* of one. But, as a living energy, it exists independently of thought, and our consciousness of it is merely a mental reflection of its activity.

Moreover, motives and emotions are elusive because they are not perceivable by the sense organs, as are their stimuli in sensation, or their effects in movement and utterance. Accordingly it is only through the behaviour or words of others that we can apprehend their feelings. But it would be ridiculously short-sighted to deny the existence of energetic conditions because the senses cannot perceive them. We have no direct perception of gravity and electricity. Yet we are assured of their existence, not merely by the material, sensible consequences that they produce, but by the fact that their operation is subject to certain laws which determine their volume or intensity. The strength of a like also varies with the attractiveness of its stimulus, and the violence of a fit of anger depends upon the degree of the injury that arouses it. These motives are, then, as actual as electricity and resemble electricity in being immaterial. The researches of modern science appear, indeed, to show that what we call " matter " does not exist as such, apart from a subtle, imperceptible, " ethereal " element, and that electricity is a condition of energetic inequilibrium resulting from the dissociation of this partnership. Nature has, then, an ethereal as well as a material side, and the actuality of the former is proved by the fact that " material " consequences may result from immaterial as well as from material causes. Heat is generated by friction or chemical action ; it is also generated by solar radiation, which is an immaterial or ethereal influence, and differs from heat in that be caused mechanically or chemically. But, under the influence of gravity, it results from a force that is beyond our powers of explanation. The weather, again, is affected by such material causes as moisture and wind movement ; but it is also changed by the action of unperceivable energies that have so far not been reduced to law. This curious duality is also to be observed in causes that affect ourselves. The activity of thought can be increased by promoting the flow of blood to the head, as by lying down ; but it is also quickened by admiration, whether of ourselves or others. An illness may be cured by a material remedy ; it may also be cured by such immaterial means as a sudden shock to the nerves, or the influence of faith or of suggestion. We are exhilarated by alcohol ; we are also exhilarated by a compliment.

Life and electricity may, accordingly, both be termed " dematerialized " forces, and there are some curious points of contact between them. It has been proved that the nervous current set up by sensation possesses electrical affinities ; and there are creatures, such as the electrical eel and the torpedo fish, which are actually endowed with electrical generators. It is characteristic of electricity that it assumes one or other of two contrary phases. Living energy is also two-phased, moving us attractedly or repelledly, pleasurably or displeasurably. As electricity may be generated by friction or by chemical action, so the sense organs may be stimulated vibratively, as in touch, hearing and sight ; chemically, as in smell, And protoplasm, from which life cannot be dissociated, appears to be characterized by an unceasing process of disintegration and reintegration, such as, we may believe, might generate electrical conditions.

Electrical energy being amenable to law, there is no *prima facie* reason why living energy should be free from it. We are inclined to repel any attempt to reduce life to rule, because the exercise of the will is one of the most prominent of our faculties, and this seems to be arbitrary, and untrammelled by conditions. But we shall find that, as a matter of fact, the will is stimulated in regular course by a shock or discord, without which there is no effort ; and that the course of volition is invariably led by ideas of success or failure that are derived from experience. In its origin, and in its course of action, volition is, then, governed by laws. That energy should be originated by discord is, no doubt, in flat contradiction to the theory of the Conservation of Energy, which until lately was accepted as an axiom of science. But this assumption has now been shaken may stray for a moment from the domain of this book, it seems clear that in the inanimate world also energy is developed by the shock of discord. For shock is involved in the friction which originates heat and electricity ; and heat, the cause of explosion, certainly appears to introduce an element of discord into the things which it affects.

The internal energies to which we were referring are often spoken of as *subjective*, and since frequent use will be made of this term, and of its contrary " objective ", it is necessary to define them. Our *subjective* activities are those which elude the senses but become apparent to us through consciousness. They comprise our motives and emotions. These are what we mean when we speak of " ourselves ", and our consciousness of them is " self-consciousness ". In the *objective* class are included the sensations which reach us through the senses of touch, smell, taste, sight and hearing, or through the sense of internal touch that brings before us our muscular movements and bodily injuries. A " sensation " it may be explained, is a sense-impression of which we are conscious. Consciousness is not, however, essential to its existence. Sense-impressions, like motives and emotions, can evidently be experienced in unconsciousness, for we can receive them when asleep. Otherwise, indeed, we could not be awakened. Sensations are primitively the stimuli of the subjective activities, of which movements and utterances are the consequences. We can, therefore, define the subjective as a condition of energy which enables an objective cause to produce an objective consequence. If this definition be extended to the external world, gravity, electricity and electro-magnetism would be *subjective* forces, and also the energy which " heats " material substances by affecting their objective condition.

The will is a " subjective " faculty. But it introduces an element of confusion into the classification, since it arises as an objective muscular effort, and, when developed into a mental effort, still retains traces of its objective origin. It can affect behaviour and thought, but is powerless over our subjective feelings. By no voluntary effort can we quell nervousness, or generate love, whereas the purely subjective emotion of love can " cast out fear ". Thought, again, introduces an element of uncertainty. For it lies across the two classes, since the ideas that it uses are derived from subjective feelings as well as from objective experiences. It is subjective when it is concerned with feeling ; objective when its materials are drawn from sensation or movement. We think subjectively of love, of its material causes ; subjectively or objectively of ourselves, according as we are occupied with our feelings or with our sensations and conduct.

As a source of information we are inclined to rank self-conscious introspection below the senses. The latter are of infinitely greater use to us in winning material success. But self-consciousness has an outstanding merit. It is the only instrument which can put us in direct touch with the immaterial forces of life. Our conscious ideas of motives and emotions no doubt mislead us as to the real nature of these inner experiences. But they are trustworthy indications of their relationships to one another. The feeling of admiration, for instance, may be very unlike the actual immaterial condition which it represents. But we can be sure that this is caused by a sensation or idea that contains an element of the successful, the strong, or the excellent, that it introduces an imitative element into the behaviour which is its consequence, and that it possesses an element in common with love and faith. Self-consciousness can, then, reveal to us truths that are hidden from the senses. We turn our attention from it to the objective life of the senses because we depend upon the latter for the material requirements of existence. In themselves, as we shall see, our objective are not more reliable than our subjective experiences. Light and sound are objective sensations ; in reality they are vibrations that are dark and silent. But our sensations, again, are correct in what they tell us as to the *relationships* between our various impressions ; and this knowledge suffices for the necessities of life. The tendency towards " objectivity "—to rate the external world higher than the internal—grows as civilization advances. It produces useful practical fruits. But it misleads us as to the true values of life, and obscures the laws by which the course of our evolution is swayed. We are, therefore, unable to resist the tendency to decadence which follows each wave of progress, so that man climbs only to fall back again. If subjective influences could withstand this reversion, their study would present us with immense practical advantages, as well as lead us to the truth.

It is only, we may repeat, by the evolutionary method of examination that one can hope to understand and classify the various faculties and activities that constitute human nature. The first part of this book is, accordingly, concerned with their simplest manifestations, and the laws which these follow. The second, third and fourth parts deal, respectively, with the energetic conditions that stimulate motives, and with the muscular activities and conduct and speech that result from them. Finally, we shall discuss the effect of experience and education in the development of the faculties, and in the acquisition of accomplishments, knowledge and bents of mind. The field that is covered by each part has been divided, as distinctly as is possible, into separate sections.

PART I

NERVOUS ORIGINS

By "nervous origins" are meant the fundamental nervous conditions and processes that are the sources from which have evolved our motives and emotions, sensations and thoughts, conduct and language. They are to be detected, for the most part, by a close comparison of various manifestations of the same kind of activity, by the elimination of differences, and the consequent isolation of a *residuum* which is common to all of them. Thus, from the comparison of different phases of ambition the fact emerges that they all involve ideas of a *success;* and we may, therefore, conclude that this idea underlies them all, and is their stimulus.

We must, at the very outset, emphasize a distinction which is likely to be overlooked. Nervous energy must not be confused with the nervous system. The cells and fibrils of which the latter is composed are *instruments* that may be compared with the electric installation of a house. Without this installation there is no electricity. But the electricity is not the same thing as the battery or dynamo which generates it, the wires that conduct it, the lamps and bells that it operates, or the light and sound that are its consequences. It is an ethereal energy which can be generated and controlled by material means.

1 Nerve-stimulation

The primitive response of a nerve to a favourable or unfavourable stimulus is a state of excitement—termed " sensory " excitement—which experiment has shown to have electrical affinities. This discharges itself in activity of some kind—by stimulating another nervous process, in movement towards the stimulus or away from it, in secretion, or in thought. Since its effects appear to be two-fold, each being the contrary of the other, we may reasonably assume that, like electricity, it is two-phased.

In nerves that are specially connected with the external muscular activities of the body, there is another development from stimulation —an energy which is not the same as sensory excitement, and is termed " motor " because it *enforces* muscular movement. It is very markedly two-phased. Its phases may be distinguished as " expansive " and " contractive " from their effects upon muscular tissue. These are easily noticeable in soft-bodied animals, such as snails, which expand under a favourable, contract under an unfavourable stimulus.

The stimulus of this *motor* excitement is a current of sensory excitement, and it is, therefore, generated only indirectly through the sense-organs. It seems that a motor nerve-cell, at its simplest, is united with the sensory nerve-cell through which it is stimulated, so that sensory is immediately and inevitably followed by motor activity. In the spinal system, however, sensory and motor nerves are distinct from one another. They are arranged in pairs, and are connected by the interclasping of branches (*dendrons*) which spring from them. Did these branches release hold, direct communication between the two would be intercepted, and an incoming sensory current would be deflected, or " switched off," to the brain. Here, then, appears a device for delaying muscular response and bringing it under control.

We have, then, learnt by physiological experiments, that nerve-stimulation generates two kinds of nervous excitement, or energy, distinguished as " sensory " and " motor ; " that nervous excitement is two-phased ; and that the stimulation of motor excitement is indirect, coming about through the stimulation of sensory excitement.

The two kinds of nervous energy correspond very curiously with two kinds of *feelings* of which we are conscious as resulting from stimuli—the practical and the emotional. The practical effect of a stimulus is to bring about conditions of attractedness or repelled-ness, of which we are conscious as likes and dislikes, or *inclinations*. Its emotional effect is to generate more or less enduring conditions of nervous excitement which consciousness presents to us as pleasure and displeasure, exhilaration and depression. Inclination and emotion are, therefore, both two-phased, each showing the contrary activities that we have distinguished as expansive and contractive. In this respect they correspond with sensory and motor excitement, and it is not a very rash inference to identify them, respectively, with these nervous conditions. This is, of course, only a *theory*, which must substantiate itself by satisfactorily explaining the origin of the complexities of motive and feeling that will come under notice in this book. But we have good reason to infer that emotion is a *surplus* product of stimulation. For it is evident that practical responses of approach and recoil can be stimulated without it. No emotion, for instance, attends movements, such as that of shrinking from a touch, of which we are capable during sleep. And we can hardly attribute emotion to such microscopic creatures as the *amœba*, which, nevertheless, moves towards the favourable and away from the unfavourable. But this surplus product is of immense evolutionary value. By means of it we acquire new practical inclinations. A like for a thing, as we well know, is stimulated by the pleasure that it affords. And, since nervous excitement must vent itself, this surplus energy actuates muscular movements of its own—" expressions of emotion," certain of which—the *efforts* which are thrown off by discordant nervous crises (such as those of discontent and antagonism)—undergo very surprising developments. For, as we shall see, they are the germs from which has sprung the will.

2 The Character of Stimuli

We ordinarily think of stimuli as sensory experiences of touch, smell, taste, sight and hearing. But we are also stimulated by internal changes, such as those which periodically excite the appetites, and by the secretions of the *endocrine* glands. And a most important set of stimuli are *relative*—that is to say, their effect depends upon their relationship to other nervous conditions—impressions, recollections, motives or moods—in being harmonious or discordant with them. An impression is harmonious when it " fits in " with its accompaniments in present or past experience, or with the feelings of the moment ; discordant when it is " out of keeping " with them. The strange, for instance, arouses the repelledness of alarm because it is discordant with past experience : the familiar is in accord with it and is, therefore, attractive. Even the dangerous does not alarm when it has become familiar. An obstacle does not annoy us unless it obstructs—that is to say, is discordant with a motive. Satisfaction and relief are plainly *harmonious* with desire. So again is success, one of the most vital of our experiences. It is a relationship between a wish and its consequence, not a thing in itself. Justice pleases because it is a harmony between what precedes and what follows : if one is good or bad, the other is good or bad also. Combinations of colours and sounds please when harmonious, displease when discordant. Harmony is, in fact, that elusive something called " charm."

The effectiveness of stimuli.—A stimulus may show its effectiveness by producing either a *practical* condition of attractedness or repelledness (which may itself stimulate either movement or thought), or an *emotional* condition of pleasure or displeasure. Attraction and repulsion are the basic elements of *purpose :* an iron filing becomes " purposeful " when it is attracted by a magnet. Pleasure and displeasure, on the other hand, primarily urge us to *expression*. But a stimulus does not attract or repel, please or displease us unless it is met by an inherited or acquired inclination, or an inherited or acquired emotional sensibility. This is a point of vital importance. If, for instance, we have no appetite, the offer of food does not tempt us. Tobacco gives no pleasure until a like for it has been acquired. The dishes of refined cookery are thrown away on an uncultured palate. Beauty makes no appeal to those who have no eye for it ; discord in sound does not displease an uncultured ear. Modern developments in music, poetry and painting are distasteful to those whose appreciative faculties have not kept pace with the times.

Inclinations and sensibilities may be established by heredity or by experience. But, when established, they may be dormant, so as to need to be awakened by internal physical changes—as in the case of the appetites—or by such circumstances as bring about the breeding season of birds. They may be restimulated by a sensory impression, or the idea of a sensory impression. A fondness for apples, for instance, may be awakened by the sight or thought of one. But their intervention remains irregular and inconstant. For they may be inhibited by a mood, or a motive, that preoccupies us. Hunger and fatigue may be inhibited by fear. If we are out of temper, or oppressed with sorrow, the amenities of life pass unnoticed, or may even annoy us by their discordance with our feelings. If, on the contrary, we are in good spirits, we disregard occurrences that would ordinarily be annoying, can even accept a snub philosophically. In fine, to render a stimulus effective a certain disposition towards it must have been established, must be awakened, and must not be inhibited. Our responses to stimuli are, therefore, exceedingly irregular.

This inconstancy of behaviour obscures the law that stimulation involves a disposition to be stimulated as well as a stimulus. Yet this is one of the profoundest differences between the production of living energy and of such inanimate energies as those of chemistry and electricity. Some insects appear to be attracted in the mass by certain stimuli, such as light and warmth, after the fashion that iron filings are affected by a magnet. Tendencies of this kind have been called " tropisms," with an implication that they are due to such material causes as chemical changes, or the expansion or contraction of tissue under the effects of moisture and heat. But, in fact, they differ essentially from lifeless movements in their irregularity and variability. The moths in a room do not fly to a lamp as uniformly as iron filings to a magnet. Indeed, at times they turn away from it. This indicates that their flight is not caused by an unvarying force, but is the consequence of nervous conditions which come and go, and may even reverse themselves.

3 Inclinations i.e. Likes and Dislikes

Dispositions to be attracted or repelled by certain stimuli may be inherited or acquired. An infant is born with impulses to suck and to hold tight ; and, later on, impulses to eat, drink, and to lie down when fatigued, develop themselves. The strange and injurious are *naturally* repellent : so also is a bitter taste. Bright colours and sweet tastes are *naturally* attractive. Our innate inclinations are, however, few and simple, and most of our likes and dislikes are acquired from experiences of pleasure and pain, or displeasure. We come to like some things and to dislike others because of their emotional effects upon us. That is to say, new inclinations are generated by surplus nervous energy. For pleasure and displeasure are not necessary for the simplest practical purposes of life. They can be dispensed with by an insect which is born with such a set of hereditary inclinations as suffices to direct its external behaviour. They are instruments for the evolution of new inclinations through experience ; and their effect is to free us, in some measure, from hereditary trammels.

We are attracted or repelled by a thing which gives us pleasure or displeasure, because its effect upon our feelings is, in fact, one of its qualities and, therefore, a part of itself. For a quality may be consequential as well as coincident. It is a quality of a wasp that it *may* sting, of a police officer that he *can* arrest. Language abounds with illustrations of this process of qualifying things by their consequences—as, for instance, when we speak of " joyful news," " anxious moments," or " wearisome conversation."

If, however, an experience of pleasure or displeasure, given by a thing, was the origin of an acquired like or dislike for it, so that, before this experience occurred, our attitude towards it was one of indifference, how, it may be asked, did we discover that it was agreeable or disagreeable ? Arguing to the past from the present, we may conclude that the discovery was made by an effort of trial, which developes a sensibility. It is by such efforts that we are constantly making new discoveries in cookery. Once discovered, a new agreeableness or disagreeableness is *learnt* by others. But learning also involves an effort—as every boy knows who has " learnt to smoke ".

It is obvious that inclinations are entirely dependent upon the organs of sense. If they are instinctive, it is through the senses that they are aroused. If they are acquired, it is through the senses that they are contracted—by experiences of the agreeable or disagreeable effects of their stimuli. The faculty of being attracted or repelled is, therefore, closely connected with that of receiving impressions of the environment. The importance of this consideration will be appreciated at a later stage.

Inclinations are the roots from which spring the great majority of our impulses—all of them, in fact, except those to antagonise, and to liberate emotion by its expression. They are the basis of our affections. For we like and dislike persons as well as things. They enter into such attitudes as those of admiration, contempt, respect, faith and pity, for in all of these feelings there are elements of attractedness or repelledness. Infused with the element of *effort* they give rise to our ambitions. So vital is the influence of an inclination in rendering a stimulus effective that if we are moved by a strong desire for a change in ourselves—physical or mental— this may be brought about by the instrumentality of almost any stimulus, however fantastic, that is accepted with unquestioning faith as capable of producing the desired change. This is illustrated by the process of " faith healing," which will be referred to in more detail at a later stage.

An inclination is primitively *passive :* it is an involuntary condition of attractedness or repelledness, and was formerly expressed in English—and is still expressed in most other languages—as the *consequence* of a stimulus ("it likes me", "*il me plait*"). It becomes a desire, or wish, when externalized towards its stimulus, a pursuit when the effort becomes physical. But we are now considering it in itself and apart from this reinforcement, which results from the intrusion of a distinct nervous process—that of "willing".

4 Emotional Sensibilities

All pleasures and displeasures are alike in being emotional conditions that may be termed "expansive" or "contractive" from their effects upon the muscles. They are differentiated into *particular* pleasures and displeasures by their origins—that is to say, by the character of their stimuli. These exhibit an evolutionary increase of complexity. Our *sensory* susceptibilities are stimulated by impressions in themselves. They afford us the various pleasures and displeasures of touch, smell, taste, sight and hearing. We commonly speak of these as "physical". Our sensibility to harmony and discord is the source of pleasures and displeasures that may be distinguished as "æsthetic". To produce harmony or discord there must be *two* sensations or feelings, for these conditions are relationships between two things. There is a further complication when nervous equilibrium is disturbed by a discordant strain or shock, which is either harmoniously relieved or occasions a nervous collapse. In this case the resulting pleasure or displeasure is "revulsive". As described in these terms, the process of revulsion may be difficult to follow. But it is illustrated by the experiences of everyday life. The nervous strain of an effort is discordant : it is dissipated harmoniously if the effort is successful, it ends in collapse if it fails. In the one case we experience the exhilaration of pride, or self-complacency ; in the other the depression of shame or mortification. The pleasure of amusement is revulsive : it always involves harmonious relief from a passing shock. The humorous and witty amuse us because they are momentarily disconcerting. The remarkable developments of revulsive pleasure will be discussed in some detail hereafter, and it suffices here to refer to them.

Pleasure and displeasure can be recalled, or restimulated by recollections, or ideas, of their stimuli.   Thoughts of a good dinner, or of a beautiful landscape, will bring back something of the pleasure that they originally afforded.   Revulsive pleasures can also be re-captured, but through a process which, owing to its incompleteness, is capable of the most amazing developments.   They are, as we have seen, the products of a shock or strain that is caused by a stimulus. But when recalled by thoughts of their stimuli, they come back to us unaccompanied by the shock or strain which preceded them. This element of the nervous sequence, or succession, is eliminated in the process of recall, so that only the resulting pleasure (or displeasure) presents itself to us.   Hence we can self-complacently recollect a successful golf stroke with no thought of the strain that preceded it.   We may laugh over old jokes although, being familiar, they are not disconcerting.   It follows that revulsive pleasures, as recalled or re-stimulated, have a peculiar character :   they do not completely represent the original experiences, and are, in fact, rather evolutions than resuscitations.   It is necessary to provide a distinctive name for them, and we may term them " ex-revulsive ". They include the pleasure that is commonly called " spiritual " ; and, as a matter of fact, the incompleteness of their presentation gives them an " immaterial " complexion.

Emotion may, then, be distinguished as sensory, æsthetic, revulsive and ex-revulsive.   Two or more of them may affect us simultan-eously.   The pleasure afforded by beauty, for instance, is a com-bination of the sensory, the æsthetic and the ex-revulsive.   For beauty always includes the element of excellence, and this is a quality of success.   All these susceptibilities are in some degree innate in man.   But they are vastly elaborated in the course of civilization by the instrumentality of persistent trials or efforts. And it is by the effort involved in teaching and learning that their developments are passed on from one generation to another.

Sensory susceptibilities.—We are born with sensory susceptibilities that render some touches delightful, others painful, that infuse hunger, thirst and fatigue with pain, and their satisfaction or relief with pleasure, that make the sweet agreeable and the bitter disgusting, and attach pleasure to impressions of colour and sound that are not too glaring or strident.   From these elementary beginnings a vast multitude of acquired tastes have evolved owing to the fact that sensory acuteness is intensified by attentive practice.   It has been proved experimentally that delicacy of sensation is increased by its conscious exercise.   One whose sense of touch is tested by a series of trials gains in tactile acuteness during the process. It is by attentive trial that fine discrimination is acquired in the flavours of teas, wines and tobaccos ; it proceeds from the appreciation of qualities that pass unnoticed in casual sensation. Once caught, they present themselves automatically on future similar occasions.

Sensibility to harmony and discord.—Rhythm is, fundamentally, harmony in movement, inasmuch as it is a succession of intervals that are equal—as are a succession of paces—however much they may be subdivided. Music is the harmonious in sound. The universality of dancing and singing, in some form or other, amongst mankind seems to show that a rudimentary susceptibility to rhythm and music is innate. But from the simplest of foundations have grown up the highly complicated sensibilities that enable us to appreciate rhythm and music in art. Rhythm is extended to sound by the drum : it is introduced into music as " time ", into speech as " metre ", and pleases us visibly in decorative repetition. From the utterance of vocal phrases expressing shades of feeling, music has developed into the complicated melodies and harmonies of the symphony, because susceptibilities have evolved that can appreciate them. The artificiality of musical taste is proved by its variation from one nation to another and at different stages of culture. Few Europeans can appreciate Indian or Japanese music. Similarly with the appreciation of form and colour. One of educated sensibility is pleased or annoyed by contrasts which make no appeal whatever to the uncultured.

Sensibility to revulsive pleasure and displeasure.—One of the most remarkable peculiarities of nervous life is its susceptibility to stimulation by shock. Indeed, it is not too much to say that energy is generally the product of a discord. It is difficulty that urges us to exertion ; and a violent shock will often have an extraordinary curative effect, bringing relief, not merely from minor troubles, but from acute paralysis. We shall treat of this peculiarity in some detail at a later stage, showing that it is the source of our various amusements. The most important of its manifestations are the exhilaration or depression that are occasioned by successful or unsuccessful effort. Of the fact of their occurrence there can be no manner of doubt. Through their evolutionary consequences they exert an influence upon life which can compete with the most imperious of our physical instincts. What is *ambition* but the desire of success ?

Ex-revulsive pleasures and displeasures.—The most impressive of our revulsive experiences are those of success and failure. These are of such cardinal importance in our lives that the mind naturally occupies itself with them, and elaborates from them a number of *qualities*, exactly as an admiring eye finds in a landscape traits of beauty which were not apparent at first sight. Success involves such qualities as power, excellence, superiority, and notability ; failure their contraries. Ideas of these qualities (as we shall see) have the same power of ex-revulsively recalling, or re-stimulating pleasure or displeasure as recollections of particular successes and failures. We know that the recollection of an exploit, or of a *faux pas* are almost as moving as were the experiences themselves. Ideas of power or excellence are equally moving, and this, too, although there is no implication of a preceding effort. When these ideas are associated with ourselves, with other persons, or with things, they inspire us with emotion which passes into admiration by stimulating the attractedness of a like.

The things with which success or a quality of success may be associated are extraordinarily various. The practice of asceticism still gives much honour to the East. It is *strong*, and therefore successful. At one time man sees power in a king—at another time in a majority of voters. Riches, titles and decorations are all prized, for the most part, because of their implications of success, power or superiority. The military profession owes its attractiveness to a similar association. Fine clothes would be nothing were it not for the " honour " or " credit " that they afford, and the changes of fashion show very strikingly how our idea of what is " chic "—or excellent—can vary from one year to another. Each change results from an inventive effort, which is eagerly adopted—that is to say, imitated—by others, if its originator is someone of repute.

5 Feeling, Thought and Behaviour

Sensation apart, the most fundamental of our nervous conditions are the internal states of inclination, antagonism, effort and emotion. which we call our " feelings ". This word is very misleading since it represents not the conditions in themselves, but their effect upon consciousness, whereas the conditions exist independently of consciousness. Indeed, experience shows conclusively that we may be affected by them when asleep. We are unconscious of vast numbers of our internal conditions—of the functioning of the liver, for instance. Were we conscious of it, we should term it a " feeling ". And a further caution is necessary. Feelings must not be confused with thoughts. Feeling and thought are distinct : for instance, we may " think in jest, and feel in earnest ". We confuse the two because they act reciprocally : each of them may stimulate the other. A feeling of pride, for instance, excites thought : the thought of a success arouses a feeling of pride. In the technical language of psychology, the two might be distinguished as " neuroses " and " psychoses ". But the words " feeling " and " thought " are more intelligible, and will invoke no misconception if it is borne in mind that the former indicates a nervous state of inclination, emotion or effort which could conceivably exist without a brain, whereas for thought a brain is essential. Under the influence of thoughts, feelings succeed one another in changes which may seem to be as capricious as those of the weather, and indeed resemble conditions of weather so closely that we use the same words to describe the two. " Misery " in one is accompanied by rain, in the other by tears. In the language of philosophy, feelings constitute our " subjective " life, as opposed to the " objective " life that is presented to us by impressions of the senses. Thoughts may be concerned with one or the other.

Behaviour is the external consequence of feeling or thought in action or utterance. It involves movement, which may be spontaneous or consciously willed. The will, as we shall see, is primarily an *effort*, and is, therefore, a link between internal energy and its external manifestation.

6 Associative Re-stimulation

Perhaps the most important of the laws that can be deduced from our experience of nervous action is that the active co-operation of two nervous conditions, processes, or " complexes ", whether simultaneously or in succession, establishes such an intimacy, or familiarity, between them, that if one of them subsequently recurs, it re-stimulates the other. This may be termed the law of " associative re-stimulation "—one of the fundamental processes upon which life's activities depend. Its action is illustrated most familiarly by the process of *remembering*. A recollection, as its name implies, is a

re-assemblage of sensory-impressions which is stimulated by a sensation or idea that has become associated with them in past experience.
The re-assemblage lacks the vividness of a sensation : it is a " sub-
repetition ", shadow or echo, of a sensation, as we can realize very
clearly if we pay scrutinizing attention to a tune that is running in
the head, or, after looking at an object, or moving the tongue or a
finger, we compare recollections of these sensations with the sensations. But a movement or a feeling (that is to say—a motive or
emotion) may be re-stimulated in *actuality*—in its full original force.
For instance, the thought of one whom we love will immediately
re-stimulate a feeling of warm affection. Associative re-stimulations
may, then, be distinguished as *actual* and *memorial*. The latter,
as we shall see, include those that are classed as *intelligent*.

Actual re-stimulation.—This may occur between one condition
of movement and another, between one feeling and another, between
a movement and a feeling, and between an idea and a movement or
feeling. The law explains one of the most difficult of problems—
how recollections and ideas can stimulate actions and feelings as if
they were actual experiences. For, since our consciousness of an
experience involves the formation of an idea of it, this idea is closely
associated, not only with the experience itself in simultaneity, but
also, in succession, with its nervous consequences, and can, therefore, become an instrument for re-stimulating them. If, for
instance, the impression of a snake has been followed by a feeling of
repulsion, the idea which accompanied the impression was also followed by the feeling and can therefore re-stimulate it. Moreover, an
idea has this power even when it does not precisely correspond with
an actual experience, if it possesses some element in common with
it. So the thought of a " snaky " movement may excite disgust.
That is to say, the idea of a *quality* is stimulating if it is an essential
attribute of something that is stimulating in itself. Superiority
is a quality of success, and since success is stimulating, superiority
is also stimulating, and so will be a person or thing to which an
idea of superiority is attached.

Actual re-stimulation of one movement by another.—This is the
origin of all our muscular dexterities. They are learnt by efforts
of will. But after practice the complicated movements which
they involve run their course automatically. Each movement of
a pianist's fingers re-stimulates the movement that follows it ;
and in walking each step is the stimulus of its successor. We may
be quite unconscious of this process, which endows us with such
automatic capacities as the lower animals owe to their inherited

instincts. Nevertheless it may be regulated by passing sense impressions. We walk automatically, but suit our steps as automatically to irregularities and turnings in the path.

Actual re-stimulation of movements by feelings and vice versa.— Feelings automatically re-stimulate actions that have become intimately associated with them. We are unconscious of our numerous " tricks of expression ", and such customary behaviour as saluting a friend and shaking hands with him, become involuntary. On the other hand, movements may re-stimulate the feelings that originally caused them—that is to say, re-stimulation may run backwards, giving rise to many of the processes that are called " auto-suggestive ". This is illustrated by the effect of a " soldierly bearing " in evoking a feeling of self-respect, of smiling or whistling in raising the spirits, and of considerate manners in breeding considerate feelings towards others.

Actual re-stimulation of one feeling by another.—In experience our admiration for a superior is followed by a feeling of respect. For we are by implication his inferior, and the thought of this tempers our admiration with an element of gravity, since inferiority is not agreeable. Respect is the admiration of a superior by an inferior. But in ordinary life these complicated interactions do not occur. Respect is automatically re-stimulated by admiration, so rapidly that we use one word—" dignity "—to express the two. A little analysis will show that dignity is self-admiration followed by respect. Pity in its origin is a complicated series of emotions, including a depressing shock caused by another's distress, a self-congratulatory revulsion that stimulates an emotional like for its object, and a feeling of sympathy. But, this sequence of feelings once established, each element re-stimulates its successor so rapidly that we use one word to express the set.

Actual re-stimulation of movements and feelings by ideas of them.— There is, in ordinary life, a radical difference between movements and feelings in their susceptibility to being re-stimulated in actuality through the mind. A movement can be re-stimulated by an idea that has been associated with it *simultaneously* in experience : a feeling can, generally, only be re-stimulated by an idea of its cause, or stimulus—that is to say, of its predecessor *in sequence*. The connection between thought and movement is more intimate than that between thought and feelings. We shall find further illustrations of this—and some explanation of it—as we proceed.

An idea of a movement or an utterance suffices to re-stimulate it automatically, when the process is not inhibited, or resisted by the will. When we are under the sub-conscious force of habit an idea of action or speech at once takes practical shape—a fact that is convincingly demonstrated by one who " talks to himself ". The routine behaviour of everyday life is " mechanically " actuated by ideas that pass in procession, each re-stimulating its successor. And behaviour is automatically re-stimulated by ideas when it is spontaneously imitative. Coughing is " infectious ", because the sensation of hearing another's cough re-stimulatively sets one coughing. It seems, then, that were it not for the control of the will, our behaviour would be swayed by the process of thought as automatically as that of an insect by its instinctive promptings.

The motives and emotions which we call " feelings " cannot, however, ordinarily be re-stimulated in actuality by mere ideas of them—that is to say, by ideas that have been simultaneously associated with them. An idea of " anger " does not make us feel angry, unless we are under hypnotic influence. An idea of a cause, or stimulus, as of a humiliation, for example, will irritate us at once. But this is re-stimulation through successive, not through simultaneous association.

In two cases, however, feelings can be re-stimulated by ideas of them. If we honestly *admire* a motive the idea of it will act as a generative inspiration. A comrade's whisper of " Courage " will strengthen a waverer's heart. So, if we admire such virtues as forbearance, mercy and justice, ideas of them will call them to life in all their energy. But, in all these cases, there must be a *stimulus* —something that our thought enables us to respond to in strength instead of weakness. In the hypnotic state, however, one can, it seems, become actuated by a motive on the bare suggestion of it— possibly because in this condition all antagonistic or inhibitive force is in abeyance, as during sleep. " Suggestion ", we can now realize, means re-stimulation through the conduct or speech of another : the process is called " auto-suggestion " when the stimulus is an action, word, or idea of one's own—that is to say, when it occurs in normal course. In the hypnotic state suggestion appears to dominate feeling, as well as action, directly—an abnormality that may be compared with the mental derangement of hallucination in which sensory conditions are re-stimulated, not merely memorially, but in actuality, through the recollections that are their consequences.

The re-stimulation of actual nervous conditions, or " feelings," by *ideas of their causes*, is the most salient feature of our " subjective " life. It is a process that hardly ever ceases. The recollection of a success, of a friend, of an adventure, conjures up emotion that is almost as vivid as that excited by actual experience. And (as we have seen) ideas of *qualities* that are derived from recollections are almost as inspiring—of the *power* or *superiority* of success, of the *kindness* of the friend, of the *danger* of the adventure. In one sense the re-stimulation is incomplete : it does not call to mind that which preceded the immediate cause of emotion. The recollection of a hard-won success does not bring before us the preceding strain of effort : the recollection of a joke does not remind us of the preceding little shock of surprise. The process of re-stimulation has, therefore, the effect of obscuring the evolutionary origin of an emotion. Since we can recollect a success without its preceding effort, success is associated with experiences that possess its qualities of power or superiority although they involve no strain or effort whatever.

Effort itself can be re-stimulated. So resuscitated, it is the energy that is involved in many of the processes to which we give the name of " willing ". But this is a point for consideration in more detail hereafter.

Memorial re-stimulation.—This is the re-stimulation of a recollection by a sensation, or by another recollection. We think vaguely of a recollection as something of the nature of a photograph which is brought forward by the process of remembering. But a comparison of memory with the phases of re-stimulation that we have been reviewing makes it clear that a recollection, when not actually " in play ", merely exists as a potentiality, left by a past sensation, of being reconstructed " in echo ". Its sensory elements are re-assembled by a sensation or recollection that has either preceded or followed their impression upon the senses. We may be reminded of lunch by the striking of the clock, or a recollection of the hour ; and the recollection of lunch may may remind us that we have asked a friend to the meal. We must infer that the sensory elements that are " shadowed " or " echoed " are contributed in part by memorial activity in the sense-organs as well as in the brain. For it is impossible that any process which is located in the brain could afford a recollection of a *movement*. The recollection of a step is an echo of a *feeling* in the leg, as the recollection of a tooth-ache is an echo of a pain in the jaw. Echoes from several sources may be combined : the recollection of a word includes its sound, its sight and the feeling of uttering it.

Remembrance is commonly considered to be a *successive* process. But when two different sensory experiences have occurred simultaneously the recurrence of one of them re-stimulates a recollection of the other *in coincidence*. In this case the two are not distinguishable apart : they merge one into the other. But we are assured that what seems to be one is in reality two, by abnormal or exceptional cases in which one fails to re-stimulate the other. Impressions of sight and of touch are intimately associated in coincidence by experiences that commence in our earliest years. An infant always endeavours to touch what it sees. And throughout life our visual sensations are incessantly associated with movements, since they vary from moment to moment as we approach or recede from objects. Consequently, the sight of an object immediately re-stimulates ideas of its solidity and distance. The connection between these ideas and its visual appearance is what we mean by " perspective ". We think that we " see " things in the solid and at different distances. But we deceive ourselves. Sight, of itself, only tells us of coloured areas and their distribution. In cases of concussion of the brain it may occur that vision ceases to re-stimulate ideas of touch and movement, and presents the outside world as a flat variegated pattern, to which the patient must gradually restore substance and distance by touching what he sees—that is to say, by reverting to the educative associations of infancy.

Words, as they are learnt, are simultaneously associated with the things or ideas that they name. Accordingly the sight or sound of a word immediately re-stimulates its meaning ; and, when memory fails, an idea re-stimulates its word-name. Words are so intimately linked with ideas that the two seem to be one ; and it has been erroneously maintained that we could not think without words. But their actual apartness is proved by the fact that we may have an idea in mind, but may forget the word that expresses it, just as we may forget the name of a plant. And, in the case of a foreign language, we not infrequently forget the meaning of a word. The evolution and use of language is, then, a consequence of re-stimulative nervous activity.

The " meaning " of a word is, then, an idea that it re-stimulates. This is so with all the things called " signs ", " emblems ", or " symbols " : they are each of them intimately associated with some particular idea—are, in fact, idea-carriers—and achieve their significance by re-stimulating it. We have seen how vast is the use made of this process in devising material forms for stimuli of pride or admiration, as, for instance, stiffness of manner or affectedness of language as well as clothes and possessions. They all have an idea of superiority attached to them, and " confer honour " upon their users or owners by re-stimulating the idea with its emotional consequences. And by a similar process they may arouse the admiration of others.

Intelligent re-stimulation.—The process of intelligence is a development of memory, and similarly depends upon associative re-stimulation. We show intelligence when we appreciate a sameness between two different things which renders them similar, or analogical, to one another. The sameness is an element or trait that is common to both, and enables us to re-stimulate the other. An idea ABC recalls or reminds us of an idea BDE, because the element B occurs in both, and acts as a " spark " for re-stimulation. The re-stimulating cause is a quality, instead of a whole idea, and it is in this that intelligence differs from memory. So a rose, by its colour, may recall a blush. The identity may be in relationship as well as in character : there is a sameness of *intention* between " going to London " and " going to speak ". Hence, when two ideas have a quality in common, the same word may be used for both—primarily and metaphorically.

Thought.—The materials of thought are ideas that are derived from sensations and recollections. Rational thought is a current of ascriptions—linkings of subjects to attributes—which are made under the influence of general laws, or " reasons ", that are either drawn from experience or dictated by intelligence. If, for instance, we think that we shall be late for dinner, or that the weather is going to clear, there is a reason, or law, in the background, so that every thought can be supported by a " because ". But the reasons would not occur were they not intelligently re-stimulated through a sameness, or analogy, between them and the conditions of each particular case.

Ideas of the future.—Evidently, then, we owe to the process of associative re-stimulation our notions of the future. For every happening immediately re-stimulates an idea of the consequence that has followed similar happenings in the past, and, until this comes to pass, we *expect* it. Without such an expectation there would be no conscious purpose in life ; and the extent to which conduct is governed by prudence, or foresight, depends very materially upon the orderliness of life—that is to say, upon the regularity of successions. There comes a wave of imprudent extravagance when a catastrophe, such as war, has deranged the successions of ordinary experience.

Associative shifts of meaning.—A curious result of the continual re-stimulation of ideas of consequences by their causes and *vice versa*, is the change that is constantly occurring in the meanings of words.

Thus " mercy " (from the Latin *merces*) originally meant a ransom ; then it came to signify the immunity that is purchased by a ransom and is its consequence, and then (in the French *merci*) the gratitude that is the consequence of the immunity. " Grace ", which primitively means thanks—the consequence of a favour—comes to mean the favour that is the cause of thanks. Owing to this shifting of meaning it becomes necessary to coin new words as language develops. " Innocent," for instance, meaning " harmless ", comes to mean without harmful feelings—the cause of harmlessness. To express its original meaning it was necessary to coin the word " innocuous ". So " frail " differs from " fragile " (both from the Latin *fragilis*) in expressing the consequence of being breakable.

Re-stimulation in instinct.—The unvarying successions of instinctive behaviour would in great measure be explained were it assumed that parents could pass to their offspring re-stimulative capacities that had been established by their own, or their progenitors', successful experiences. Such innate associations (or inherited memories) might be distinguished as " concatenations ", since their effect would be to *chain* nervous conditions together. Their disappearance from the external relations of life would be a long step towards freedom, for an animal would no longer be enslaved by habits that were contracted by its progenitors. The habits that dominated it would be at least its own.

Re-stimulation in cell-growth.—If the inheritance of memorial nerve-associations be granted, we may hazard the speculation that the growth of a living organism is the consequence of associative re-stimulation. For each nerve-cell, having within it, so to speak, an innate intimacy with the step in development that should succeed the stage which it occupies, might re-stimulate the step. This, it may be admitted, is difficult to realize and to believe. But it is not more wonderful than the continuing activity of a magnet.

7 Imitation

Our propensity to imitate is of vast and far-reaching importance. For we imitate another, not only when we follow his example, but also when we obey his commands : for we give effect to his words by imitating in conduct the ideas of conduct which they convey. An artist imitates his subject. If it is before his eyes, he transfers it to his canvas by copying it through gestures that imitate its outlines in miniature. If it is " in his mind's eye " he materializes it in precisely the same fashion. Our vocabulary is largely imitative —such words as " jump ", " sneeze ", " lick " and " kick ", for instance. An idealist imitates his ideal by translating it into action. For it is a law that we imitate what we admire. So it is that a popular sportsman or artist can set a fashion in hats or neckties.

It is then not surprising that a faculty which attains such important and dignified developments appears to us to be inherently voluntary or " willed ", and that we should feel some reluctance in admitting that its origin is a spontaneous action of the nerves. Yet there is conclusive evidence to show that it is fundamentally automatic. It is well known that coughing and stuttering are " infectious " : so is a smile, which can spread itself round a table without a trace of voluntary effort. Members of a family not infrequently have little tricks of manner which have been imitated from one another. But the strongest of all proofs is the use in hospitals of the sound of running water to relieve a patient of urinary difficulties. Spontaneous imitation is, in fact, a striking illustration of the law of associative re-stimulation. For we unthinkingly imitate another when our sensations of his gestures or utterances provoke similar gestures or utterances in ourselves. When we cough we hear ourselves cough, and the action and the sound are, therefore, intimately associated. Consequently, when another coughs, we are apt to cough also.

What is called the " psychology of the crowd "—as if a crowd had a personality of its own—is really the consequence of this imitative propensity. A few professional " claqueurs " can lead an unenthusiastic audience into applauding. Surrounded by a cheering crowd we cannot help cheering, although the object of our shouts may not particularly excite our admiration. And if we imitate the gestures and cries of others, we become gradually infected with their feelings. For such gestures and cries, when made spontaneously by ourselves, are associated with certain emotions, and they therefore automatically (or " auto-suggestively ") re-stimulate these emotions. So panic is infectious. One runs because others are running, and, as he runs, his fear increases. This connection between action and feeling enables one, by whistling, to " keep his spirits up ".

8 Individual Duality

Each of us is convinced of the " one-ness " of his individuality, and is disposed to ridicule the notion that his personality is actually double.   Yet we habitually admit our duality.   We speak of " loving ourselves ", " antagonizing ourselves " and " controlling ourselves "—conditions which would be impossible were there not two elements in our constitution.   Our doubleness is strikingly manifested in our ability to " think in compartments ", so as to hold at the same time two contrary opinions—the practical and the emotional—one based upon experience, the other upon sentiment. Thus our reason may accept the existence of a pitiless " struggle for life ", while we emotionally believe in a benevolent Providence ; and one who preaches the inevitability of economic laws may still be devoutly convinced of the efficacy of prayer.   No life is so prudent as to be undisturbed at times by romantic enthusiasm. This curious inconsistency between reason and emotion is in itself proof positive that we are possessed of a double nature.

We have learnt from experience that every individual—whether an animal or a plant—that is produced sexually is formed by the combination of two distinct living creatures—the male and female germs—that are different in their appearance and in their apparent activities.   It must consequently be endowed with two distinct natures.   This duality is recognized in the terminology of Mendelism which calls an individual a " zygote "—that is to say, a *yoke*, as of oxen, that may work together in harmony, but may at times " fall out " and antagonize one another.   We are aware of it in our consciousness of the difference between the " body " and the " spirit ", between our physical and our animative natures.

It follows that an individual contains both female and male elements.   Individuals differ in gender according as their function[1] is to produce female or male germs for the succeeding generation. Gender accordingly involves a slight excess of one or other sexual element which marks itself in character and appearance.   Women are more feminine than men, and men more masculine than women. But the degree of excess varies, and hence there are " masculine " women, and " feminine " men.   As regards the external marks of sex, it has been proved by experiment that a cock will assume the

[1] Hence females may be termed " physiogens " and males " psychogens ".

plumage of a hen if it be engrafted with tissue from a hen's ovary.

Now, quite apart from these considerations of duality in constitution, we have found two different basic elements in our motives —the inclinational and the emotional—and we may reasonably connect these two dualities. We may identify the inclinational with the feminine, and the emotional (or animative) with the masculine element, since, on the whole, the effects of physical inclination are more noticeable in woman than in man. She is the more *practical*, and less liable to lose sight of life's essential requirements in emotional aspirations or phantasies. Further, we may bring into connection with these dualities the two-fold nature of nervous excitement, as sensory and motor ; and, since motor excitement and emotion are both distinguished by their energy, we may regard motor excitement as typically masculine, and sensory excitement as typically feminine. It will follow that the masculine (or animative) element of our nature reacts to the influence of the feminine (or physical) by the generation of a condition of activity that is distinguished by its *forcefulness* from the element to which it owes its birth.

Emotion shows its influence, not only in pleasure and displeasure, exhilaration and depression, but in the continuing nervous states of which, during our waking hours, we are conscious as our moods, " spirits " and " states of temper ". It seems clear that motor energy is generated in surplus—in excess of the requirements of the moment—and can in some fashion or other be accumulated, as electricity is accumulated by a storage battery. There is a fact which indicates that in the case of vertebrate animals the " storage-battery " is the highly complicated appendage to the spinal cord known as the " cerebellum ". For this organ is specially well developed in birds, and of the vertebrates, birds are undoubtedly, as a class, the most active. Their flight demands immense energy ; and their song is a manifestation of acute emotion which must be liberated.

Kinetic and tonic energy.—Accumulated as a reserve, motor energy develops a variety of functions. Its primary use is to increase the force of muscular movements, and to enable us, with the help of ideas, to graduate its amount according to requirements. In lowly organized creatures the muscular response to a stimulus is " all or nothing " ; and physiological experiments have detected a similar lack of proportion in the response of certain of our own nerves that are uncontrolled by the brain. For the graduation of effort a reserve of energy would be necessary. And such a store would be of vital service in keeping a certain number of muscles braced, as is essential for the maintenance of an upright position. Its primary functions would, then, be " kinetic ". From these could be evolved the " tonic " functions which are manifested by the effects of our moods upon our general disposition. Kinetic and tonic functions are evidently connected, for in good spirits we are muscularly stronger than when depressed, and the weakest of men becomes dangerous when he is angry.

Harmonious reaction and discordant resistance.—Nervous excitement being two-phased, it follows that the physical and the animative sides of our nature may be in accord or discord. Both may be in a phase of expansion, both in a phase of contraction, or their phases may be different. It may be objected that nervous contraction or depression is not excitement, but its absence. Apathetic neurasthenia may, it is true, be the consequence of a failure of tonic energy —a reduction of current, so to speak. But misery, fear, shame and sorrow involve so much nervous force that they must often liberate it by cries and tears. That the physical and the animative may be in contrary phases results from the fact (of which we are quite conscious) that our moods are more constant than the immediate effects of passing stimuli, so that they can maintain their phase against experiences the physical effect of which is contrary to them. Were we not sustained by a stable condition of tension we should be at the mercy of passing impressions ; life would be a hysterical succession of " ups and downs ". If we are in good spirits we make light of troubles that would ordinarily be annoying, and would depress us greatly were we " out of sorts ". On the other hand, if we are depressed, the pleasantest experiences lose their savour. This antagonism is generally that of animative expansiveness to physical shock. For, fortunately for mankind, animative excitement is not only more stable than physical but is naturally disposed to the expansive phase.

There is harmony between the physical and the animative elements when a physical like meets an animative mood of expansiveness, or a dislike meets a mood of depression. We all know from experience that in this case the mood is intensified in phase : its gaiety or dejection is enhanced. Indeed, a like or dislike may find a vent for itself in this intensification, so that it loses its *practical* bent. If a sensation, or an idea, stimulates a like that is not strong, the inclination passes off in a course of " sentimental " thinking.

It is, however, in the introduction of *discord* into life that duality produces the most momentous of its consequences. For discord is a source of living energy, emotional and physical. It is a condition which could not possibly occur in the life of a *monad*. There is discord between the two elements of our nature when the phase of one is contrary to that of the other, as when natural gaiety is " shocked " by a sensation of pain or by alarm. The discord may be a continuing conflict, or may result in the dominance of the animative, or of the physical. These three conditions are illustrated very clearly by anger, spontaneous courage and fear. Anger is a continuing conflict—spiced with pleasure, since it involves expansive resistance. In spontaneous courage the animative overcomes physical shock : it is, therefore, a condition of unmixed exhilaration. Fear is so miserable because the animative is overcome by the physical, and both become contractive. These motives must be sharply distinguished from the conscious voluntary efforts that a restimulated by ideas. That they are purely nervous re-actions is proved by the fact that they vary automatically with the tension of our spirits. Fear can hardly be resisted when the nervous tone has been lowered by hunger or fatigue : it is irresistible when tone has been lost as from " shell-shock ". On the other hand, courage if assisted by anything that stimulates the spirits—by love, by patriotism, by pity, by music and by alcohol. Anger cannot be altogether stilled, as fear is by courage, because it is aroused by an *actual* injury, obstruction or humiliation, whereas the danger that causes fear in only the *possibility* of these misfortunes. Resistance can, consequently, be only partially successful, transforming depression into irritation. That anger involves resistance which is dependent upon nervous tone follows from the facts that one may be too ill or depressed to be angry, and that, when the misery of prolonged illness becomes irritable, we know that the patient is recovering strength.

The effects of this spontaneous internal antagonism are to be discovered in other less noticeable directions. An arresting impression causes a slight nervous shock. This is antagonized in spontaneous attention—the focussing of our perceptive faculties upon an object that actually occurs before we are consciously aware of it. The disconcerting effect of the strange is resisted in curiosity, as that of the dangerous is in courage. It is animative antagonism that limits the shattering power of physical pain, and enables us to endure it. Should the general nervous tone be lowered, as by illness or shell-shock, one loses these resistant powers. The attention will not fix itself ; the patient becomes nervous and incurious and succumbs unresistingly to his troubles.

Subjective and objective antagonism.—The conflict between the emotional and the physical is primarily internal. That, however, of which we are most conscious is to persons and things of our environment—the opposition that manifests itself in emulation, irritation, quarrelling and war. It is "objective" instead of "subjective". But it has its origin within us. When we suffer from an injury, difficulty or humiliation, we primarily resist the depression, confusion or shame that is its internal consequence. Our antagonism becomes "externalized" by being transferred from the consequence to its cause—by extending its aim from the immediate to the proximate. Anger is but internal irritation projected outwards ; and, when there is no outside cause upon which it can be projected, it remains directed against ourselves. Resistance of this "subjective" kind is also illustrated by self-control, which is a conflict between an inclination and an *idea* that excites emotion —as, for instance, an idea of success, dignity or strength. In this form antagonism is of mental origin : it is evolved through thought, and is not an unconscious automatic struggle between the two sides of our nature.

The source of animative energy.—It seems clear that our activity of mood must arise from the effect of impressions upon certain nerves, causing sensory excitement that passes into motor. Of the nature of these impressions we are for the most part unaware. For they may be internal as well as external : of the former we are unconscious when they are normal ; and it seems probable that we appreciate but a small proportion of the impressions that we receive externally. The effect of weather and of sunlight upon the skin is only perceived by us through its *consequences*. Moods, or tempers, would be expansive or contractive according as the impressions that are received are preponderately favourable or unfavourable ; and it is obvious that if the former is not generally the case, life could not continue. There is, moreover, evidence to show that moods are very dependent upon the secretions of the " endocrine " glands —a fact which explains the remarkable effect of alcohol upon the spirits.

So far of *physical* stimulation. But the spirits, as we all know, are also stimulated mentally. A thought of our own success, power or superiority inspires us by re-stimulating a feeling of pride : a similar effect can be produced by one of the artificial re-stimulating instruments that have come into use—a compliment or a prize, for example. Hope inspires and strengthens because it is an expectation of success. On the other hand we are depressed, and weakened by recollections and anticipations of failure. It is when emotional conditions are stimulated by ideas—as of the power of our King, our country, or of virtue—that we give them the name of " spiritual,"

Effect of duality upon evolution.—Duality of constitution must have momentous consequences in promoting the variation of off-spring upon which evolution depends. For the two elements, although distinct in themselves, are so connected in the constitution of the individual that it is reasonable to suppose that one could be affected, and in some degree changed, by the influence of the other. Hence the sex germs produced by each generation will differ in some respects from those of the generation preceding.

Duality in the nervous system.—In the nature of things there is no reason why the two elements should not be intermingled without loss of their identity, as, to make a homely comparison, sugar is mingled with tea—undistinguishable but still separable. There are, however, some reasons for concluding that, in vertebrate animals each element has its own mechanical equipment, so to speak—the feminine, inclinational or practical, operating through the sympathetic nerves, and the masculine, emotional or animative through the nerves of the spinal cord. For these two systems are very strongly contrasted. They develop in the embryo after as distinct a fashion as the two growing points of a germinating plant seed, one of which tends downwards, the other upwards. Speaking broadly, the sympathetic system innervates the interior, the spinal the exterior of the body. The seat of the animative energy which reinforces or antagonizes physical promptings appear (as we have seen) to be the spinal cord and its extension, the cerebellum. It would follow that the promptings which are reinforced or antagonized are connected with the other system—the sympathetic. This is the primary regulator of our internal organs ; and, in terming likes and dislikes " physical ", we recognize that there is an analogy between them and such processes as the beating of the heart or the operations of the stomach. Both sympathetic and spinal nerves contribute to the brain, which may be likened to a highly complicated knot formed by strands from both systems, which in the course of their detached lengths are further united by numerous junctions, or *plexuses.*

The source of our sensory and reflective capacities.—The processes of sensation and thought are known to us through our consciousness of them. But they can proceed in unconscious darkness. It has been established that we can receive sensory impressions of which we are unaware—as during sleep ; and that we can think in some fashion when asleep, is recognized in the saying "*La nuit porte conseil*". Perception, it will be shown, becomes conscious when it is infused with emotion—that is to say, when masculine energy unites itself with perceptive activities. These include, not only the reception of sense-impressions, but the associative re-stimulations which link sensory experiences into a connected continuity. Since these processes become conscious under masculine influence, we may conclude that, in themselves, they are of feminine origin ; and this inference is borne out by the consideration that it is through sensation that our conduct becomes " practical ", whereas emotional enthusiasm is indifferent to its actual surroundings. Thought, we shall see, is evolved from sensation, and is therefore, ultimately, a feminine capacity. This, indeed, follows from the fact that effort is undoubtedly stimulated by discord between thoughts and masculine energy, and there must be two different things to produce a discord. And a further argument which indicates that perception and thought, are essentially feminine attributes, is that, when not interfered with by inclination or emotion, they run their course on the *practical* lines that we call " rational ", interpreting what is new in the light of past experience. Both processes are turned from this course if an inclination develops itself or an emotion is excited. When we like or dislike an object we see qualities in it which would otherwise pass unnoticed ; and, if we are prejudiced on a subject, we are unable to think rationally concerning it. On the other hand, under the influence of enthusiastic emotion, both perception and thought become idealistic or imaginative.

It may be observed that the faculties of sensory susceptibility and associative re-stimulation must be possessed by both the masculine and feminine germ-cells, since in their independent life they manifest activities which would be inexplicable were they not endowed with these fundamental nervous aptitudes. But, when united in an individual, masculine sensibilities are, so to speak, enveloped by the feminine element : they are aroused, not by sensory stimuli, but by the effect of sensory stimuli on the feminine side of our nature. We can find traces of this masculine subordination in the very beginning of nervous life. For physiological experiments seem to show that motor nervous energy can only be excited through sensory energy.

There is nothing is the constitution of the brain which contradicts the separate existence of feminine and masculine nervous elements, and the occurrence of interactions between them. It is a composite organ, deriving materials from both the sympathetic and the spinal systems ; and its extreme complexity testifies to the multitude of fashions in which the capacities that are elaborated on each side of our nature can affect one another.

Duality and sleep.—The duality of our constitution leads us to an explanation of the mystery of sleep. This may very well be the consequence of the disuniting of the two elements. Sleep is a condition of unconsciousness, and we are rendered unconscious by such shocks as would naturally derange connections between the sympathetic and the spinal nerve systems. One of the largest of these uniting junctions is the *solar plexus* in front of the abdomen. A blow on this spot will knock a man " out of time ". The brain is a still more important point of union, and a violent concussion— or a sudden emotional shock—reduces one to the unconsciousness of sleep. Soporifics, such as opium, would send us to sleep by their chemical effect in interrupting connection, or, so to speak, " breaking circuit ". During sleep the sympathetic nerves continue to function, so that the interior processes of the body follow their course without interruption. But the spinal system is out of action, since it has been severed from the sympathetic chain upon which it is dependent for stimulation. Such consciousness as makes us aware of our dreams may be attributed to a " break " in the severance—to a thread which allows some emotional energy to filter through. Owing to the lack of resistant energy, one is more liable to contract illness—to catch cold, for example—during sleep than in waking hours. Orientals, when sleeping out of doors, carefully cover the face.

9 Externalization

What we call our " sensations " must actually be conditions of our own sensory nerves. Our impressions of the bite of a mosquito, of its appearance and its buzzing, are really the effects of the insect upon our nerves, just as the pain of a toothache is the effect of an internal derangement upon them. Why do we " externalize " the one by attaching it to an outside " objective " cause, while we accept the other as arising internally within ourselves ? The answer that is commonly given to this question is that we assign to an external cause any impression that reaches us through the external sense organs. But this explanation is not satisfactory. For the most fundamental of our senses—those of touch and taste— act internally as well as externally. It is by internal touch that

we feel pain and the movements of our limbs : our taste may be
affected by internal derangements of our own, and our senses of smell,
hearing and sight may also be stimulated internally, producing
more or less vivid sensory hallucinations. Moreover, it is not at
all clear why the mere fact of certain sense organs being situated
on the surface of the body should have the effect of isolating from
ourselves the impressions that they receive—of attaching them to
things that are outside us.

There is another phase of the same problem. Inclinations may
be turned inwards as well as outwards. The strongest of them all
is self-like, and this is to be attracted by oneself. We may like
an *idea*, and this is part of ourselves. Our dislike of the mosquito,
on the other hand, is to something external. How do we know
that it is outside us ?

This question must not be confused with another one—whether
our sensations are reliable indications of what causes them. Our
sensations of a mosquito bite and of a toothache may or may not
correctly represent the actual nature of these conditions. But
their reliability or unreliability is irrelevant to the present issue,
which is why one is externalized and the other not.

The problem has been one of the stock playthings of philosophy.
Its solution seems to be that we derive our ideas of an external
world from movement, and that we place in this world the causes
of all sensations that are instinctively and primitively accompanied by movement. Movement is, in fact, an essential element
of our perception of outside things. In *feeling* a thing we combine
touch with movement. Sensations that come from outside, and
inclinations that are stimulated by outside causes, are instinctively
accompanied by movements of approach or recoil, or by tendencies
to make them. Lowly organized creatures respond by movement
to every impression that strikes them ; and we can see illustrations
of this tendency in the behaviour of little children. In ourselves
these active responses may dissipate themselves in thought : the
brain, as we shall see, acts as a " shock-absorber ". Nevertheless
touches, smells and tastes ordinarily provoke muscular movements
of some kind, and impressions of hearing and sight become closely
associated with ideas of movement because we so often touch the
things that we hear and see. As we have seen in Section 6, it is
owing to the concurrent re-stimulation of ideas of touch and movement that the things which we see present themselves as material
objects. It is, then, movement that reveals to us the actuality of
our environment. Our external senses tell us of the world outside

us, not because they are external, but because their use is fundamentally associated with movement. The two are linked together by innate and inherited instinct so that we cannot be convinced that there is no material world, apart from our sensations of it, however logically philosophy may maintain this paradox. By kicking a stone Dr. Johnson roughly but effectually answered Bishop Berkeley's doubts as to the actuality of external things. His argument lay in his *movement*.

10 Effort and the Will

The will is one of the most mysterious of our faculties, because it is the product of a succession of nervous activities, some of which will reveal themselves to consciousness only if carefully searched for. We may clear the ground by commencing with some definitions to which our analysis will lead us. Willing is an *effort ;* we habitually speak of an " effort of will ". Effort is our response to a discord, such as annoyance, discontent, or doubt. Willed differs from spontaneous effort in that it is guided by ideas of successful or unsuccessful possibilities. Moreover, owing to the intervention of the brain between motive and action, muscular effort can be separated from the discord which prompted it, so that its execution may be suspended or " inhibited " until an occasion occurs which promises success. It is, then, re-stimulated, or " released ". Willing may affect thought as well as conduct. We may will to think on a particular subject during a walk as well as to take the walk. This illustrates the close connection—seemingly so paradoxical—between thought and movement.

Origin of effort.—We make no effort when all goes well, and it is, therefore, a law that effort is primitively the outcome of discord—a truth which is obscured by the fact that effort can be associatively re-stimulated without the preceding discord, in a form which, in the case of emotion, we have styled " ex-revulsive ". But we can verify from experience that all *spontaneous* effort arises from a condition of discord. We make efforts when in pain or distress, and when alarmed or surprised. They are primitively purposeless changes of feature, or gestures which liberate an emotional strain, as when a sudden noise makes us jump even before we realize our alarm. Spasmodic muscular reactions of this kind are exhibited

by all living things that are sexually generated when suddenly
confronted with a strange experience. These random efforts
become *purposeful*, because a discord generates an apprehensive
dislike, and this has an *object*. The sting of the whip stimulates
a horse to purposeful effort, instead of a plunge or a kick, because
it arouses an apprehension of its repetition. Hence the mere crack
of the whip may be equally effective. The efforts of courage,
curiosity and anger similarily become purposeful because these
conditions stimulate a desire, and this is discordant until it is satisfied.

Desires and apprehensions, then, invariably include an element of
discord which acts as a stimulus of purposeful effort. These
motives are likes or dislikes that are reinforced by emotion—
feminine inclinations strengthened by masculine energy. They
are followed by a discord, because they are not immediately
satisfied or stilled—a discord that is felt as discontent or impatience.
We call it a " want ". An apprehension is, of course, discordant
in itself. But it is also *followed* by a discord, arising from difficulty
or delay in escaping from it ; and there is a similar *following* discord
in desire caused by difficulty or delay in achieving it. No effort
attends a desire that is satisfied as it arises. The discordance of
desire is manifested by its restlessness : it is not a happy feeling.
It is, no doubt, owing to the intervention of a discord between a
desire or apprehension and the effort which follows it, that the
latter is separable from the motive of which it is the instrument,
and can be re-stimulated by itself.

Effort is, then, a useful fruit drawn by Nature from what is evil.
We spring out of the way of a threatening motor-car because it
produces the discord of apprehension. It is the discord of hardship, or of unfulfilled desire that is the ultimate stimulus of industry.
It must be remembered, however, that, since the *force of a desire*
is increased by hope, man may be strengthened by optimism as
well as by adversity.

The education of effort.—Our response to a desire or apprehension
is purposeful. But, until it is educated by successful and unsuccessful experiences, it is only a vague effort of trial, such as is
made by a baby that wants something. It is man's peculiarity
that his efforts are not directed by inborn instinct. To this he
owes his " freedom ". In animals of lower type—the insects for
instance—efforts are hereditarily adapted to the particular purposes
which they serve. But in man—and in a less degree in the higher
vertebrates—methods of action must be *learnt*. They are taught
by success and failure. For an effort, however vague, may succeed ;

and since success is attended by vivid emotional consequences, the experience is remembered, and its method will be repeated on a similar subsequent occasion. We illustrate this educational experience when we proceed " by trial and error ". Methods that are discovered by one generation are handed down to its successors by instruction. It is obvious that man is more dependant than any other animal upon the instruction that he receives. He is helpless until he *learns*.

Willing as a physical effort.—An effort may be postponed and be re-stimulated by ideas that involve possibilities of failure or success. Since failure and success are the educators of muscular effort, they become intimately associated with it as its past consequences and future possibilities, and can therefore either inhibit it, or re-stimulate it " ex-revulsively "—that is to say, without a preceding discord— and regulate it. They present themselves as ideas of unpromising or promising possibilities of action—in time, place and method— that is to say, as possibilities that are qualified by failure or success. The former inhibit, the latter re-stimulate and guide. Illustrations of this suspension and " release " of effort are offered in abundance by the ordinary course of life. If, for instance, we are engaged for a round of golf, the striking of the clock may set us on the road to the links, since it recalls the idea that to be " in time " we must start at once. When we make a " resolution ", effort is suspended until it can be effectively acted upon. If one " bears a grudge " towards another, a favourable occasion is awaited for carrying it into execution.

This re-stimulation of effort must be sharply distinguished from the re-stimulation of a desire or an apprehension in itself. We all know well that these impulses can pass out of mind, but will be re-stimulated in full force by an idea of their object. But it does not follow that effort will be re-stimulated along with them, unless a favourable possibility presents itself forthwith.

Willing as a mental effort.—When ideas of success or failure are forced aside by the urgency of our motive, our action is impulsive, and does not differ in character from the spontaneous. It rejects the lessons of experience. A mental effort is involved when these ideas are able to stay our action, by setting up the discord of doubt, either because they are not very clear, or because two or more compete with one another. For ulterior as well as immediate possibilities may present themselves in mind, and the two are generally incompatible. We may evade the difficulty by a vague effort of trial, or by referring its decision to chance, as in " tossing up ". But we can only " settle " it by a mental effort—by a decision or choice. We reach a decision through the process of *deliberation*, in which the various possibilities are balanced one against the other with reference to the prospects they hold out of success or failure. We finally adopt the one which promises best, either from a practical or an emotional point of view.

The delay involved in deliberation is caused by the fear of failure. Ideas of success beckon us onward ; but apprehensions hold us back. They manifest themselves very clearly in the anxious expression of one who deliberates : indeed, those of nervous disposition may be so deterred by possibilities of failure as to be quite unable to " make up their minds ". On the other hand, those of sanguine temperament are notoriously hasty in their judgments. But, it must be remarked, we should not be embarrassed by conflicting possibilities—could not hesitate between them—were it not for the re-stimulating activity of reflection in suggesting ideas of them. This is increased by habit—that is to say, by practice. It is also increased by experience. Adults are more deliberate than children. The practice of deliberate willing is called prudence, or " providence," because it involves the rejection of immediate for ulterior possibilities.

A deliberate decision may take the form of an effort of trial. So haphazard endeavour evolves into ordered experiment. And action upon it may be suspended to be re-stimulated by a favourable occasion. In this case a decision is a resolution.

The alternatives between which we hesitate may be objects as well as methods. We may deliberate between two dishes at table. And they may be questions of what we should think, as well as what we should do or say. When we are confronted with a difficulty as to the ascription of a quality to a subject—as for instance, whether depreciation of the currency stimulates industry—we proceed exactly as if we were concerned with a question of conduct. We may decide impulsively under the influence of a prejudice. Or we may deliberate and adopt the idea which accords most generally with experience—that is to say, in a fashion of speaking, is most " successful."

It may be observed here, in passing, that, since the will, whether as a physical or mental effort, is stimulated and guided by experience, the faculty of volition must be acquired after birth, and is not an inborn endowment. The efforts of an infant cannot but be spontaneous.

Willed desires and aversions.—We now come to a new phase in the effect of success and failure. They act, not as re-stimulators and regulators of action, but creatively in stimulating desires and aversions of a particular kind—those which have as their objects phases or symbols of success or failure. A desire to win distinction is on a different plane from a desire to revenge oneself : the former is volitional, the latter is spontaneous. So an aversion for untidiness differs from an apprehension of illness : the one is artificial (or acquired) the other natural. To a desire which is focussed upon a phase or symbol of success we give the name of " ambition."

The effort that attends these willed motives may be stimulated by the discord of dissatisfaction or restlessness that is caused by contradictory circumstances, as is the case with spontaneous motives. But it can also, apparently, be re-stimulated ex-revulsively by its object, since, as a phase of success or failure, this is intimately associated with effort. For efforts of ambition have very commonly an optimistic complexion, very different from the nervous anxiety which is associated with an impulsive desire.

Their active execution may be suspended, or inhibited, precisely as that of spontaneous motives. It may be re-stimulated impulsively, or tentatively, or be stimulated through the effort that is generated by a doubt and follows the process of deliberation.

The phases of success and failure which are the stimuli of these volitional motives, and may act as re-stimulators of effort, are extraordinarily numerous and diverse. Success and failure are not, of course, " things in themselves." They are qualities or " conditions " of certain methods of conduct and things. Ideas of them are highly elaborated : they include a number of *deduced* qualities which are in fact the antecedents or outcomes of success and failure, such as power, superiority, excellence, peculiarity or their contraries. We may win success by achieving things through talent or industry, by skill in sport of all kinds, by gaining power or authority over others, by attaining distinction whether through our abilities or our clothes, by impressing others—that is to say, through public esteem or popularity—and even by associating ourselves with the great, the rich, or the notorious. And since the success of victory may be won over ourselves, we are induced consciously to antagonize physical responses, such as fear or submission, which are tinged with failure, and so deliberately to act courageously, or " wilfully " to assert our independence. These self-assertive reactions may, as we have seen, come about spontaneously : the will calls them voluntarily into effect. We can go further. Led by the glamour of success man can voluntarily restrain physical inclinations that are pleasurable, and deny himself everything beyond the bare necessities of life. We may smile at these self-repressive efforts when carried to excess. But amongst them are the virtues of patience and self-control.

The success at which ambition aims may, then, be self-repressive as well as self-assertive. The latter, when impulsive, is the wilful vindication of our own dignity or independence : it takes a higher flight in the pursuit of liberty. The will acts self-repressively in the deliberate adoption of the conduct that is called " virtuous ", or manly—conduct which after a time becomes established by habit but needs an initiatory effort. So it enables one to repress cowardly behaviour while quaking with fear, and to stifle all manifestations of anger although trembling with irritation.

Free Will.—When we will impulsively or optimistically, we are obviously " carried away " by the idea that is before us. But a decision, choice or resolution, made after deliberation seems to be " free " or arbitrary. For it has exercised the power of rejecting possibilities ; and the considerations that have determined it cannot without some difficulty be identified as qualities of success. But, in fact, a choice resembles a desire in that it involves a yielding to the attraction of its object. There is nothing arbitrary in the judgment of one who, hesitating over an appeal for charity, yields to the thought that his subscription will be published in *The Times*.

Scope of the will.—Effort primarily affects *muscular* activity, and it is therefore over our movements—our conduct and speech— that the influence of the will is most obvious. It is the origin of all our varied dexterities of action and speech ; they are learnt by efforts of will, although with practice they become habitual and effortless. But, looking further, we are confronted with an apparently inexplicable problem. The will extends its authority over the brain. By an effort of will we can change the current of thought into any channel that suggests itself. This remarkable inconsistency bears out the contention of some authorities that thought has evolved from movement ; and we shall find some reason to believe that the development of thought owes something at least to one kind of movement—that of tentatively " feeling " with the fingers. And it is to be said that the brain is so far related to the limbs in that it is an " appendage " to the body. On the other hand, it is a notable fact that the will has no control whatever over the elemental forces of inclination and emotion. By no effort oan we rid ourselves of a desire, or a passion, subdue a thrill of fear or fit of anger or conjure up admiration or pity. We can control their external manifestations—that is all. It is the same with the internal organs of the body : no amount of willing can enable us to interfere with the working of the heart or the kidneys. The will, it seems, has no power over the internal feminine or masculine components of individual life : its jurisdiction is limited to the external organs which are built up as a kind of living machinery, around them.

It is not inconsistent with these conclusions that the will can influence feeling indirectly, through voluntary manners or speech. For this is an auto-suggestive process—the consequence of associative re-stimulation. So polite manners may bring into existence some real consideration for others, and manifestations of reverence may call up reverential feelings. It is in this fashion that discipline affects the character. But in this case the will influences feeling, not directly, but through a subterfuge. Moreover the feelings that it can so conjure up in this manner are seldom strong ; and the process ceases altogether when the conduct has become habitual.

The ability of the will to control conduct and speech without affecting feeling endows us with a faculty of immense importance— that of deceiving others. For the instruments of deception are deeds and words that misrepresent feeling. Experience shows that this misrepresentation may *succeed*, and there is accordingly a strong motive to elaborate it.

Spontaneity, deliberation and habit.—In the development of behaviour the course of evolution has been from the spontaneous (or impulsive) to the deliberate, and from the deliberate to the habitual. This is clearly traceable in the growth of morality, and in the replacement of the spontaneous (or " heart-felt ") by the deliberate in attention, courage and curiosity. It is strikingly illustrated in the growth of children. At first their conduct is impulsive : it is gradually steadied and educated by willed endeavour, or prudence, and finally becomes habitual or conventional. We may detect similar changes in the development of a nation as a whole. This results, not from any real analogy between the growth of an individual and that of a multitude of men and children, but from the tendency of civilization to stimulate the prudence which is its cause. Each elder generation tends therefore to become more prudent, and therefore more conventional, than its predeces sor ; and its character influences that of the younger generation which learns from it.

11 Success and Failure

The process of evolution is illustrated with extraordinary force
by the influence of ideas of success and failure upon our aims,
emotions and drifts of mind. Success is harmony between an
effort and its consequences : it is rewarded by a surge of emotional
exhilaration. There is failure when the consequence of an effort
is discordant with its aim ; it is punished by a nervous collapse.
These emotional crises are plainly of a revulsive character. For
effort involves a strain which is suddenly released by either success
or failure. But their revulsive character is disguised by the incompleteness with which they are re-stimulated by recollections of their
causes. For they are re-stimulated in themselves, as " ex-revulsive "
emotions, without any presentment of the effort that preceded them.
The recollection of a hard-won victory is altogether pleasing, and
includes no memento of the strain that it cost. Accordingly, the
exhilaration of pride and the dejection of shame become isolated
from the effort that was their original begetter.

We shall discuss in Parts II and III the effect of ideas of success
and failure in stimulating ambitions, in arousing admiration, and
kindred emotions, and in firing the imagination. Our present
concern is with nervous origins. Nevertheless, it will be convenient
at this point to indicate in bare outline the history of the developments that we owe to these poignant experiences. It will suffice
to refer to the consequences of success, for those of failure are their
precise contraries.

Success is so delightful—and so necessary to life—that the mind
dwells upon it, and extracts from it various ideas of its *qualities*, as
that it involves power, superiority, excellence and peculiarity, or
distinction. Ideas of these qualities are as effective in re-stimulating
emotion as ideas of success in itself. Nor is this surprising. For
we only know of things through their qualities. Apart from their
qualities, their substantive existence can only be vaguely inferred.
And, since these qualities have the power of re-stimulating emotion,
we may be exhilarated by ideas that have no connection with effort
—such as by ideas of the superiority that is given by birth, fine
clothes or good luck. We may even be stimulated by an idea of
popularity, since this establishes our superiority by recognizing it.

Ideas of success, or of its qualities, may present themselves as
future possibilities or as present actualities. In the first of these

phases they are (as has just been shown) the stimuli of conscious willing. They are also the incentives that urge our ambitions— those inclinations that arise from the pleasure of success. Ideas of *present* success, or of its qualities, also stimulate inclinations—those of admiration and respect. These are highly emotional since they are suffused with the exhilaration which the ideas re-stimulate. When these ideas are associated with ourselves they inspire us with self-admiration, pride or self-complacency ; and, since we must have some successes in order to continue alive, our ordinary frame of mind is that of self-satisfaction. When the ideas are associated with others, our admiration goes out to them, unless it is inhibited by dislike.

Perhaps the most influential of the ideas that are derived from success is that of *superiority*. This is a correlative : it cannot exist unless there is inferiority in some other quarter. Hence, if we appreciate the superiority of another, a thought of our own inferiority obtrudes itself upon us. Another's inferiority, on the other hand, gives us an agreeable feeling of superiority. We are dominated by these ideas to an extent that we do not realize. They lurk in the background of our thoughts, insensibly influencing our attitude towards others. It is their rapid alternation that gives its spice to gossip. They mark themselves upon the most trivial and the gravest of our motives. A boy's " pinch for new clothes " is a protest against another's superiority : jealousy of another's superiority is the moving spirit of the anarchist. They sway the course of our emotions. It is a sense of inferiority that converts admiration into respect—a sense of superiority that stimulates our pity for others. We cannot pity one who self-assertively resents our compassion.

We have still to arrive at the climax of this remarkable evolution. Admiration and pity are amongst the emotions which transform the character of thought into the imaginative phase : they are the particular emotions that inspire the imaginings that bear fruit in the drama, fiction, poetry and painting.

This brief outline is unconvincing until it is completed in detail. But, by including it in our preliminary review, we shall facilitate the understanding of much that follows.

12 Consciousness and the Mind

The researches of science appear to show that our environment affects our sense organs through its vibratory activity—through a complexity of vibrations that vary in kind, rapidity and amplitude, and in the medium that they agitate. It can be demonstrated that what in consciousness is sound is in actuality the vibration of matter or air : it can be inferred from experiments that light and heat are also vibratory conditions, and that matter which appears to be solid is actually in a condition of violent internal movement. We are, then, surrounded with movements such as those which are detected by wireless receivers, and the explanation of our sensory capacities that is most closely supported by experience is that the sense-organs of touch, sight and hearing are collections of " receivers " each " tuned " to respond to a definite rapidity or " length " of a particular kind of vibration. It responds by vibrating sympathetically, as a violin string will vibrate in sympathy with its note if struck upon a piano. The sense nerves of smell and taste appear to be similarly susceptible to chemical changes on the impact of certain substances. Whether the nervous response be vibratory or chemical, it generates a current of an electrical character. Electricity may, of course, be generated either mechanically (through vibration caused by friction) or chemically, as in a galvanic battery.

These impressions of the senses bear, however, no resemblance to the conscious presentments of them which we call " sensations " and " recollections ". Sound and light are vibratory conditions. But as sensations they appear to us in quite a different guise. Their conscious apprehension must, therefore, be a different process from their sensory reception : it must result from a faculty which stands apart from the sensory organs, and can take their impressions as materials for the development of conditions that are active as well as passive, including, as they do, the activity of " awareness ". Moreover, our consciousness is not limited to sense-impressions. We are also aware of our motives and emotions, that is to say, of subjective experiences which are unperceivable by the sense organs.

Unless we recognize the fundamental duality of our nature, it is impossible to arrive at even the vaguest comprehension of this " awareness ". For a condition cannot obviously be aware of itself. But, if there are two elements within us, it is conceivable that one should influence, and be influenced by, the other, and should, not merely suffer, but *manifest* the effects of this influence. Conscious-ness would be this manifestation. The unconscious processes that underlie perception and thought would be emotionalized : emotional energy would be "impressionized." Such an evolution can be traced to its primitive origin. Perception and thought are, as we shall see, evolved from sense-impression, and sense impression is the conse-quence of sensory nervous energy. Emotion is the consequence of motor nervous energy. Consciousness would, then, be ultimately traceable to action and reaction between these two nervous forces. Their reciprocal influence would not result from the mere fact that sensory energy is the generator of motor energy. For in this case the two energies do not act together but in succession. That they should act simultaneously upon one another it is necessary that sensory energy should meet a standing " head " or " charge " of motor energy, so that the two can operate in coincidence. There must, then, be a store of motor energy before consciousness can come into being. We have already reviewed the facts which prove the existence of such an accumulation.

The two elements would be *unified* by their reciprocal action, each upon the other, and we can therefore understand why our essential duality is concealed from us. How this unification comes about must remain a mystery. For consciousness is the ultimate observer, and cannot, therefore, itself be observed. We can, however, verify by experience that it does not come into existence unless perceptive (or reflective) and emotional conditions are in active operation together.

Before, however, going further on this point, it may be remarked that consciousness must exist in germ before it can be evolved. It is impossible to watch a butterfly fanning its wings in sunlight without inferring that it has some awareness of its well-being, how-ever dim this may be. But the fact that insects, when severely injured, will continue to feed in apparent contentment, seems to show that they are not conscious of pain as we feel it. And such consciousness as they possess must be vague and indefinite. It cannot take the form of definite ideas of their sensory or emotional conditions. For ideas, it is generally agreed, come into existence through the action of the cerebral hemispheres.

The brain, it appears, may be likened to a telephone exchange. The sensory changes that originate in the sense-organs are trans-mitted to it, and are co-ordinated by it. Sense-impressions become, in fact cerebral-impressions which are elaborated by the memorial re-stimulation of a number of past sensory experiences. So the sight of a flower recalls its name, and various unseen qualities, with, it may be, a feeling of like or dislike ; and the sound of its name has a precisely similar effect. These co-ordinated and amplified brain-impressions become, it seems, " mentalized " as conscious *ideas* when they are emotionalized. If, as appears, the cerebellum is an accumulator of emotional energy, the brain is in intimate connection with an instrument for emotionalizing its reflections. And, through the same instrumentality, there is a means for the accomplishment of the contrary process—that of registering emotional conditions and bringing them within the scope of consciousness as mentalized " feelings ". The conscious presentments of these emotional (or subjective) conditions would, however, differ from objective sensations and recollections in possessing no sensory basis. They are, therefore, less arresting than objective sensations ; and oscillations in our spirits are often manifested to others by the expressions of our features more clearly than they are realized by ourselves. Inclinations, it may be added, would become conscious through the emotion which accompanies them. We should become aware of a like through its pleasure.

Now it may be objected to this conclusion that consciousness is not, in itself, marked by the pleasure or displeasure that we associate with emotion. The things of which we are conscious may stimulate these feelings. But, on first thoughts, we should not say that our mere awareness of them has this effect. On further self-examination, however, we shall find that sensation and feeling is always tinged with the agreeable or disagreeable—an accompaniment which has been used with effect in the arguments of some eminent psychologists. The tincture is, no doubt, faint. But it is not unreasonable to suppose that emotion, in its inter-action with reflection, loses something of its poignancy.

Experience shews that consciousness vanishes if there is no co-operation between the sensory organs and emotional energy. The cerebral hemispheres appear to be the link between the two, and the behaviour of dogs that have been deprived of these organs leaves no doubt that they have lost consciousness in the ordinary sense of the word. They continue to be influenced by sense-impressions, and can exercise the functions of automatic life : they can " see " their food, will reject it if made bitter by quinine, will sneeze under the effects of tobacco smoke, and growl if roughly handled. But their conduct exhibits the unwavering, mechanical responsiveness of a somnambulist. We all know that consciousness is lost if the brain is injured by a violent concussion.

There is again no consciousness without emotion. Habitual impressions become unemotional. We are, therefore, unconscious of the continuous ticking of a clock, of the movements of the tongue and lips in speaking and the movements of the legs in walking, unless they are accompanied by the unpleasantness of fatigue. Our inclinations are not realized by us unless they are attended by emotion : they are motives of the " subconscious self ", as hidden from us as is the functioning of our internal organs. The most probable explanation of sleep is that it results from the " short-circuiting " of the brain—and its reflective activities—from the influence of emotion. It is our emotional—and volitional—energies that suffer from fatigue and need the rest of sleep. The " practical " side of life, such as is involved, for instance, in the functioning of our internal organs, does not require periodical rest. Our emotional susceptibilities are rested by their severance from the brain, since its ideas are their most continuous stimuli. In the absence of emotion sleep is unconscious. We may dream. But this involves consciousness of a far less active type than that of our waking hours. We shall touch on this point again. It is probable that fainting, whether from shock or debility, results from the brain's loss of its emotional connections, and that this is also involved in the stupefying influence of anæsthetics, and certain drugs, and in the effect of a " knock-out " blow on the important junction between the sympathetic and spinal nerves, called the " solar plexus ".

These experiences bear out the conclusion that consciousness is the product of interaction between the two elements of our nature. The feminine is affected by the masculine, so that it receives emotional as well as sensory impressions : both kinds of impressions are mentalized through emotion, and so become conscious. The " Mind " is a construction in which reflective activity and emotion are combined. It brings a third influence into life, by which the feminine and the masculine—the Body and the Spirit, so to speak—are overshadowed.

Dreaming.—In sleep, we have inferred, emotion is cut off from the brain. If the brain continues to act, we are unconscious of its accomplishments until they are presented to us on awakening. But when its activity takes the form of dreaming, a peculiar kind of consciousness comes into being. This must, it seems, be the result of an escape of emotion into the brain. For dream-thoughts invariably take the " sensory ", concrete, forms that characterize imaginative thinking; and we shall find that it is under the influence of emotion that thought spontaneously assumes an imaginative quality. But the connection between the brain and emotional energy is only partial. It does not expose the brain to the influence of the energy of effort that is stimulated by the shock of discordance, and there is, therefore, an absence of will-power and consequently of the possibility of any voluntary external movement. The dreamer cannot *escape* from the frightful. Dream images are, then, isolated from external, objective life, and possess a subjective quality that may be described as " weirdness ". In forming them the brain can use both memories and intelligent analogies. But its processes are fantastic and incoherent because they are undirected by any motive, and are uncontrolled by the influence of the will.

In somnambulism there is also an escape of masculine energy. But it is of a different kind—kinetic instead of tonic—and seems to produce movements that may be guided by the senses but are quite unconscious. A sudden shock restores complete connection, and the sleep-walker awakens to find himself in surroundings of which he was completely unaware.

13 The Nature of " Ideas "

Consciousness manifests itself in *ideas* of such of our sensory and mental experiences as are attended by emotion. We think of ideas as ethereal existences that are different and distinct from sensations and recollections. But these only become conscious experiences, because ideas contribute to their constitution. Sensations and feelings are nervous experiences that are associated with ideas of them, and recollections are " echoes " of them that are similarly associated. The study of " subconscious " activities shows that we can receive sense-impressions, and even recollect them, without attendant ideas. But in this case we are unaware of them.

Ideas can exist independently of sensations, feelings and recollections, because they can be detached from them. Their detachment, we shall see, is affected by a mental operation of refinement, the instruments of which are processes of combination, comparison and deduction, that can be traced back to the associative restimulation that is one of the fundamental characteristics of nervous activity. Their effect is to isolate qualities—that is to say, attributes—or combination of qualities, from the things that possess them. These qualities may be of *character*—as of the colour of a table cloth, for instance—or of relationship, as that the cloth is *on* a table. An idea of the table itself is, indeed, only of certain combined *qualities* of sight, touch, and usefulness which are attached to an indefinite " substance ". Our idea of a particular word is a combination of certain qualities of hearing, sight and feeling. By comparing different men we isolate the idea of " men " as a quality of *kind* : by comparing courage and generosity we isolate the idea of manly resistance, or virtue, because this is an element possessed by both of them. We similarly form an idea of the relationship of " succession " by isolating this quality from sequences of different particular kinds.

A quality does not, of course, exist in actuality apart from the thing which possesses it. But the mind, by isolating it from its possessor, gives it a separate *mental* existence—an appearance of independent apartness. It is a quality or attribute of a dog that it is *running*. The running does not exist apart from the dog. But, since it is mentally distinguished from the dog, it can be ascribed to a multitude of other objects—to a stream, for instance, or a railway train.

These mental processes of refinement find their way very gradually, and hence ideas grow in number and in elaboration precisely as the organs of a living creature develop from its germ. We are well aware of the difference in complexity between a savage and a civilized vocabulary. But we need not go far afield to find illustrations of a gradual development. An adjective expresses the *possession* of a quality—a " virtuous " man is one who possesses virtue. In English the possession is itself abstracted, and expressed by the suffix " ness " (virtuousness). This refinement has not, as yet, come about in French.

Ideas may be distinguished as objective or subjective according as they are derived from external impressions that are received by the sense-organs, or are the mental impressions of emotional conditions. In the former class are included the impressions of our own bodily activities, and of derangements of tissue, which we receive through the sense of internal touch. The organic and muscular tissues of the body are external to the nervous system, and impressions that come from them are, therefore, objective. But under the name of " feeling " we confuse objective impressions of ourselves with mental impressions of our subjective emotional states. We speak of a " feeling " of movement, or of pain, as if it were of the same kind as a feeling of admiration.

Qualities are immaterial, and ideas of them are, therefore, of an etherial character. But this does not necessarily put them outside the domain of natural laws. Electrical conditions are unsubstantial. But they can be traced to their origin, can be brought about artificially and made to do work for us—can even be measured. There are, as we have seen, some striking analogies between electrical and nervous activities. The mere fact that ideas are etherial does not, then, necessarily imply that they are beyond the reach of science.

Some of our ideas seem to be so remote from any actual experiences as to be quite untraceable to them. It has consequently been held that they are innate—that we are born with them. But this doctrine fails if it can be shown that there are, in fact, no ideas, however transcendental, which cannot have been gathered from experience through the action of certain definite mental laws. Their evolution in this fashion will be traced in detail. It may be observed here that man would not be so wonderfully plastic— would not have his marvellous capacity for development—were he not born absolutely free from hereditary preconceptions. We are disposed to think that our ideas are innate, because we forget the events of our infancy, and amongst them the process of acquiring the primitive materials of thought.

The reliability of ideas.—The processes by which ideas are evolved will be considered in Part III. But we may refer here to a question of intriguing interest. How far do the sensations and feelings from which ideas are derived, correspond with the actualities from which they spring ? Do they give us reliable information as to the nature of the things which they present to us ? Or are they deceptively symbolic ?

There appears to be nothing more certain—however difficult it is to believe—that our ideas of our surroundings and ourselves are quite misleading as to their real character. The hues of a rainbow, the notes of a skylark's song, are ethereal and atmospheric vibrations: as colours and sounds, they are created by ourselves. The " feel " and taste of a peach are our ideas of material and chemical conditions which are analysed by science into molecular or atomic movements or changes. It is as if when firing at a target our idea of a hit was the ringing of a bell. The ringing is not the hitting. But it is a lively symbol of it, such as we use imaginatively when we speak of a road as " running ", of fields as " smiling ", of the sky as " angry ", and of Nature as " benevolent ". And, indeed, since our sensations and feelings are in part the products of emotion, it is unlikely that they should be " matter of fact ". For the effect of emotion upon the brain is always to give an *imaginative* complexion to thought. There seems, indeed, to be no escape from the seeming paradox that our sensations and feelings deceive us in regard to our surroundings and ourselves.

But we must not exaggerate the unreality of our knowledge. Our sensations and feelings give us correct indications of the relationships of one thing to another, in qualification—that is to say in " belonging " to one another—in space, in time, and in being identical, similar, or different. We misapprehend the colour of a rose : but it is something that *qualifies* the flower. Consciousness does not disclose the real nature of whiskey and water : but one is certainly *mixed with* the other. It gives us wrong ideas of thunder and lightning : but one must come *after* the other. Movement is a change of relationship : our ideas of vibration are therefore trustworthy. Change itself is a relationship in succession. Shape is the relationship of points on a surface to one another. It follows that our notions of *form* do not mislead us. A leaf and a spear-head must have a resemblance to one another however much they may differ in nature from our ideas of them. The analogies upon which reasoning is based are, therefore, real.

Accordingly our lives are not prejudiced by the unreality of our sensations and feelings. For the relationship between two things is not affected by error as to their nature. We may mistake the nature of tea and sugar without affecting the fact that one is *changed* in taste by the other. And it suffices for the needs of existence that our knowledge of relationships should be correct. In avoiding a motor-car, for instance, it is its movement, direction and weight— all *relative* qualities—that are of vital importance to us—not the precise nature of its composition or construction. Knowledge advances by the use of inferences, drawn from experiences of relationships, to correct the " imaginative " errors of sensation. So it was discovered that sound is a vibration, and that what seems to be continuous substance is in reality a sieve of interstices.

That we should persist in contradicting scientific experience, and in holding that our ideas of things correctly represent things in themselves, illustrates the " thinking in compartments " to which we have already referred. The philosopher who *knows* that his senses deceive him can hardly bring himself to feel actual distrust of them, although he may argue at length on the illusiveness of sensation. And, in taking this line, philosophy has commonly " pushed beyond the mark ". It has confused our notions of relationships with our notions of *things*, and has impugned the reliability of one as well as of the other. But, if relationships were not substantially as we conceive them, it would be certain death to cross Oxford Street. Intervals of time and distances of space must exist according to our concepts of them. Our knowledge of them is, however, based upon our ideas of them ; and any attempt to define them must begin with the experiences from which these ideas are derived.

Ideas as stimuli.—The evolution of ideas and thought has endowed us with a supplementary stimulating environment—a miniature world within ourselves—which maintains our motives and emotions in an unceasing state of fluctuating activity. For, owing to the process of associative re-stimulation, an idea is almost as exciting as a sensation, and no experiences of sensation can be as rapid and as changeful as the procession of thoughts. The ideas that come to us, or are brought to the front by the conversation of others, are followed by changes of nervous tension and phase, so that our spirits are constantly rising and falling, like the jet of an ornamental fountain. The charm of poetry is that it plays upon the spirits—like a pianist upon his instrument—through the sentimental—that is to say, stimulating—quality of the thoughts which it calls up. But the most exciting of ideas are generally those of our own superiority and inferiority, and, since these are correlative conditions, another's superiority gives us a feeling of inferiority and *vice versa*. Changes of feeling manifest themselves in facial expression, as well as in words, and we have only to watch the features of one who is interested in conversation to appreciate the energy of the fluctuations which occur in his moods, and the rapidity with which one succeeds another.

From another point of view the mind may be likened to a picture or sculpture gallery, exhibiting to us excellencies that excite our admiration. When we admire a virtue, we admire the *idea* of it, that is presented in thought, which exists as actually as a symbolic representation of it in colour or marble. To ideas that arouse our admiration we give the name of " ideals ".

Ideas and words.—Generally speaking, ideas can only be expressed through the words that signify them. But we must guard ourselves against the mistake of confusing words with ideas. The two are fundamentally distinct. An idea is an existence of nervous life : a word is an utterance that is used to signify this existence. Words being the *expressions* of ideas, it is obvious that an idea must exist before a word for it can be invented. We can have ideas without words, as when we hunt for a word to express a thought. And we can have words without ideas, as when we are addressed in a language which we do not understand.

14 Emotional Reaction to Shock

The shock of discord, as we have seen, stimulates the energy that is involved in effort. We are now concerned with its effect in producing emotional revulsions in what we call our " nerves ", " moods " or " spirits ". This introduces us to the nature of *amusement*, and of our appreciation of the humorous and witty.

Nervous elasticity.—We commonly speak of nervous " elasticity ", meaning a tendency of the spirits to revert to a normal. Fortunately for mankind this normal is the moderate exhilaration of which we are conscious as " cheerfulness ", and acute exhilaration or depression tends itself to revert to this condition. Joy loses its first ecstasy and sorrow " wears itself out ". This recovery is greatly assisted if emotional excitement, whether joyful or sorrowful, vents itself in muscular movements, utterances or tears. In the undemonstrative this safety-valve is obstructed ; and they are generally recognized to possess " deep feeling ". Tearless grief is persistent, and may be dangerous. But recovery, whether aided by expression or not, is dependent upon nervous tone. Nerves that have run down lose resistant energy. We are " fatigued " when nervous elasticity fails us, and discords affect us without occasioning rebounds.

The experiences with which we are now concerned are very striking developments of this elasticity. They are nervous explosions and collapses that follow a condition of discord and owe their intensity to it. If, for instance, we find that we have been causelessly alarmed, our relief is " revulsive " and we " smile at our fears ". A burst of laughter is a sign of a sudden nervous explosion the violence of which is imperfectly shown to us by our feelings. It can always be traced to a preceding discord. Nor is it *prima facie* unlikely that a discordant shock should have an intensifying effect upon emotion. For it has (as we have seen) a similar effect upon motives. It is the stimulus of effort and of the will : it converts a like into a desire. A discordant shock appears, in fact, to generate energy ; and there are some curious anomalies in the generation of radiate energy by different " frequencies " of light that this law would seem to explain.

E

Whether the shock is succeeded by relief or by discomfiture, there follows a nervous crisis of far greater intensity than a stimulus, of itself, could produce.

The effects of tickling illustrate in a homely fashion the pleasure that may be given by a discordant experience. To be tickled is disconcerting : it gives a succession of little shocks to the nerves. But they fall short of physical pain, and consequently produce a succession of revulsions that must often be vented in screams of laughter. Pleasure is extracted from displeasure, just as amusement may be distilled from the disagreeable by those who are blest with the spirit of cheery contrariety that Dickens personified in Mark Tapley.

Joy and Sorrow.—These, we can feel, possess a revulsive quality. They are caused by pleasurable or displeasurable experiences, but are very much more intense than the emotions that would result from the experiences in themselves. The discord which precedes and intensifies them is that caused by the unexpected or surprising. This clashes with the expectations that are presented in the course of associative re-stimulation. Joy and sorrow lose much of their poignancy if their causes are anticipated. We are over-joyed at meeting a close friend unexpectedly : were the meeting arranged, it would please but not transport us. So a death that has been foreseen does not arouse the depth of sorrow into which we are plunged by a sudden bereavement. When, however, joy or sorrow is re-stimulated by a recollection of its cause, its revulsive origin is obscured. For our memory does not repeat the shock which preceded its original onset.

Pride and shame.—These are forms of joy and sorrow that are stimulated by success and failure. The discord that precedes them is that of effort, which, as we can feel, involves a strain. This is " resolved " expansively by the harmony of success, contractively by the discordance of failure ; and there follow revulsions of exhilaration or depression which become pride and shame by stimulating, respectively, like and dislike. Pride is, of course, self-admiration, shame self-contempt. These feelings are experienced quite independently of any preceding discord when they are re-stimulated by ideas of our own or another's success or failure, or by concepts, such as those of power and superiority, that are deduced from ideas of success and failure. Hence we do not appreciate their evolutionary connection with effort. They take the form which we have styled " ex-revulsive " and become parted from their evolutionary origin. But they owe their existence to it none the

less. And, when actually stimulated by the successful or unsuccessful consequences of effort, we can feel their revulsive
character.

We shall find that the emotion of pity also arises as a revulsion
from the shock of another's distress, stimulated by a self-complacent
thought of our own superiority.

Amusement.—It is obvious, then, that an excellent expedient
for extracting mirth from life is to bring about discords that can
easily be relieved, and will rarely end in complete discomfiture.
This source of pleasure has been exploited in the devising of artificial
means of amusement. These all involve discordant shocks, as those
of danger, difficulty, apprehension, humiliation or surprise, which are
relieved by successful effort, by luck or by a mental process that
harmonizes the discordant. They have been elaborated in immense
detail as forms of " play ", or of humour or wit. They begin in
children's games : " playing at bears " is amusing because it conjures
up apprehensions which are relieved by the thought that all is
" make believe ". In Blindman's Buff there is the fear of being
caught which is continually relieved by escape ; and if one is caught
it is, after all, only " in play ". The " switch-back railway ", and
similar contrivances, tickle the sensibilities through a little alarm.
Adults are not content with these simple excitements. Their games
must be spiced with ambitions of victory or of gain, as in football,
gambling and betting. But, to be amusing, these must have " down
and ups " which are continually generating discords and relieving
them. The effect of a reverse can always be mitigated by ascribing
it to bad luck, while one takes credit for success as obtained by skill.
There are no such fluctuations in chess. This is purely a means of
winning success. One does not turn to it for amusement.

Fiction and drama that are amusing are similarly diversified by
sharp contrasts. The hero's triumphs must be intensified by difficulties or misfortunes. Shakespeare's comic interludes are rendered
amusing by the intensity of the feelings which they interrupt.
Fiction and drama, of course, need not be amusing to be attractive.
There is " human interest " in everything that happens to another.
For we realize his feelings and thoughts through ourselves. Admiration and pity need no adventitious shocks to inspire us. But
a tragedy such as *Othello* would be almost unbearable were our feelings
not relieved by the thought that it was unreal. There are some,
it is true, who revel in horrors. But only because they are relieved
by the thought that they themselves are not concerned.

The humorous and facetious.—These differ from one another as

" fun " does from " wit ". The one momentarily shocks our memorial associations ; the other our understanding. In both cases the discord is dissipated by " second thoughts ". That which surprises because it is out of accord with convention is immediately recognized as, after all, *natural*, and therefore accordant with experience. If it were miraculous, it would not amuse but astonish. It frequently involves another's humiliation, and it has been suggested that this is amusing because it reassures our feelings of superiority. But we are not *amused* by flattery. And incidents may be humorous without any reflection upon another's dignity. In the *facetious* the intelligence is confused by a discord between a word and its application. But the confusion is dissipated by the detection of a sameness, or analogy, which harmonizes the two. In both cases, therefore, the revulsion is sudden and, therefore, energetic. Humour and wit break upon the staid interests of life like patches of sunlight.

Incidents are humorous, or funny, when they are out of accord with expected routine. Thus we are amused when we and our fellow travellers are discomposed by a sudden jerk of the train. The incident is unusual. But it is quite natural. Its strangeness simply lies in its attendant circumstances. Hence decency may be humorous in an indecent, as indecency in a decent atmosphere. For the same reason we are amused when adults behave childishly, and when children ape " grown-up " manners. We call such incidents " ludicrous " or " ridiculous " because of their consequences upon us. The sudden discomfiture, or humiliation, of the great is entertaining because its incidents are out of relationship with expectation. In themselves, they are natural enough. A practical joke is amusing for the same reason. The humorist takes advantage of this sense of pleasure to give amusement artificially. This is well exemplified by Dickens. We are amused when Simon Tappertit reflects that he should have been born a corsair, when Mr. Micawber professes the heroic, at Mrs. Nickleby's absurd inconsequencies. The operettas of Gilbert and Sullivan are so entertaining because they associate dignity in musical style with flippancy in thought and word. Humour can enliven the dullest of subjects, and may even make science amusing.

The facetious, or witty, plays upon our understanding, as the humorous upon memorial association. The witty is an analogy which gives a momentary shock, because it is not immediately assimilated by the intelligence—because, for an instant, a sameness is not recognized and appears to be an incongruity. We are not seldom momentarily disconcerted by failing to identify a person who is familiar and testify to our relief by a smile. Wit similarly amuses us through a discord that vastly intensifies the feeling of relief. If there is no relief—that is to say, if the intelligence cannot assert itself, wit is not amusing ; and consequently to the stupid jokes are merely confusing. Many people take time to " see " them, and show by their features that they are puzzled and disconcerted meanwhile.

We may be affected humorously by circumstances or by ideas : wittily by ideas or by words. There is wit in the lines of Hudibras :

> For rhymes the rudders are of verses,
> By which, like ships, they steer their courses.

because the sameness of function between rhymes and rudders is not patent until intelligently appreciated. There was something comic—an element of wit—in many of our metaphors until they passed into the habitual. To speak of the " rising of the wind " was vulgarly witty until it became commonplace. There is a subtle sameness between contraries—since one becomes the other if reversed—and hence we are faintly amused by the innocent pleasantry which calls a disgusting day " charming ". But it is in words that wit most commonly finds its instruments. It plays upon double meanings punningly, and we are disconcerted until we appreciate them both. When Dickens wrote that " Miss Bolo went home in a flood of tears and a sedan chair ", he played upon the double meaning (temporal and spatial) of the word " in ".

The re-stimulation of amusement.—The law of associative restimulation explains the remarkable fact that we may be intensely amused by a good story time after time, although in its repetition there is nothing that is unexpected or surprising. This experience obscures the essential necessity of the element of shock in the humorous and witty. We can enjoy the comic although we know what to expect. But this merely illustrates the connection between memory and feeling. It does not affect the fact that on our first experience of the ludicrous there was something which would have consciously " taken us aback " had it not been immediately thrown off.

The amusement of the interesting.—The law of intensification by shock will lead us to the solution of a very curious problem : What is the pleasure that is given by the observation of others, by " news " of them, by the ordinary incidents of social life, by gossip and by the happenings of which we learn from the newspapers ? What, indeed, is the pleasure afforded by information, or knowledge, of any kind that is not concerned with our personal interests ? Our interest, it seems, is of a " revulsive " character, arising from contrasts between the effects upon us of the familiar and the strange (or new), of the harmonious and the discordant, and of that which is com- plimentary and derogatory to ourselves. From the first of these contrasts springs our interest in what is new or strange in the familiar, and what is familiar in the new or strange. If the strange cannot be linked on to the familiar, it is confusing and repellant— an effect that is marked on the features of those of non-mechanical bent who wander through galleries of complicated machinery. But we are pleased by a lesser discord—that which resolves itself by connecting the new with the old, and the old with the new, for this excites our curiosity. It is the spice of gossip. And it follows that the wider is our knowledge the more varied are the novelties that can give us pleasure. Animals are interesting because they are unlike and like ourselves : Zoological Gardens are therefore popular. There are contrasts between harmony and discord in the " impro- prieties " which amuse us under protest. And an abounding source of interest is the oscillation which is constantly occurring between our self-assurance and our self-distrust. Superiority and inferiority are correlatives : an idea of one recalls an idea of the other, and consequently our self-esteem may be flattered relatively as well as absolutely—by suggestion of another's inferiority as well as of our own excellence. Another's superiority similarly implies our own inferiority, and is displeasing unless we are moved to admiration. But thoughts come in abundance to reassure our dignity, and it is positively accentuated by the shock it has received. In conversing with another we are constantly assailed by little depreciatory shocks which have the effect of enlivening the conviction that we are " not so bad after all ". There is pleasure in repeating gossip to another, quite apart from any desire to gratify him, in that the repetition of the interesting re-stimulates the pleasure that it afforded. When relating an amusing incident we experience our amusement over again. So a child likes to recount its experiences at the Zoo.

Other developments.—The law of intensification by shock is Nature's expedient for producing pleasure out of pain, good out of evil. It is utilized very largely in music : discords are introduced because there is pleasure in resolving them. There are other more serious developments. It is the discord of self-denial that infuses self-control—and even the extremes of asceticism—with their energy.

This discord of hardship, as is well known, may have a marked effect in strengthening the character. Moreover, the law seems to have some quite material bearings. It is likely that many stimulating drugs that are poisonous—strychnine, for instance—invigorate us by giving shocks to the nerves. This clearly seems to be the case with such irritant remedies as mustard plasters, blisters and the electric current.

15 Emotion and Emotional Expression

When discussing our emotional susceptibilities (in Section 4.) we insisted upon the point that feelings of pleasure and displeasure are *emotions*, and differ from the feelings that are commonly called " emotional " only in their origin, their intensity and their accompaniments. All these feelings are in their essence one and the same —conditions of animative excitement that may take one or other of two phases. This conclusion is out of accord with common ideas : we are disposed to think of each kind of pleasure as distinct in its nature from other kinds. We, therefore, revert to the point—passing on to review a set of characteristic activities which arise from the necessity that emotion should find a means of discharging itself.

Emotion may be sensory, æsthetic, revulsive or of the " exrevulsive " type that is called " spiritual ". That of the first class is excited by pleasurable or displeasurable impressions of the senses. It is differentiated into *kinds* of pleasure and displeasure by its sensory accompaniments. The " pleasures of the table " are actually one and the same pleasure that is given by and associated with various stimulating tastes. Æsthetic pleasure is aroused by harmony in sight and sound, in feelings, and in manners. Revulsive pleasure is the exhilaration of relief from conditions of discord or effort—exhilaration that is intensified by the discord. It enters into the delight of triumph and into the thrills of amusement. When re-stimulated, its character is changed by the elimination of the preceding discord. In this form it has been distinguished as " exrevulsive ", and is generally identical with the emotion called " spiritual ". Its re-stimulation may be exceedingly vivid. The recollection of a triumph is almost as inspiring as the triumph itself : the recollection of an amusing incident, or a joke, may make us laugh aloud, and this, although the memory does not recall the discord to which the original pleasure owed its origin. The pleasure is re-stimulated purely and simply.

Sensory and æsthetic pleasure stimulates a like for its cause. Revulsive emotion acts in precisely the same fashion. By stimulating inclinations it disposes us towards or away from its causes in the active feelings of love and hate, admiration and contempt, respect, faith and pity. When it is excited by an idea of success and is reinforced by the will, it becomes energetic as ambition. In itself it is passive, and in terming emotions " passions " we correctly interpret their original nature.

But emotion possesses a characteristic activity of its own. It actuates movements and utterances through its urgent need of liberating itself in muscular expression. Nervous excitement must find a vent. If it is imprisoned it may even endanger life. If we are prevented by convention from liberating feelings of amusement, they may become unbearably acute—as may happen, for instance, in church. We recognize the need of an outlet in such expressions as " I cannot contain myself ". And we have all experienced the relief that is afforded by the venting of emotion in gestures and action, and in the utterance of exclamations, or expletives, of some kind or other—the relief that comes to excited children when they " jump for joy ". By muscular activity we can even lessen the intensity of pain.

The movements that liberate emotion are manifested by infants, and must, therefore, in their simplest forms, be inherited, or " instinctive ". They are gestures of the arms and legs, crowings and cryings, the facial movements of smiles and frowns, the explosion of laughter, the secretion of tears. Yawning is also instinctive : it gives relief to feelings of hunger, fatigue or " boredom ". Facial expression becomes elaborated with advancing years. It may grow into a permanent manifestation of emotional tendencies (such as cheerfulness or peevishness) that combines with inherited facial dispositions to give an " expression of countenance " which (if we come to think of it) is the principal element in our idea of another's personality. It may become elaborated into *nuances* of expression which flit across the face, as clouds and sunshine across a landscape, revealing to us the succession of emotional thoughts that are passing within. In this form it manifests thought as well as feeling, and enables us to understand and sympathize with the actors in a wordless drama—as in the cinema.

In the muscular effects of pride and shame we have excellent illustrations of unconscious emotional expression. Pride braces the muscles : shame relaxes them. A cock that feels masterful, or a dog that feels heroic are models of highly-strung rigidity. Similarly automatic is the stiffness of deportment and manner which characterizes a man who is well-satisfied with himself.

Thought has some curious affinities with movement, and it is, then, not surprising that emotion should find in thought an outlet for its relief. The more active is the reflection which a feeling stimulates, the less immediate is the need of a physical vent. Imaginative thought—perhaps the most remarkable of all human capacities—is, as will be shown, the effect of emotion upon the brain in assimilating reflection to sensation—that is to say, in giving an objective form to the subjective, and in endowing the objective with subjective qualities. But imaginative thought only affords temporary relief. The images that it creates excite fresh emotion which must be liberated by their active expression in movement or utterance.

Emotional expressions are, then, primitively spontaneous. But, in so far as they involve muscular movement, they come under the control of the will and become " willed " or voluntary. We can smile or frown deliberately if we please, although we cannot *force* ourselves into tears. Gestures and utterances can all be voluntarily imitated. This development of the willed from the spontaneous makes its mark upon imaginative art. The skill with which artistic imaginings are expressed must always be acquired by voluntary effort : it is the emotion which inspires the skill that is primitively spontaneous. But, since the will can influence thought, we can force ourselves to imagine in cold blood, and may succeed in the production of poems, pictures and music which commend admiration by their ingenuity or audacity, however much they may lack emotional vivacity.

This subjugation of spontaneity by the will illustrates the law to which we have already adverted as the passing of the spontaneous into the deliberate, and the deliberate into the habitual. The expressive evolves into the purposeful, the emotional into the practical. Gestures and ejaculations which originally were merely emotional safety-valves, develop into purposeful manners and language. And imaginative art, which is fundamentally as spon- taneous as the song of a bird, becomes practical as a calculated means of gaining a livelihood.

PART II

MOTIVES

The subjective energies which we call "motives" are aroused by stimuli that may be outside us or within ourselves, presenting themselves in the one case through sensation, and in the other case in thought. A motive may be either purposeful or expressive. When it is *purposeful* it renders us attracted or repelled by its stimulus, sets us in antagonism to its stimulus, or provokes an effort. That is to say, it is "directive". The attraction or repulsion need not manifest itself in movement : it may affect us mentally as a "turn" of thought, for reflection can take the place of action. An *expressive* motive is a condition of excitement that has its end simply in liberating itself—as by tears, laughter or expletives. "Unpractical" emotions of this kind are (under the view which we have been developing) the products of the masculine side of our nature. On the other hand, every *purposeful* motive includes the feminine attitude of *inclination*. In antagonistic and effortful motives the masculine and feminine elements co-operate : antagonism and effort are, in fact, reactions of one element against the other.

Our essential duality is obscured from us by the fact that in most of our conscious motives the two elements are blended. For one element tends to stimulate the other. Conscious inclinations—that is to say, likes and dislikes—are attended by emotion : indeed, it is through the emotion that we become conscious of them. On the other hand, emotion stimulates inclination. A "taste" for a thing is generated by the pleasure that it affords ; and the "ex-revulsive" emotion that is excited by ideas of success and failure generates the inclinations of admiration and contempt.

The two elements of our nature are thus usually so closely associated that their diversity escapes consciousness. It is, nevertheless, possible to find experiences that isolate them. There are purposeful motives that are emotionless. Such are the force of habit, and the energies that drive the functioning of our internal organs. We are affected by physical inclinations during the unconsciousness of sleep. And experiments with dogs and pigeons, whose upper brains have been excised, show that, in this unconscious condition, the animals are still moved by alarm, hunger and sexual instincts. On the other hand, emotion occurs, apart from inclination, in the exhilaration of joy and amusement, and in the depression of misery. And when it is associated with inclination in the impulses of admiration and contempt, we can still appreciate its distinctness. We recognize the two elements of admiration when we speak of its " inspiration " and its " attraction ".

In classifying our motives we must first of all distinguish the force of habit, which differs from all others in that it is simply urged by familiarity—-that is to say by an associative re-stimulation of actions or ideas that runs of itself. It is the case, however, that familiarity is *liked*, and this contributes to its influence. Habit apart, motives are emotionally *impulsive*. The impulses that direct our behaviour and thoughts may seem to be so numerous and complicated as to defy any attempt to classify them simply and intelligibly. We shall, however, succeed in doing so by working from below upwards. If we realize the existence of two activating elements, and their distinctiveness, we can apprehend the various interactions and reactions of which our conscious motives are the products. The most distinctively feminine of our impulses are (as we have seen) our inclinations, or likes and dislikes, urging us towards or away from their stimuli. These inclinations may be inborn. But, generally, they owe their origin to the effect of the pleasure or displeasure which is generated by their stimuli, that is to say, to the effect of emotional conditions of expansion or contraction. The vast majority of our likes and dislikes are not innate but acquired through experiences of the agreeable or disagreeable. They are evolved from emotional consequences. When they incline us towards persons, likes are termed " affections " or " attachments ". When intensified by emotion inclinations become " loves " and " hates ": but the former are properly so-called only when they are infused with admiration. These motives need not impel us to actual movement, since their activity may be dissipated in thought. One may satisfy a liking for music by thinking of it.

A like becomes a *desire* when it is reinforced by the masculine effort which is stimulated by its non-appeasement—that is to say, by its non-realization. It is, in fact, energized by the discord of discontent ; a desire presses us to *pursue* its object. A dislike is similarly energized into an active aversion (or " fear ") when it threatens us with realization. A desire expands into a *hope* when it is accompanied by a thought of the possibility or probability of its realization. When its realization is impossible or improbable, it contracts into a feeling, which is called a " fear ", because it is an apprehension of non-fulfilment.

In the generation of *antagonistic* motives, masculine emotion plays a more critical part, since antagonism, in its subjective phase, is a *conflict* between one element and the other. A displeasurable physical shock, arising from an unfavourable stimulus, is opposed by expansive emotion ; and a condition of discord results in which —to borrow the terms of Mendelism—either element may be dominant or recessive. There is feminine dominance in fear, doubt and distress, masculine in spontaneous courage, curiosity and anger.

We may also ascribe to masculine energy, in its " kinetic " phase, the *effort* that springs from a condition of discord. This becomes purposeful when the discord arises from the non-appeasement of a desire or an apprehension. The effort may be absorbed in thought. But when it retains its muscular character, it is brought under the control of experience by ideas of successful or unsuccessful possibilities that are presented by thought. So effort becomes " willed ". It is inhibited by possibilities of failure, and re-stimulated by possibilities of success. Uncertainty in these possibilities, or clashes between alternative possibilities, set up discords which result in efforts of decision or choice. Success and failure, from being the guides of effort, become objects in themselves, stimulating volitional desires and apprehensions which may be distinguished as ambitions and aversions.

Accordingly we owe to success and failure the genesis of the incentives that sway our voluntary life. Nor is this all. Through their emotional consequences they are the origin of the feelings with which we regard persons, things and qualities that are associated with conditions of success or failure. The motives of admiration and contempt, faith and respect, pity and jealousy are phases of expansive or contractive emotion " ex-revulsively " re-stimulated by ideas of success or failure—in themselves or in comparison with our own conditions—which are given an inclinational bent by the practical influence of the feminine element. We may style these motives " appreciative emotions ". And ex-revulsive emotion has a further astonishing development. It is the origin of our imaginative activities. We imagine when we invest a *quality* with living individuality. This, as a spontaneous " creativeness ", occurs when the quality arouses emotion, and reaches its artistic climax when the emotion so aroused is that of admiration or pity—that is to say, is a response to qualities that imply success or failure. Finally, emotion is in itself a motive in so far as it obliges us to *express* it. We express appreciative emotion in our manners and conduct, imaginative emotion in art, a blend of one and the other in religion.

It may be observed, in passing, that " instinct ", being effortless, cannot win the exhilaration of success. An instinctive process can, therefore, lead to none of these emotional developments.

Following our analysis we may classify impulsive motives as (1) inclinations, (2) affections, (3) antagonisms, (4) efforts of will, (5) ambitions, (6) appreciative emotions, (7) imaginative activities, and (8) emotional expression.

1 Habit

If we attempted to compute the total of our daily thoughts and actions we should be surprised to find how largely habit ordinarily contributes to them. It is unemotional, and we are consequently unaware of the strength—indeed, of the existence—of its energy. It is an obsessing force—the begetter of everything that is regular and conventional. In fact, as a guide to everyday life, it takes the place of the instincts which so unerringly control an insect's activities. Its influence, like that of instinct, is automatic. It results from a procession of ideas and movements that associatively re-stimulate one another in familiar sequence. But, unlike instinctive promptings, habits must be *learnt*. Man is more dependent than any other animal upon the instruction that he receives. Beasts and birds come into the world endowed with nervous concatenations that guide their impulses. These inherited aptitudes diminish as we ascend the animal kingdom until in man they almost wholly disappear. To compensate for this deficiency children are endowed with extraordinarily quick memorial powers, both of body and mind. And through the lack of hampering instincts, their mental and bodily activities are plastic and capable of artificial development. They are free to acquire memorial associations, however strange, or even *unnatural*, these may be. We owe to these acquirements our muscular dexterities, our habits of body, and our habits of mind. Our dexterities are exercised, for the most part, unconsciously : our habits consciously. Once acquired all three are almost as compulsive as instinct, and are, indeed, often miscalled " instinctive ". But their extraordinary variation from nation to nation, and from one period to another, proves that they are artificial and not innate.

Dexterities.—We become dexterous when complicated muscular movements follow one another automatically—that is to say, without the intervention of ideas. We think of dexterities as of capacities for skilled creative or expressive effort, such as painting, or the playing of musical instruments or of games. But actually they include everything in action or speech that distinguishes an adult from an infant : eating must be *learnt*, as well as walking and speaking, and the playing of golf or the violin. Orientals who take to European customs find it difficult, at the outset, to " hit off " the mouth with the end of a fork. Dexterities are acquired for the most part by imitation, and this sometimes involves the use of intelligence, since the analogy must be perceived between the visual impression of a movement and the tactile feeling of it in oneself. But, once learnt, they pass into automatic life. They are initiated by general ideas of what we mean to do or say, and pursue their course in complete unconsciousness, although their course may be controlled and guided by visual and other sense impressions. We may be quite unconscious of our steps in running upstairs. But they automatically follow the turns of the staircase. There is a similar connection between the notes of music which a pianist sees and the movements of his fingers on the keyboard.

Habits of body.—Our habits are also memorial associations, but on the conscious plane. That is to say they are impelled or guided by ideas that re-stimulate one another in sequence and also re-stimulate the nerves of muscles. We are borne along by the force of custom, but are aware that we are carried. Habit goes much further than to regulate the routine of life. It governs our manners and in a great measure our morals. The former are customary methods of expressing *feelings* of respect or affection for others, or of self-respect. They are so far spontaneous in that submissiveness of itself tends to relax the muscles, whereas self-respect naturally braces them. But they are for the most part artificial inventions, as is shown by their diversity in different countries. Orientals show respect by uncovering the feet : Europeans by uncovering the head. In Tibet one salutes a friend by putting out the tongue at him. Manners become so conventional that they are used without reference to actual feeling, and even in contradiction to it, as when one signs oneself as " your obedient servant " in addressing an authority which in fact he despises. Morals, other than the idealistic, are rules of behaviour that conduce to the stability of the government or the welfare and dignity of the community. They are in some measure derived from successful experience. But they vary extraordinarily with the locality. Polygamy is moral in Asia, immoral in Europe. The rules of decency and modesty arose out of antiphysical repugnances to physical functions that seemed to humiliate human dignity. They are, however, in great measure arbitrary. In the East it is still indecent to wear a short coat. But they become so firmly rooted in us by habit that they seem to be instinctive. Discipline is habitual self-control. It begins with the repression in infancy of physical promptings that are inopportune, but grows into an automatic self-restraint that can mask the existence of fear and angry feeling. It is developed by practice which may consist in little acts of self-victimization that have no intrinsic value, but are educative means to an end.

Habits of mind.—Habit is mental, or " subjective ", when it consolidates and preserves the acquired associations of ideas that set us towards or against other persons or things in like or dislike. Our acquired affections and attachments, aversions and hostilities rest upon the connection of their object with ideas of kindliness, fellowship, power, excellence or their contraries. These connections may be formed by actual experience of these qualities. But they may be learnt through being instilled into our minds by instruction. Thus a child may learn to love a father whom it has never seen. In either case it is a habit that supports them and protects them from disillusionment. Loyalty to established authority is very largely conventional, as is appreciated very clearly by those whose business it is to inculcate it. Each nation is habitually inspired by its peculiar flag. Also conventional is the respect for old age, which originates in the days when we are dependent upon our elders, and subsists as a habitual attitude of mind. It is to be noticed amongst beasts and birds and is by no means an exclusive attribute of humanity.

Ideas and associations of ideas, such as the possession of a particular quality by a person or object, are amongst the things for which we contract habitual likes and dislikes. We dignify them by the names of " beliefs ", " opinions ", " prejudices " and " convictions ". The etymology of the word *belief*, it may be observed, appears to indicate that it originally meant a view that was supported " by like ". Devotion to particular religious dogmas and ceremonies is sheltered by habit from the effect of criticism. Hence argument can seldom deflect a man from the conviction that his religion is unassailable, and that all others are obviously false. Scientific beliefs are similarly protected, and new conclusions have, therefore, to fight for acceptance. Franklin's discovery that thunder-storms were electric was rejected by the Royal Society ; and the law of evolution was received resentfully and adopted with reluctance, since it conflicted with the idea of man's inherent nobility. So again, in reasoning as to the conduct of others, habit blunts our appreciation of analogies. We cannot put ourselves in their place, and see ourselves with their eyes.

Education is largely concerned with the formation of habits of mind and may, therefore, actually lessen one's capacity of testing statements by referring them to experience. It is a fact, acknowledged by schoolmasters, that boys on leaving school are not uncommonly less intelligent than when they entered it, however much may be the knowledge that they have acquired from their lessons.

2 Inclinations

We pass to motives of impulse, the most fundamental of which are the inclinations which set us towards or away from persons and things. We are conscious of them as likes and dislikes. They are conditions of attractedness and repelledness, which urge the humbler animals to " tropistic " movements of approach and recoil. But with the development of a brain another escape is provided for them. If not strong, they expend themselves in developing appreciative thought which re-stimulates emotion of the mild type commonly called " sentimental ". That is to say, in virtue of its intermediary position between sensation, or feeling, and behaviour, the brain can act as a " shock-absorber ". Otherwise our behaviour in response to sensation would be as restless and inconstant as that of a butterfly. With thought as a safety-valve, mild likes and dislikes merely set us thinking, with sentiments of pleasure and displeasure.

A strong like or dislike cannot be dissipated in this fashion. Whether it is stimulated by a sensation or a thought, there must be an interval between its inception and its realization. There is a delay which sets up a discord that is felt as discontent, impatience, or " longing "—a discord that results from contrariety between the like and the effects of its non-fulfilment. This stimulates *effort*. There is no desire in an inclination which satisfies itself forthwith.

Since it involves a discord, desire is not a happy feeling; indeed, amatory poetry drips with tears. An aversion is discordant in itself: it "threatens" us. And it is irritating, because it sets up emotional resistence to its effects, which is materialized against its object. Desires and aversions pass into pursuits and avoidances when the effort that they stimulate passes into the muscular activity of behaviour.

An inclination becomes *prudent* when it is directed by deliberation —by the comparison of alternative possibilities that are suggested by experience. We speak of it in this case as "reasoned". Mere inclination is superseded by volition. These various developments are not, however, in point at present. Our concern is with the simple likes and dislikes that dispose us towards or away from certain experiences and certain persons, or, in sentimental fashion, towards or away from ideas of those experiences and persons. Inclinations that are stimulated by persons may be conveniently considered apart, as *affections*. We are now concerned, therefore, with our inclinations towards or away from *things*—that is to say, objects, conditions, actions and utterances, or towards or away from ideas of them.

The appetites.—We are hereditarily—or instinctively—inclined to certain things by the appetites—sexually by lust, to food when we are hungry, to drink when thirsty, to repose when fatigued. It has been proved that in vertebrate animals these instincts survive the extraction of the upper brain; and they can evidently act independently of consciousness, for they are experienced by the humblest of living organisms. But the guidance which they afford man is general, not particular; and hence we can acquire tastes for any kind of food and drink which has satisfied our needs and is not actually harmful. It is liked because the pleasure of satisfaction is associated with it. Judging from his teeth and the length of his intestine, man is naturally a vegetarian. The discovery of fire and the art of cooking brought a flesh diet within the range of possibility. The very precise information given by Herodotus shows that cannibalism was at one time wide-spread; and he is corroborated by the fact that in burials of the Neolithic period, the flesh was not uncommonly stripped off the bones before sepulture, since parts of the skeleton are decorated with red ochre. It is in the last degree improbable that this troublesome dissection should have been undertaken with the rough flint knives of the time, unless the flesh was turned to useful purpose. Cookery affords innumerable possibilities in human diet, and tastes have developed and changed as it has

F

extended its range. We cannot understand, in these days, how the Romans could have relished the marine curiosities, such as the octopus and jelly fish, which they esteemed as delicacies. The taste for alcohol is plainly acquired. Its properties were discovered, in all probability, through casual fermentation. In many parts of India fermented porridge is still used to hearten the labouring man ; and, to preserve the ferment, a careful housewife will leave the porridge-pot uncleansed for years.

The familiar and the strange.—A like for the familiar and a dislike of the strange are instinctive, for they arise from the effect of the accordant and discordant upon established memorial associations : the former " fits in " with them, the latter disconcerts them. It is obvious that these effects are independent of consciousness, for the humblest organisms are disturbed by a strangeness of environment. The inclinations that result from them are consequently very strong —much stronger than is commonly realised. The attraction of the familiar is illustrated by the compelling force of habit ; and it is likely that familiarity is the foundation of the " gregarious instinct " so strikingly illustrated by insects.

The harmonious and the discordant.—The harmony and discord with which we are now concerned are those which affect us through sensation, not those which result from states of internal feeling· They so far resemble the familiar and the strange in that harmony is intrinsic familiarity between two things, discord intrinsic strangeness. The harmony or discord may be between two sense impressions, between a sense impression and a recollection, or between a sensory experience and a desire—that is to say, a like which is energized by effort. Thus we like a combination of colours that " go together ", and musical notes, in a coincidence or sequence, each of which leads to the other through a harmonic. We like the helpful and dislike the obstructive and injurious. But a sensibility to harmony may be artificial, for anything we become " used to " is, in fact, harmonious. The order in which the various courses of a meal are served, which seems to us to be inevitable, may be quite incongruous to the tastes of an Asiatic. And a child is quite indifferent to the sequence in which it eats what it likes. It is possible, therefore, that the most startling passages in modern music may be harmonious to ears that are " up-to-date ".

Two of the most admirable of human motives—gratitude and justice—spring from the like of harmony. For acts that are grateful and just are harmonious in that they requite good with good and bad with bad. They introduce harmony into a sequence, and therefore influence our inclinations. All men like them in the abstract and as applied to themselves. But they unfortunately cannot compete with the stronger motives of self-interest, *esprit-de-corps*, and antagonism.

The fearful.—Fear is the acutest of all discordant dislikes—and naturally, for an animal that was absolutely fearless would have no chance of survival. It is stimulated, not by a thing in itself, but by the relationship of a thing to experience—by its strangeness, or its discordance with motives of self-care. Actual injury causes, not fear, but pain. Fear is a " presentiment " of injury, pain, difficulty, loss or humiliation—that is to say, it is stimulated by an *idea* of harmfulness or failure. It is the response of our purely physical side to danger or difficulty ; and accordingly, during sleep, when the animative spirits are in abeyance and no antagonism can develop, a very slight noise, if it is strange, will awaken us with a momentary thrill of terror.

Sensory likes and dislikes.—We like certain touches and dislike others. Pain, whether internal or external, seems to be caused by injurious pressure. A like for the sweet and a distaste for the bitter and acrid are so universal that they must be innate. Dogs whose upper brains have been excised will reject food that is flavoured with quinine, and sneeze under the effects of tobacco smoke. But, for the most part, our dispositions towards odours and tastes must be acquired, since they vary so extraordinarily from one people to another. In regard to pleasures of sight and hearing there is, again, such diversity and discrepancy that our instinctive sensibilities must be of the very simplest. Colour and rhythm appeal to all men. But, for the rest, our appreciation of tints, and their combinations, of the complexities of rhythm or " time ", and of the musical arrangement of notes of sound must be acquired. We owe them, it appears, in great measure to the sharpening of sensibility which comes from the attentive exercise of the sense-organs. But an important contributory element is the development of associations which offer new possibilities of harmony.

The amusing.—Those who are either depressed, or " superior ", may have no liking for amusement, the former because their nerves have lost revulsive elasticity, and the latter because it is undignified, and accordingly unseemly, to " give way " to excitement. The generality of mankind are devoted to it, whether it comes from the varying circumstances of life and manners, as in the drama, from the successes and failures of playful emulation, as in games, or from the ups and downs of luck, as in gambling. The strength of its attraction is demonstrated by the immense popularity of the cinema, of football matches and the race course. Most men respond to jokes and witticisms, and extend their liking to those who can invent these instruments of gaiety.

The pleasure of society.—A very remarkable liking is that for the society of others, since it is quite independent of any attachment to or affection for them. It is obviously an acquired taste, for it may be lacking entirely amongst country people ; and, indeed, experience shows that one can live contentedly in solitude. Mankind is not instinctively gregarious. A liking for society is acquired by experience of it. But it may grow into an obsessing habit, so that, without this excitement, life seems intolerably dull. Social intercourse offers a variety of pleasures. Those of superior rank or fortune feel assured of their superiority in the company of their inferiors : those who are inferior are flattered by being associated with their superiors. Conversation with others must be interesting in that it exercises one of the most important of our faculties—the divination of their real feelings and thoughts from their manners and language. Personal gossip pleases by exciting at times admiration, at other times pity or a feeling of our own superiority : also by giving shocks—accidentally or " in chaff "—to our dignity, which if we are in good spirits have the revulsive effect of reinforcing our self-esteem. We are naturally pleased by talk which ministers to a like or prejudice. And the words of others may amuse us through their humour or wit. So it comes that for a vast number of persons one of the chiefest pleasures of life is to be with others.

Rhythm and dancing.—Rhythm is the succession of *equal* intervals, which may be sub-divided at pleasure. It may, then, be defined as harmony in movement. Men's fondness for it, whether in movement, as in dancing, in sound, as in the drum, in poetry, in music, and in decorative pattern, is impossible of explanation if we look for its origin outside us. For what is called the " rhythm of nature " makes, in fact, no rhythmic appeal to us. Its intervals are too long, and are, moreover, irregular. In ourselves, however, we have two perennial sources of rhythm—in the beating of the heart and in the steps of walking. The former is generally hardly noticeable, but in walking and running rhythm is innate and makes a forceful impression upon us. Its appeal is instinctive : in our method of progression we are rhythmic animals. Dancing is derived from walking by the more or less complicated sub-division of a step. The extension of rhythm to poetry and music is an elaboration which will be discussed when we come to treat of Art.

The influence of success and failure.—These, as we have seen, stimulate admiration and contempt—for ourselves and for others. But there is a like in admiration and a dislike in contempt, and it will be convenient to make a passing reference to them here. Success and failure influence our inclinations more through the concepts that are deduced from them than in themselves. They generate in the mind, as their qualities, ideas of power, skill, excellence (or superiority), and peculiarity (or nobility) which by their association with particular things render them attractive, and enter very largely indeed into our notions of the " beautiful ". A vast number of the objects that we like are in reality symbols of these qualities— fine clothes, decorations and titles, for instance. On the other hand, we dislike the inferior or " common ". We like conduct or words with which power, excellence, or nobility are associated, or which associates them with ourselves. So we are attracted by compliments and, through association, by those who pay them to us. The like for popularity, or the esteem of others, is a like for success that is attributed to us by the conduct or speech of others ; and, since it is stimulated " objectively " through impressions of the senses, it is valued even more than the consciousness of one's actual success which comes to us subjectively, through feeling.

The effect of association.—It is, then, obvious that many of the things that we like are attractive simply because certain pleasing ideas are associated with them, and are re-stimulated by them. A tall hat, for instance, is singularly unattractive apart from the sense of dignity that it confers. If we follow this clue we shall realize that all inclinations, other than the instinctive, are stimulated associatively—that is to say, not by things in themselves, but by the qualities that they possess. For if a thing loses its pleasing quality, it ceases to attract us. The association between a thing and its quality is natural if the quality is perceived by the senses. We imitate it artificially when we connect the pleasure of success with a piece of coloured ribbon.

3 The Affections

We give affection the name of " love " when it includes an element of pride or admiration. *Love* always implies this, and may mean little else, as in the " love of justice " ; the kindred words " laus " and " lob " express in Latin and German the praise that is admiration's consequence. Three of our affections are plainly urged by instinctive promptings, self-love, sexual love, and maternal love. And the effects of familiarity and strangeness instinctively dispose us towards acquaintances and against strangers. But, for the rest, our affections are the consequences, not of inherited inclinations, but of mental processes—of the associating or connecting of certain ideas with particular persons or classes, or of identifying particular persons or classes with ourselves. That this is so is proved by the fact that our social dispositions depend for the most part upon the education that we receive, and can be changed by a change of ideas, as by " conversion ".

Self-love.—The inclination towards oneself, which becomes self-care when confronted with discordant experiences, is so necessary for the preservation of life that a creature which lacked it would very soon perish. That an individual should be attracted by itself would be impossible unless its nature were dual. But, given a duality of constitution, it is conceivable that one element should be attracted by the other ; and, since to be attracted is, as we have seen, a " feminine " characteristic, it follows that egotism is the attraction of the " feminine " by the " masculine ". We can, indeed, feel that this is so. For our egotistical feelings are aroused by emotional qualities, such as courage and success, which result from the victory of masculine over feminine proclivities, whereas in such processes as enjoying our food, we are not egotistical but absorbed. It is hardly necessary to explain that in drawing this distinction we are referring not to men and women, but to the male and female elements which both possess.

Sexual love.—This is called " love ", par excellence, because it illustrates the power of admiration with extraordinary force. Mere sexual desire inclines an individual of one sex towards any individual of the other. It is by admiration that the inclination is focussed upon a particular person. Hence it is dangerous for a man to admire a woman ; and his wife is well aware of this. Admiration, as we shall see, transforms the character of thought. It converts the dull appraisement of a like into an enthusiastic appreciation which stimulates the decoration of its object. And, when under its influence thought flies from the material to the immaterial—from a person to the *qualities* of a person—it creates images which personify these qualities. Accordingly, a lover's idea of his mistress's appearance and personality may differ very widely from the truth. For she is " transfigured " in his eyes.

Hence we say that "love is blind". By these mental processes sexual love is etherealized into an ecstasy which is reluctant to own its connection with the earth. Love fades as imagination is disillusioned. It is more enduring in women than in men, because, in her case, it is blended with the maternal instinct.

Maternal love.—The love of a mother for her child is the strongest —and therefore the most admirable—of all the affections. It is quite regardless of merit. A father will shut his door against a son who has disgraced him : his mother cleaves to him throughout. A woman is destined by nature to cherish another, and is condemned to produce more nutriment than suffices for herself. But her instinctive promptings must be directed by the mind. A mother has no innate recognition of her baby, and will adopt a changeling as her own, if she is ignorant of the change. Hence the cuckoo can find a foster-mother anywhere, a hen contentedly accepts a brood of ducklings, and a woman's maternal affection may expend itself upon a doll, a lap-dog or a husband.

Affections of association and unification (or identification).—These may be distinguished as attachments and unions. The first result from the attaching of a pleasing idea to a person—as of helpfulness or good-will : the second from the identifying of another's origin, attributes or feelings with one's own. These are mental processes. For the kindly idea that attaches us to a friend may be detached by his behaviour, or even by the slanderous words of another ; and we regard him as a friend no longer. And the feeling that we are related to another by "one-ness" of family, disappears if we learn that he is actually of different blood. Since the days of Aristotle man has been regarded as *innately* social in his habits. But as a matter of fact his sociability is acquired, and it is by no means impossible to be happy in solitude.

Attachments.—The ideas which attract us to others are those of indulgence, protection, helpfulness or good-will. These qualities stimulate a like which is extended to their possessors. They are our *friends*. In the face of ill-will friendship is impossible. The love of children for their parents, which seems so "natural", will not develop if the parents be unkind. An inclination, in itself, is a passive, not an active, condition—a fact which is illustrated very patently by the short-comings of friendliness. It is often content to receive without giving. We may entertain our friends liberally, but there are frequently thoughts of social prestige in the back-ground. Children are seldom disposed to "help mother" in preference to playing. Active good feeling is the result of stronger motives than a like : it is the fruit of sympathy, gratitude, admiration, pity or generosity.

Unions.—The notion that one may be mentally united with another—or, put more precisely, that the idea of oneself may be united in some respects with the idea of another—is difficult to realize. Yet we habitually use words that imply it—such as " at-one-ment ", " assimilation " and " unity ". That we are hardly conscious of this mental process is no proof that it does not occur. We are not conscious of the digestion of food by the stomach. The assimilation of two ideas through a quality that is the same in both—or common to both—is as we have seen, the fundamental process of *intelligence*. Affections of union are intelligent, whereas those of attachment are memorial.

The actuality of this process of unification and the strength of its influence, is proved by its effect in barring the rise of sexual feelings between members of the same family. Sexuality implies the existence of a difference of " gender "—that is to say of *kind*, and this difference is lost in the close union of the family—a natural consequence which is reflected in the marriage laws of all peoples throughout the world.

The effect of mental union with another is to render us altruistic—ready to help him or to give him pleasure. For, if he is one with us, in pleasing him we please ourselves. We may, it is true, give him pleasure by an effort of will. But this is a complication with which we are not at present concerned. We have in mind not forced, but spontaneous kindness. And this, we know very well, may be as pleasing to the giver as to the receiver. We are inclined to gratify him, not simply because we like him, but because to gratify him is to gratify ourselves.

We may be united with another in origin—that is to say, in family—in belief, in manners and speech, in occupation, in environment, and in feeling. Any of these samenesses has the effect of grouping us in the same " kind-class " with him. For we are of the same " kind " with another whether he is a cousin, a fellow Christian, a fellow-workman, a fellow-townsman or a comrade. Hence come the words " kinship " and " kindness " : the former is commonly, but not universally, limited to blood relationship : the latter has come to signify the behaviour that is the *consequence* of kinship. The various phases of union, which have knit individuals into societies, have been determined by the distinctive samenesses that have, from time to time, seemed to be so important as to be bonds of fellowship, or *esprit de corps*. The family, which was the first of all unions, still retains its solidarity in India, China and in France. Tribal cohesion rests upon ideas of sameness in racial descent which may be illusory but are none the less effective. Identities of language and religion can unite peoples of very different races. Community in domicile was the origin of the Greek and Italian " city-states ", and, when extended to a country, contributes to the feeling of national patriotism. But the idea of nationality includes other important elements—subjection to the same government, and community in traditions which foster collective sentiments of pride. In competition with national unity are the numerous " fellowships " which arise from unity of sectarian, social, professional or occupational interests, such as maintains the distinctness of the Jews, knits together political parties and clubs, and unifies the members of a Trades Union. National solidarity may be completely undermined by these fellowships, since they tend to group the people of a country into fraternities that may be as indifferent to one another as if they were distinct peoples. They become in fact distinct " species ", for a species is a *kind*. They may endeavour to maintain their exclusive self-importance by the prohibition of outside marriages. So they develop into hereditary castes, as in India. The simplest, and the most portentous, of these uniting distinctions is that which draws the poor against the rich—an antagonism which threatens the existence of our present economic civilization. It can be effectively countered only by feelings of respect, or of sympathy for which the persuasiveness of political oratory is a very ineffective substitute. But it is mollified if the poor are admitted to political power. For this has the effect of assimilating them to the rich.

Unity, as already noticed, prompts us to active benevolence, since we must feel a glow of pleasure in obliging those who are one with ourselves. But its promptings become less and less urgent with the widening of our fellowships : their intensity varies inversely with their extent : political and industrial strife shows that there is no great warmth in our feeling for a fellow-countryman, as such, unless our unity with him is accentuated by a common danger or enthusiasm, as during a war, or by a common feeling of strangeness, as in a foreign country. Sympathy is at its strongest when our unison is only with an individual—that is to say, when we are united to a particular person by sameness of aims, interests and tastes. This begets the sympathy of comradeship—the warmest of all. The " pal " is nearer than a brother.

So far of the sympathy, or fellow-feeling, that comes from identity. But there may be sympathy from an entirely different source. It may be the outcome of admiration or pity for another. For these emotions stimulate imitation, and imitation in feeling—that is to say, " subjective " imitation—is in fact, sympathy. It is an indisputable fact that we are impelled to imitate one whom we admire, be it only in dress and manners ; and it is obviously by feeling with one whom we pity that we realize his necessities. The sympathy which comes of admiration or pity will, however, be discussed most conveniently when we are considering the origin of these feelings. And sympathy assumes a third form when it is idealistic, when, that is to say, it is inspired by admiration for the harmony which sympathy represents. This is the comprehensive " loving-kindness " which is the Christian ideal. We shall refer to it in more detail hereafter.

4 Antagonisms

The effect of a nervous shock, or of a dislike, is not always overwhelming because it may be antagonized. This capacity proves the duality of our natural constitution : " it takes two to make a quarrel ". Its utility in the struggle for life is self-evident. It is this internal antagonism which makes life a struggle instead of a funeral procession—with interludes of dancing, perhaps—but none the less submissively bent towards the tomb. The outcome of antagonism may, it is true, be defeat. A fear may utterly subdue us. But it may be the victory that triumphs in courage, or the resentful energy of irritation. Without antagonism, there could be no anger. That there is self-antagonism in courage is less evident. But we may feel sure that a slight shock of fear precedes and provokes it. For, when there is no fear, as when one has become accustomed to a danger, fearlessness is a matter of habit, and is of a quite different character to courage of the animated, bright-eyed type.

A shock, or dislike, is antagonized by the spirits because it is discordant with their expansive tension. If they are at a low ebb, resistance fails. Hence anything that raises the spirits increases resistant strength. For the antagonism to which we are now referring, is, so to speak, functional and quite independent of ideas. It is exhibited very plainly by many of the insects. This opens the question why some animals are more resistant than others—and why, amongst men, we find such differences in resistant—or as it is

commonly called " nervous "—power. The explanation seems to
be that the development of the masculine element may be dis-
proportionately weak, or may be postponed for a period. In the
insect world we find striking illustrations of this delay in development. In a caterpillar, for instance, animative energy seems to be
atrophied. But it " comes into its own " through the metamorphoses that take place in the chrysalis stage.

The discord of antagonism is, as we have seen, the ultimate source
of willing. But the will is a later development. The reaction with
which we are now concerned is the automatic stimulation of resistance by conditions of discord. There is a discord when a like is not
immediately satisfied. An effort is consequently stimulated. When
the discord arises, not from dissatisfaction, but from dislike that has
been stimulated by injury, difficulty or opposition, emotional
antagonism energizes the dislike into anger or hate. When the
discord is that of apprehension or doubt, it may be antagonized out
of apparent existence by an effort which overcomes it in courage or
curiosity. These may be voluntary or deliberate. But we are not
at present concerned with voluntary, but with spontaneous nervous
resistance. There can be no question of " willing " in the audacity
of a wild boar, in the curiosity of a monkey, or in the endurance or
perseverance of a worker-bee. Moreover, the will cannot affect the
feelings : by no effort can we make ourselves *feel* angry, or subdue
a feeling of nervousness.

Anger.—The resistance of which we are conscious in anger is a
struggle, not a victory, because the stimulus of our dislike is not an
apprehension as regards the future, but a present fact. It may be
the ill-will, or " contrariety " of another, the idea of which sets up
opposition in ourselves. It may be an injury, hindrance or humiliation that has been actually experienced, the effects of which the
spirits can combat, but cannot entirely overcome, whereas they can
wholly stifle the shock that is caused by an apprehension. Anger
is, then, necessarily bitter. But the nervous energy that generates
it spices it with pleasure. For the same reason anger gives strength.
Being the consequence of opposition or actual injury it cannot be
conjured up voluntarily. But it can easily be re-stimulated by a
recollection of its cause, or the idea of a similar provocation.

Anger differs from simple irritation in that it is influenced by an
idea of another's personal ill-will, or malevolence, which makes him
our " enemy ". Consequently, when out of childhood, we cannot
be *angry* with the inanimate, however irritating it may be. An idea
of another's ill-will may be gathered from the words of others. We

may, therefore, be infected with the war-fever by propaganda, which may lead us to hate a nation which has in fact done us no harm. For if another's ill-will be figured as enduring, anger becomes hate. We cannot, then, be angry without a mental operation, whereas irritation comes automatically. It is noteworthy that the distinction between a malevolent injury and an injury that is simply irritating is recognized by the law. A harmful act is not " criminal " unless it is done with criminal intent : if this is lacking, its commission merely involves a liability for civil damages.

The antagonism of anger is primitively internal, or " subjective ": we oppose the *effects* of ill-will or injury. It may remain internal as when we are angry with ourselves. It is externalized by being directed against him who causes these effects. For they present themselves as his *qualities* and, therefore, as belonging to him. And the character of our responsive movements is changed : instead of shrinking from the cause of our distress, we throw ourselves against it. The actions to which we are prompted are suggested by the injuries that we have suffered. In their simplest forms they are retaliative—" an eye for an eye, a tooth for a tooth ". But, through analogies, the mind can devise more elaborate methods of revenge. Idealistic morality apart, the demand for vengeance is insistent. The history of criminal law shows that, in punishing offenders, its object was not merely deterrent, but sought to obviate civil disorder by satisfying the injured person's desire for vengeance in an orderly way. For, since the judge has no ill-will, the punishment that he inflicts excites no desire for vengeance in the offender.

Indignation.—Amongst the causes of irritation is discord between the character of an intent and the character of the results which follow it. If one is good and the other bad there is a discordance that shocks us. It defeats an expectation that is based upon our own subjective experience, inasmuch as a successful effort is followed by pride—both good ; whereas failure is followed by shame— both bad. We look for a similar correspondence outside us, calling the harmony " justice ". We are very generally disappointed, for the course of worldly events shows but the most casual correspondence between merit and reward. The irritation caused by this injustice is called " indignation ", because its *cause* is " unworthiness "—another curious illustration of the substitution of cause for consequence.

Courage.—We may be courageous naturally (or spontaneously), voluntarily, that is to say, by an effort of will, or idealistically, when we are inspired by admiration for the quality. We are now concerned with the spontaneous kind, the most salient peculiarity of which is its variability from man to man—not only in general strength, but in regard to the particular kind of shocks which it is able to subdue. Some children, from the earliest age, are more courageous than others, and the scope of their courage may vary : one can resist pain, another danger, another, almost from infancy, shows the " moral courage " which renders it almost indifferent to the neglect or contempt of its companions. These peculiarities persist into adult life. The boldest riders may be terrified of precipices : the hardiest of mountaineers may utterly break down under the stress of illness.

It is, then, obvious that the " nervous tone " of individuals may differ innately in degree, and in its bearings—differences that support the conclusion that the development of the masculine element may be stunted, or retarded in regard to particular sensibilities. The feminine element appears to over-ride it. This defect may be remedied in regard to a particular kind of shock by frequent exposure to it, for as a danger becomes familiar it loses its sting. It may also be remedied, with a more general application, by the education of the will. This, being fundamentally of muscular origin, can undoubtedly be strengthened by practice (as the muscles can be strengthened) or by the discipline of hardship. But although an effort of will may enable a nervous man to face danger manfully, it will not enable him to face it without feeling nervous.

It may be added to these comments that the masculine element is certainly more delicate than the feminine. For it is liable to fatigue ; and it may be completely disabled by an over-violent strain. The victim of " shell-shock " is in this condition. His physical functions may not suffer in the least. But he has lost all resisting power. It is in curious accordance with this reflection that male infants are more delicate than females.

Curiosity.—As courage resists fear, so curiosity resists doubt ; there is probably an affinity of origin between the words *cor* and *cura*. A doubt is mental confusion that is caused by an impression or idea of what is unaccountable or " unplaceable ". When curiosity is *willed* it is " scientific " : when it is prompted by an idealistic admiration of the true, it is the " spirit of enquiry ". But as we see it illustrated by the persistent " why ? " of childhood, it is clearly a spontaneous reaction.

With advancing years this spontaneous curiosity declines. A schoolboy is much less inquisitive than a child : indeed, he despises curiosity as a sign of childishness. We might be inclined to attribute this loss of edge to the blunting influence of rebuffs : for a child's curiosity is annoying and is reproved. But its more probable cause is the formation of habits of mind—beliefs and prejudices which stifle doubts automatically. For one has no doubt as to the origin of a thunderstorm if it can be assigned to the Almighty, or as to the cause of the earth's attraction if it be formulated as " gravity ".

Perseverance and endurance.—These are resistances to disappointment and fatigue. By means of them the attention is kept fixed upon an object, and is not permitted to wander. They are, moreover, the mainsprings of industry. We generally conceive of them as voluntary efforts. But there must be something of the spontaneous in them, as they are exhibited so forcibly by the conduct of quite inferior animals. It must be admitted, however, that they produce but little effect during the first years of life. Childhood is characterized by its volatility and impatience. This may, perhaps, be attributed to its acute sensibility to fatigue. Children require far more sleep than adults. And it is indisputable that their nervous sensibilities are abnormally acute, as is proved by their excitability, the vivacity of their imagination and the retentiveness of their memory. Their lack of application may, then, be ascribed, not so much to a lack of resisting power, as to an excess in that which has to be resisted.

5 Efforts of Will

The faculty of willing, we have seen, is the use of experience to guide effort in the successful realization of our motives, or in the attainment of success or avoidance of failure. An effort is fundamentally an energetic muscular reaction from the nervous strain of a condition of discord. It becomes purposeful, or practical, when the initiatory discord is generated by the non-appeasement of an energetic inclination—-a desire or an apprehension. Through the intervention of the brain the effort can be divorced from its motive, since the brain, lying between the nerves and the muscles, can be influenced by the motive but delay the effort until the occasion for it has arrived. This presents itself as a successful possibility, and the idea of success, being closely associated with effort, is able to re-stimulate it, and regulate its action. Moreover, the idea of success in itself suffices to generate effort. For it stimulates desire, and this involves a following effort.

Effort can influence thought as well as movement : it can initiate or control a course of reflection as well as a course of action. It is remarkable that energy which is primarily concerned with the muscles should extend its influence to the brain. This seems to indicate the existence of some kinship between movement and thought—a point to which we have already referred. We shall touch upon it again in the succeeding section.

There is the energy of discord in fear, doubt and distress, and that of contrarified discord in spontaneous, or unthinking, courage, curiosity and anger ; and this frees itself in effort. But there is no *volition* unless the effort is re-stimulated and guided by ideas of successful and unsuccessful possibilities. This can only occur when the effort is *purposeful*—that is to say, when it is the consequence of a like or dislike, animated as a desire and an apprehension. But all emotional conditions tend to develop into one or other of these motives, since the disagreeable stimulates a dislike, the agreeable a like.

If our motive over-rides ideas of possible contingencies, and adopts the first idea of action that presents itself, our volition is *impulsive*. It is *tentative* or *deliberative*, when doubt is developed, either by the absence of clear ideas of possibilities, or by conflict between various possibilities. Trial may be combined with delibera- tion. In this form volition has been the most fruitful of all the causes that have contributed to material civilization. For it is to intelligent experiment—to experiment that has been guided by past successes and failures—that we owe the great mass of the inventions which have made civilization what it is. We attribute these discoveries to " science ". But science for the most part merely explains them. If we follow the development of the steam and gas engines, or the various uses to which electricity is put, we shall find that they represent the results, not of abstract reasoning, but of a vast number of trials—made, it is true, with a purpose, and by men of intelligence—but trials none the less.

In deliberate volition, effort is inhibited for a time by the doubt that is caused by a conflict between various possibilities. There is a period of hesitation during which they are balanced one against the other ; and the discord is terminated by an effort, choosing the course that *promises* best. That is to say, our behaviour is influenced by ideas of future, or ulterior consequences, and is accordingly called " provident " or " prudent ". We think that our willing is " arbi- trary ". It may perhaps be called so, if it is simply made at random, in despair of decision, since in this case it is merely an expression of discordant feelings. But, when we deliberately choose, we follow the line which appears to be the most advantageous. A choice is, in fact, a prudential inclination that governs our conduct exactly as does an impulsive inclination. It is ridiculous to attribute " free-will " to one who chooses a taxi-cab instead of an omnibus because he is late for an appointment. The success or failure which influences us need not, of course, be material. We may refuse a glass of wine because it would be undignified to accept it.

It may be urged that a choice cannot be attributed to the will at all, if it simply results from the attraction of an advantage. But it requires an effort to rid oneself of the impulse that first presents itself, and to " make up one's mind " amidst a number of conflicting inducements, each of which, if given time, will develop almost endless possibilities. It is by an effort that we select the course, which is, " on the whole ", the best, within the time that is practically at our disposal.

A choice, or decision, endows us with a " purpose " to which we give a number of different names. At its simplest, it is an *intention*. It is a *resolution* when it is a decision to make a certain choice on a particular future occasion. An intention becomes an *obligation* when it is " bound " to its object by the contingency of failure, shame or punishment. We are " obliged " to leave in time to catch a train because if late we should be punished by missing it. We are " obliged " to a person when his conduct to us is such as to make ill-will or indifference on our part shamefully discordant. An obligation becomes a *duty* when it is in pursuance of a general rule of conduct. It is our duty to pay our bills because dishonesty is condemned by society as well as shameful in itself.

We are only " responsible " for our actions when choice is possible —that is to say, when an idea of consequences presents itself. It may fail to put in an appearance because we have not had sufficient experiences of consequences to be impressed by them, or because, owing to a derangement of the nerves, ideas follow one another in wrong connections. Children illustrate one of these cases : the insane illustrate the other. Both are absolved from the penalties of the criminal law. With advancing years ideas of consequences *must* present themselves, since they are memorially re-stimulated by every idea of action that occurs to us. In persons of emotional disposition they may be over-ridden by impulses. But this occurs because they are not sufficiently certain, or sufficiently serious. No one would steal if it was certain that what he stole would be recovered from him. And it has been proved by experience that the fear of flogging will deter men from crimes that would defy thoughts of imprisonment. This is the argument in favour of capital punishment.

Willed thought.—The influence of effort upon thought will be discussed when we are concerned with the process of thinking. But we may touch upon it here. The ordinary procession of thoughts is disturbed when a doubt occurs, since this occasions a confusion that arrests us. It may be as to the identity of something unknown that is in relationship to something known—as to the *reason* why the behaviour of a friend has been so chilly, for instance. Doubts of this class are expressed by interrogative pronouns and particles. It may be as to the existence of a certain relationship between two known things : for example, whether strikes will *continue* to be frequent—a doubt which is put as a question by reversing the order of the subject and the verb. We hunt for *clues* which will connect the problem with a " law "—that is to say, a general relationship of succession that is based upon experience or upon the authority of one whom we trust. We find a clue to our friend's chilliness in some incautious words that we have spoken of him, which a tale-bearer must have repeated, for it is a *law* that friendship is cooled by criticism : a similar clue to the continuance of strikes is given by their profitableness, for it is a *law* that men continue in a course which they find to be profitable. An effort is involved in tracing the clue and hence we give it as the " reason " for our decision, omitting to state the law to which it has guided us when the law is well-known. If a clue is self-evident no reasoning effort is required : we still refer to a law, but so naturally and spontaneously that we are hardly aware of the reference. When we infer, for instance, that a man who wears a white tie is a clergyman our inference is based upon the law that " all men who wear white ties are clergymen ". But when a clue must be searched for, an effort is required ; and those who are dis-inclined to exert themselves leave it unsought, and accept, as a *belief*, the opinion of another which is in accord with their likes or prejudices.

The will and the future.—Our idea of the future is, as we have seen, owed by us to the process of associative re-stimulation, since this presents to us a thought of the consequence of everything that we do, or that happens. But our view of future time is extended and clarified by the process of willing, since this is directed by thoughts of consequences which are often not immediate but ulterior, and lie, therefore, in a future that is at some distance from the present. We may, for instance, decide to please another, because he has amongst his friends one who may possibly do us a service. We acknowledge the effect of willing in bringing the future before us when we use the word " will " to indicate future time. Our idea of the future is then strengthened by the exercise of the will. But the exercise of the will is, on the other hand, strengthened by the clearness of our idea of the future. There is reaction as well as action. For the greater is the possibility of remote consequences actually happening, the greater will be their effect in guiding us to particular decisions or choices. If the future is quite obscure, we act upon impulse—a tendency that is illustrated very strikingly by the change of popular character which is brought about by the disturbance of war. Hence voluntary behaviour gains upon impulsive as society becomes more and more orderly—that is to say, with the advance of material civilization. In other words, a nation becomes more *prudent* as it becomes commercialized.

The educability of the will.—Our muscular movements are extraordinarily educable. We owe to their plasticity all our various dexterities or " accomplishments ", of action and speech. The will, being evolved from movement, is also educable. The more we practise the making of efforts, the easier they become—indeed, in time it becomes habitual to make them. When they are concerned with behaviour, their practice is *discipline*, which amongst the Spartans was brought to a fine art, and contributed vastly to the success of the early Roman arms. There is also mental discipline—that of facing mental difficulties and thinking for oneself, instead of accepting the views of others—which immensely increases one's ability to solve the problems that present themselves. And, just as we may learn particular kinds of muscular dexterity, such as those of playing different instruments or games, so we may learn to deal effectively with particular kinds of problems. " Business ", for instance, develops an extraordinary aptitude for rapidly making up one's mind on questions of profit and loss. The study of mathematics similarly sharpens a capacity for deciding problems connected with numerical, or proportional relationships. We can, then, cultivate the use of the will in forming decisions upon various kinds of difficulties such as those presented by politics and the different sciences. We call this " cultivating the intelligence ". But the process is actually one of training the use of the will. It is, indeed, very doubtful whether either the memory or the intelligence can be " cultivated ". They are the results of nervous activities that have no connection with muscular movement. And, generally speaking, they are amazingly acute during childhood, and only fail in results because experience is lacking. With whatever architectural ability, one cannot build without materials.

6 Ambitions

We have seen that volition becomes " ex-revulsive " when the effort that it includes is re-stimulated by an idea of success. Desire becomes ambition, excited, not by a thing but by the success, power or superiority that will be involved in obtaining it. An ambition includes an inclination : that is what incites us to *pursue*. But the inclination is energized by voluntary effort : it affects us through reflection, whereas the effort that converts an inclination into a desire is an automatic reaction.

The objects of ambition are so numerous and diverse, firstly, because the mind deduces from the idea of success a number of concepts, each of which is as stimulating as the idea of success ; secondly, because success can be won in a vast number of different methods ; and thirdly, because it may be won indirectly as well as directly. We will consider each of these complications in turn,

Stimuli derived from success.—In deriving concepts from the idea of success, the mind works on lines which will be discussed when we are concerned with the evolution of our ideas. The process of derivation is influenced by our experience of the current of changes that attends life, and is, indeed, an essential feature of life itself. Everything that happens in a current must have a predecessor, or antecedent, and a successor, or consequent—a fact that is impressed upon us by the process of associative re-stimulation. For this brings before us recollections of what has preceded and what has followed every action that we have taken, and every experience that we have undergone. Consequently we deduce from success that it must have been preceded by strength or power, and is followed by the superiority, or excellence, of achievement. We naturally associate these qualities with " greatness ", as their cause. Excellence " stands out ", and is therefore *peculiar*, or notable. Hence the peculiar is successful—even when it simply amounts to eccentricity or rarity. It follows that we are successful when we are powerful, superior or peculiar.

Methods of achieving success.—We may win success against ourselves, against other persons, or against things and circumstances.

We conquer ourselves *self-assertively* when we demonstrate our power by subduing a dislike, or by restraining its consequences in conduct or language. Thus we win success when we " fight down " fear, or control the expression of nervousness or anger. We may also conquer ourselves *self-repressively* by withstanding a like, or " temptation ". This ambition contributed to the ascetic self mortification which was so esteemed in the early days of Christianity, was the motive of Puritanism, and is still of much account in the East. Self-repression bears more wholesome fruit in such virtues as sobriety, sincerity and humility, and it is an important element in all such " magnanimous " feelings as those of generosity, tolerance, and mercy. It should, however, be observed that, although these self-repressive virtues may be practised ambitiously—with the idea of winning success—they may also proceed from the sublimer feelings that we call " idealistic ", the motive of which is not a desire for personal success, but an inspiring admiration for these virtues in themselves. For, being *strong*, they are admirable.

More obvious, because more " objective ", methods of achieving success or superiority are through conflict with others. Emulative ambition is the spirit of competition. It gives strenuousness to school, professional, and business life, and is so attractive that it has prompted the invention of games that afford artificial occasions for it. It can even render war attractive. The lust for possessions is very largely the desire for excelling others. Emulation takes another form in the hunting spirit. This is commonly attributed to " instinct "—a view which is quite untenable, since the character of man's teeth and the extraordinary length of his intestines demonstrate that he is naturally a vegetarian.

We win success against *things* by industry, as in gardening : it is by this ambition that labour is sweetened. Ambition is reformative when the success in view is that of improving things, whether by beneficial legislation, social service, or such administrative efficiency as prompts a Cromwell or a Mussolini. Explorative ambition is, in great measure, the desire of surmounting difficulties, whether they be such as oppose themselves to travel, or the ignorance and misconception that prevents us from understanding the origin and causes of things, and their relations to one another. But here again we must make a qualification. Reforms and explorings, whether geographical or intellectual, may be inspired by an admiration of goodness or knowledge which compels its service. In this case their motive is ideal. It is a disconcerting reflection that one may win success over things by destroying them—an ambition that is naively illustrated in the nursery, but moved such conquerors as Attila and Nadir Shah, and is not unknown to literary critics.

This catalogue of methods is, of course, merely illustrative, not exhaustive. It indicates but a few of the victories that present themselves, as possibilities, to an ambitious mind. Success may be won in love, and even in the service of idealistic morality.

Direct and indirect success.—Actual success can only be won directly—by achievement. But a *feeling* of success may be obtained indirectly through the esteem or admiration of others, or through mere association with the powerful, great, excellent or peculiar. For the lack of better words we may distinguish these two indirect kinds of success as *re-stimulated* (or suggested) and *reflected*. We feel successful when admired by others because the feeling is re-stimulated by their admiration, inasmuch as in ourselves success is associated in sequence with admiration—the admiration of self that is pride. And we feel successful when we are associated with the great, because persons and things are invested with qualities by being associated with them, and we are accordingly invested with the quality of greatness.

Success through re-stimulation or suggestion.—This is very lucidly expressed in French as *succès d'estime*, since it is the outcome of our popularity or of the esteem in which we are held by others. The difference between it and actual success is brought out in the words "dignity" and "honour". Dignity is a feeling of distinction followed by the respect of others : honour is the respect of others followed by a feeling of distinction. *Succès d'estime* is one of the very strongest of lures : it is even more attractive than actual success, inasmuch as it comes to us, objectively, through sensation, whereas the pleasure of achieved success can be only subjectively appreciated. For the same reason failure which is implied by the contempt of others, is even more bitter than failure in itself.

We may be inclined to scoff at this tender susceptibility to *succès d'estime*. But it is the foundation of conventional morality. For, by inspiring us with a desire to be popular, and "respectable", it renders us amenable to the force of convention. Man's likes and dislikes are in great measure habitual, and hence we can earn the esteem of our fellows by behaving conventionally, as well as by talent, energy, heroism or riches. It follows that a respect for public opinion is the force that keeps society together. But we respect it only when it is the opinion of our *fellows*—of those who are identified, or united, with us—since it is only in this case that their approval or disapproval associatively re-stimulates our pride or shame. The opinion of " outsiders " affects us no more than the chatterings of a monkey-house. An Englishman in the tropics troubles himself not at all over the feelings with which the natives regard his conduct. Hence the importance of social *solidarity* in preserving conventional morality. The criminal disposition, which it is fashionable to attribute to irregularities in the functioning of the endocrine glands, really arises from the criminal's idea that there is nothing in common between him and respectable society. And the curious fact that cats are shameless, whereas dogs will betray their misdeeds by their apologetic behaviour, may be attributed to a difference in breadth of identifying, or classifying, intelligence—in the faculty of appreciating analogies. A dog thinks of itself as identified in fellowship with its master. A cat always remains in a class apart.

Success through " reflection ".—We may gain this indirect success through an association, or connection, with either things or persons. Things afford it when they are the consequences or the symbols of success, power or excellence, and are possessed by us, since our proprietorship links them to us, and is itself a form of power. Hence wealth, imposing houses, equipages and furniture " reflect " dignity upon those who own them, and titles and decorations, as symbols of success confer honour. We are also honoured by acquaintance with persons who are great or powerful, or are renowned for their skill. Many people " dearly love a lord ", although profoundly convinced of human equality ; and there are few who are not pleased to have influential friends, while protesting that they would not go out of their way to make them. For the ambition to shine by the brilliancy of others involves a loss of personal dignity which renders it somewhat contemptible. It implies an acknowledgement of our own inferiority, which is not in question when the source of our honour is not a person, but a thing. Consequently, there is a general feeling that success which is won merely by " reflection " is too unreal to be estimable ; and one who prides himself upon it is called a " snob ".

7 Appreciative Emotions

Evolution, as we have seen, works by developing causal activities out of consequences. Effort is a revulsive response to the shock of discord— a consequence of the duality of our nature. If successful, it is followed by a flush of emotional exhilaration ; if unsuccessful, by depression—nervous crises which, originating as the after-effects of a discord, can be restimulated "undiscordantly " by ideas of success or failure, or of any qualities of success or failure. Under the bent of feminine inclination, the glamour of prospective success affects us *ambitiously* : actual present success or failure—or ideas of them—move us *appreciatively* to admiration or contempt. These emotions affect us far more acutely than we consciously realise. They must be liberated physically in facial movements, gestures, utterances, or in tears. They touch the very depths of our nervous susceptibilities, impressing upon the memory occurrences that would otherwise escape it. Outstanding successes or failures are never forgotten. And emotion is almost equally energetic when ex-revulsively restimulated by ideas. How masterfully do admiration and contempt manifest their power in the roars of applause or execration which the mere name of a politician will provoke !

Admiration takes a subjective form as pride—that is to say, emotional exhilaration aroused by oneself passes inclinationally into self-love. Its converse is shame. We are attracted by ourselves when proud, repelled by ourselves when ashamed. We recognize the dual composition of admiration when we say that it may be " inspired " or " attracted ". In the first case we stress its masculine *exhilaration :* in the second, the feminine *inclination* to which this gives rise. These remarkable transformations are inexplicable except through the duality of our nature, which renders it possible for one side of us to be attracted or repelled by the other. The physical side is attracted by the animative when this is exhilarated ; it is repelled by it when depressed. We admire ourselves in success, despise ourselves in failure. Pride and shame are, then, " subjective " like and dislike that are strongly emotionalized.

We think of admiration and contempt as stimulated by individuals —by persons or things. Actually they are stimulated by certain qualities or conditions that are associated with individuals. When we admire an eloquent speaker it is not the man, but his eloquence, that appeals to us. Accordingly we admire other persons—and also ourselves—because admirable qualities are associated with, or possessed by them or by us. Our admiration passes from possessed to possessor—or, as we might express it, from a consequence to its cause. It is " objectified ". It is necessary to stress this point since it affords us a clue to the development of idealistic appreciation and of imaginative activity. These are stimulated by qualities in themselves, that are unattached to things or persons. Imagination subjectively personifies them.

The conditions, or qualities, that attract or inspire admiration are all derivatives, or attributes, of success that are deduced from it by the mind with exceeding subtlety. The conditions of power, strength, superiority (or excellence), and peculiarity, have already been noticed. We must add to them skill, value, beauty, harmony and elegance. Skill is, of course, dexterous power. Value is also a kind of power : a thing is worth a sovereign when it overcomes the reluctance to part with this sum. Beauty includes excellence and harmony as well as mere pleasingness. Harmony is strong because it resolves discord—one of the most disturbing of life's experiences. This is the " beauty of peace ". Elegance is strong because it economizes material, and is also harmonious in outline. There is strength in all emotions that can gain victories, as that of courage over fear, self-control over irritation, mercy over revenge. Loving-kindness is strong because it produces the harmony of unity. And, finally, the idea of success is widened so as to include good birth and good luck. For since the exhilaration of success may be re-stimulated without the effort that preceded it, anything that possesses a *quality* of success will serve as a restimulant. Accordingly, we admire persons and things with which any of these conditions or qualities are associated.

We must pursue our analysis one step further before beginning to apply it in practical fashion. In all cases when a success is actually achieved it involves a struggle and a victory, and there cannot be a victory unless there be a defeat on the other side. Victory and defeat are correlatives, in that one cannot exist without the other. Consequently, most of our ideas of the admirable are correlatives. There can be no superiority or excellence without inferiority, no peculiarity without a contrasting " commonness ", no value without something that it " commands ". Skill implies the possibility of awkwardness, beauty that of ugliness, harmony that of discord. We shall see that this correlation plays a part of notable importance in the genesis of such emotions as those of respect and pity, which arise from admiration and contempt through the interaction of ideas of superiority and inferiority.

It may be repeated that since all these conditions and qualities exist in idea, thoughts that " remind " us of them are as potent stimuli as ideas that are gathered from actual perception. Success and failure are actual happenings. But they are accompanied by ideas of them, and, consequently, under the law of associative re-stimulation, an idea of success is exhilarating, and one of failure depressing, in itself. We are elated by the thought of a past exploit, depressed by the recollection of a *faux pas*.

The emotions that are excited by these ideas may move us either appreciatively or imaginatively. We are now concerned with motives of the appreciative kind. But it may be remarked that both appreciation and imagination are characterized by an *enthusiasm* which is lacking in our more sedate desires, affections and ambitions. And they show the preponderance of masculine influence in being fundamentally *unpractical*. They develop useful fruits in such virtues as devotion, loyalty, obedience and sympathy, and material fruits in the accomplishments of Art. But these consequences are expressive rather than purposeful—not so much *intentions* as *manifestations* of the enthusiasm which inspires them, and uplifts them above the plane of physical life.

Admiration.—We may admire either ourselves, other persons, or things. In the first case, our feeling is called " pride " or " self-satisfaction ". It is the foundation of conscious egotism. For it as an abiding complacency, being continually re-stimulated by ideas of success or superiority, if this be only in the extent of one's losses, or in one's power of drinking beer. Our admiration of other persons may be inspired by ideas of their power or excellence that have been impressed upon us by instruction, as well as by actual perception of it. Hence our feelings are liable to be disillusioned by the discovery that their objects are not as admirable as we thought. Admiration for skill is on a firmer footing, since skill is demonstrated to the senses. Consequently one who has lost all admiration for the Government may still be devoted to Charlie Chaplin.

Our admiration for another, whether it be spontaneous or implanted, produces a momentous effect upon our practical feelings and behaviour towards him. Admiration expresses itself by imitation. The leaders of society are imitated in their tastes, manners and fashions of dress. So a popular colonel " sets a tone " to his regiment. When an artist embodies an inspiring idea in a painting or sculpture, he *imitates* the idea in material. Imitation may take the form of sympathy : we sympathize with another when we imitate his feelings. Consequently, we sympathize with one whom we admire, and sympathy, as we have seen, is the source of *active* affection. It makes us wish to do something for him. It is the source of all obedience other than that dictated by fear. For we *imitate* the wishes of another when we obey them.

We have already noticed the influence of admiration upon sexual feeling. It transforms an instinctive physical like into an ecstatic passion. With all justice, then, we term admiration "intoxicating". Love is, in fact, three parts admiration, and hence we use the word "love" to express admiration pure and simple, such as is aroused by the majesty of God, or by the more excellent virtues.

In things, including actions, speech, and circumstances, we admire the large, the strong, the swift : the pleasure of motoring consists very largely in the exhilaration that is stimulated by the "power" of velocity. The beautiful is the pretty that is also excellent and harmonious. But, since our standards of excellence vary, ideas of the beautiful are inconstant, changing in the course of time and often differing very greatly from one people to another.

It is to be added that admiration not only sets us imitating. It has a further effect in urging us to embellish, decorate, or "glorify", its object. We admire an individual because of his qualities, and we are therefore disposed to express our admiration by exaggerating them. A man ornaments with jewellery the woman of his heart. We glorify the king. We decorate a motor car. And this propensity takes a self-regarding turn in the boastfulness of self-conceit. If one has caught a large fish, his pride makes it larger.

Shame.—This is self-dislike, one of the bitterest of human experiences. It is a catastrophic reversal, since every conscious effort has the intention, or hope, of success before it which failure, not merely denies, but *contradicts*. If there is no intention, there is no shame, and in this case failure is merely a regrettable incident. Shame is so poignant a distress that we fend it off with any excuse that can soften it into regret. If we cannot lay the blame on others we endeavour to palliate our failure by ascribing it to such causes as the state of our health, or bad luck, or even to the weather. Yet it is wholesome to feel ashamed. For shame is a necessary prelude to repentance, and without this there can be no improvement.

We owe to the fear of shame one of the most imperious of motives —that of conscience, the sense of obligation or duty. An obligation is an intention which cannot be forsworn without shame, or its objective equivalent in a legal penalty, material loss, or the disapproval of our fellows. It becomes a duty when it is prescribed by a rule of morality. Duty is safeguarded by the whisper of impending shame. This is what we mean by the "voice of conscience".

Appreciative emotions objectively derived from ex-revulsive emotion.—The emotions of respect, faith, jealousy, disdain and pity spring from ex-revulsive emotion through the influence of certain ideas upon this nervous condition. They differ from admiration and contempt in that they primitively arise from our *objective* relations to others, and are afterwards *subjectively* extended to ourselves, whereas admiration and contempt are fundamentally subjective (as pride and shame) and become objective by being extended from ourselves to other persons and things.

Respect.—We can feel that respect is admiration with which a consciousness of personal inferiority is associated. Inferiority—the correlative of superiority—is suggested by admiration, when the qualities that are admired are superior to our own. A sense of inferiority cannot but be tinged with unpleasantness, since it involves something of the nervous depression that is the consequence of failure. Accordingly respect contains an element of gravity that is lacking in admiration pure and simple. Having become accustomed to associate respect for another with our admiration for him, we make the same association in regard to ourselves. Consequently self-admiration is followed by self-respect.

It seems, then, that the feeling of respect has an objective origin, and would not be experienced by one who had always been isolated in solitude and had never been confronted with one who was his superior. It is essentially a *social* emotion. One might, no doubt, argue that, since one side of us can admire the other it could also feel itself inferior to the other, so that respect, like admiration, might originate as a purely subjective feeling. But this, it must be felt, puts a strain upon the possibilities of duality. And, in favour of the objective origin of respect, there is the unquestionable fact that jealousy—which is akin to respect—arises objectively ; and, moreover, cannot be experienced subjectively. One cannot possibly be jealous of himself.

Respect becomes awe if it includes an element of fear. But, quite apart from this, its influence upon us is immense. It is the mainstay of the State, since it can be inculcated through the propaganda of teaching. For this can impress upon us that certain persons, or authorities, possess qualities that are admirable, and are our superiors. That the feeling of respect is the foundation of State authority is proved by the fact that unrest and disaffection thrust up their heads immediately a people becomes dis-illusioned—that is to say, so soon as they realize that their ideas of the power of the State are not warranted by facts. There remain for the support of the government only *prudential* considerations—that it would be *disadvantageous* to rebel. These may suffice to hold in check a commercialized people—one that is accustomed to appraise conduct by its consequences. But, for the impulsive or idealistic, a government that has lost respect has practically ceased to exist.

It is through a similar association, made by experience, that we respect age. This feeling, which contributes so forcibly to maintain the authoritative order of society, arises from childish impressions of our elders' power. Being received at the most impressionable age, they produce a habit of mind that is so involuntary as to appear to be instinctive. It is by a curious extension of this association that we respect the antique.

Faith.—When we are assured that he whom we respect means well towards us our feeling becomes that of faith or confidence. Faith is, then, a combination of affection and respect, and is, therefore, more powerful than either of them alone. Being re-stimulated by every thought of its object, it has the effect of investing him, as its cause, with an enduring halo. The strength of faith's influence can hardly be exaggerated. Those who can follow a leader (or an ideal) in unquestioning confidence are untouched by the hesitations which come from fear or the balancing of consequences. They will face anything, dare anything at his command. We read with astonishment of the courage of martyrs, of the mental exaltation which enabled delicate girls to encounter the most appalling and degrading forms of death. And faith gives happiness. There is cheerfulness in a regiment if the men " believe " in their colonel, and despotic rule is contentedly accepted if the ruler be loved and venerated.

Faith, like respect, engenders sympathy and obedience. Both these conditions are " imitative "—the one subjectively, the other objectively—as was realized by the author of the *Imitatio Christi*. Faith is the sheet-anchor not only of religion, but also of education. For we cannot possibly verify for ourselves all the events that have occurred in the past, and there are limits to the possibility of verifying those that are capable of being verified. All the experiments of chemistry, for instance, cannot be repeated in a class-room. Consequently we must trust for much of our knowledge upon others, in the belief that the information which they impart to us is well-meaning—that is to say, is meant to conduct us to the truth and not to lead us astray.

When faith is accompanied by a strong desire, its power over body and mind is miraculous. If one ardently desires a change, mental or physical, within himself, and has complete confidence in the ability of a certain thing to effect it, the thing may produce the desired consequence, however fantastic and imaginary may be the connection between the two. Faith in the touch of a king's hand will enable it to cure scrofula, just as admiration for an idealized virtue will generate the virtue in ourselves. In both cases the real stimulus is the nervous impulse of a like, reinforced by the energy of strong emotion. The nature of the external cause that is relied upon is of little importance. Its use is simply to stimulate faith, and so long as it does this it may be the magic of a " medicine man ", the incantations of an exorcist, a holy shrine, image or picture, the sacraments or supplications of a priest, the prayers of the brother-hood, or a medical prescription. Doctors are well aware that very many of the medicines they employ are efficacious only if they are believed in, and that they must assume an air of pontifical authority in order to stimulate this belief.

Jealousy.—Respect becomes angry or jealous when it is embittered by feelings of dislike, or is jangled by a discord between an affected superiority and a real inferiority. Many will deny that respect enters into jealousy. But we cannot possibly be jealous of one who is altogether our inferior. Nor can we be jealous of the dead, since their superiority has been vanquished. Jealousy is the outcome of a feeling of being " outbid " by another through a superiority of some kind, be it only in dress. When good is corrupted it be-comes worse than evil, and jealousy is the meanest and the most dangerous of all emotions, insidiously setting us against every one who is not our inferior, if he is in no way identified with ourselves. It is an illuminating fact that we cannot be jealous of children. They do not irritate us by any suggestions of rivalry, and there are few who have not smiles for them. " Little " is a term of endear-ment because it waves jealousy aside.

Disdain and Pity.—These are contraries—differing from one another as dislike differs from like—and may, therefore, be con-sidered together. Both are stimulated by another's failure or dis-tress, which should give us a depressing shock, since another's success excites us. Yet both of them are agreeable, self-complacent feelings, because they arise from *revulsions* of the kind described in Section 14 of Part I. The revulsion is caused by the self-congratula-tion of superiority. For the object of our feeling is our inferior, inasmuch as we are unaffected by the misfortune which he experiences.

If we are antagonized against him, our self-congratulation passes into disdain—the attitude of a superior towards an inferior who is disliked. Being associated with failure—or a mental derivative of failure—it can be extended to ourselves. Shame generally includes a feeling of self-contempt.

If we are drawn towards him by a like, our attitude becomes pitiful. His misfortune may of itself suffice to attract us, since it emphasizes our superiority, and hence we can pity the unfortunate although we have no personal acquaintance with them. Pity is uncorrupted by any trace of bitterness, and is, therefore, as inspiring as admiration. Consequently, it acts like admiration in setting us in sympathy with its object—in rendering us one in feeling with him : we feel his misfortune almost as if it were our own, and our self-congratulation is therefore tinged with sadness.

Experience enables us to verify the steps of this complicated series of transformations. It is evident that pity contains an element of nervous expansiveness, or exhilaration. For one who is moved by it is so strengthened by the feeling that he may disregard death in his effort to succour the object of his compassion. And the feeling contains so much that is agreeable as to be one of the most powerful *motifs* of the drama and fiction. It has, indeed, been well said that there is something not wholly disagreeable in the misfortunes of our dearest friends. That this element of exhilaration is the revulsive consequence of an idea of our relative superiority is shown by the fact that one in distress will alienate our pity if he antagonizes us by self-assertively putting himself on a level with us, and disputes our right to " patronize " him. Moreover, we know very well that it is easier to pity our inferiors than our equals. The cause of " distressed gentlewomen " does not open our purse-strings so readily as that of " waifs and strays " ; and there are thousands of good people whose hearts are touched more nearly by the sufferings of dogs and cats than by those of hungry and neglected children. That exhilaration must stimulate a like in order to pass into pity is demonstrated by the pitilessness of war. To our enemies —to those who are antagonized to us by feelings of ill-will—our hearts are closed, and their miseries are consequently a source of disdainful triumph. The passage of self-congratulation into pity is, of course, easier when the sufferers are our friends than when they are strangers. But misfortune of itself can attract us. Our hearts go out to entire strangers if they are in affliction, and there is no antagonism to withstand our like.

It shocks one as outrageously cynical to ascribe to such origins one of man's noblest feelings. But, evolution being what it is, humbleness of descent is no reproach to any of our faculties. Pity must be judged in itself, not in its origin ; and we do it no dishonour, if in extolling it, we appreciate the homeliness of the sources from which it springs. Indeed, on the contrary, we may gratefully marvel at the evolutionary process which has blessed us with the capacity of being aroused to pity by a stimulus that primarily generates contempt.

Pity is, then, fundamentally a *social* virtue. It arises from objective experience and is subjectively extended to ourselves through its association with failure or distress. So we come to pity ourselves and to extract some pleasure from our misfortunes whilst re-stimulating a very lively sense of them. Indeed, a sensitive child will actually pity itself into tears if this feeling is excited by injudicious expressions of compassion.

Pity, it follows, resembles admiration in springing from nervous exhilaration. But it differs from admiration in that the exhilaration is a " correlative " revulsion from the emotional effects of another's failure, not *directly* stimulated by success. Like admiration, it arouses sympathy with its object—altruistic because imitative— that manifests itself in an active desire to help him—a desire which may render one quite indifferent to danger. Pity inspires the stretcher-bearer with a courage that owes nothing to personal pride, the lust of conflict, or the hope of glory. Pity and admiration are the strongest of the ties which bind us to our fellows. Amusement apart, they are the instruments which the dramatist and novelist principally use to move men attractively.

Pathos.—Pity becomes pathos when the exhilarating revulsion proceeds from a contrast, not between ourselves and another, but between the actual circumstances of life, and the " might have been ". There is no pathos when failure or misfortune is the result of character—that is to say, of a fault—and not of circumstances. Cowardice and jealousy may be pitiable : but they are not pathetic. When, however, confronted with the unhappiness of another—or of ourselves—a thought occurs of the happiness which might have ensued had things turned out better, we experience a revulsive glow which draws us sympathetically towards the subject of our thoughts —a sentiment which, however mournful, contains a gleam of the agreeable, a ray of sunshine through the clouds. Pathos differs from pity in that no thoughts of personal superiority are involved. But it contains a similar element of revulsion.

Idealistic appreciation.—The motives which we have been considering are aroused by particular qualities or conditions. But, since these qualities are possessed by individuals, their effect upon us is directed to the individuals that possess them. We may, however, be moved by admiration for qualities in themselves when they are of the " subjective " kind—that is to say, are internal conditions, or feelings, that are apprehended, not by sensation, but by our own consciousness. They inspire admiration if they are *strong*. Courage and self-control are obviously strong and we

admire them whole-heartedly in themselves.   The self-assertive re-
pudiation of inferiority is strong.   We admire it under the name of
Liberty.   But Charity, Mercy and Forgiveness are also strong, since
they involve the repression of egotistical feelings.   If we admire these
qualities, they become " ideals ", and our appreciation of them is
" idealistic ".   We are affected by them exactly as by an individual
whom we admire.   We are impelled to imitate them subjectively—
that is to say, to experience them ourselves sympathetically—to have
faith in them, to be loyal to them and to glorify them.   Our imitation
of an ideal is then subjective.   In this Idealism differs from Art.

Ideals affect us, not through the will, but through the spontaneous
force of admiring enthusiasm.   This is what we mean by saying that
they are " heart-felt ".   An ideal is therefore a motive of tremendous
power—as strong as is loyalty to an adored king.   Ideals of asceticism have driven multitudes—Buddhists as well as Christians—to
forego the pleasures of life in desert hermitages or monastic prisons ;
and, in later days, have disciplined society generally with the
morose rigours of Puritanism.   The ideals of Muhammed—the unity
of God, the brotherhood of the faithful, and the predestination of
the hour of death—enabled their devotees, within the space of a
century and a half, to establish an empire from Bagdad to Cadiz.
What vast changes the ideals of Liberty and Equality have been
able to bring about !   To what *unnatural* innovations the ideals of
Socialism are leading us !

There is a halo about the word " ideal " which inclines us to assume
that the thing which it represents cannot but be good.   We are
misled.   A hero is not necessarily good because he is strong.   Idealism
in some forms, and carried to extremes, may be exceedingly pernicious.   Ideals of the self-assertive class have brought incalculable
miseries upon mankind.   Liberty and Despotism, for example, which
idealize respectively freedom from another's power and power over
another, rapidly degenerate into license and tyranny.   The French
Revolution was inspired by an ideal of personal equality : the
Bolshevist revolution in Russia extended this equality to possessions.
Both ideals are inspiring : both degraded their acolytes to bestial
depths of cruelty.   So-called " Christian " ideals have actually
afflicted mankind like plagues : through persecutions, massacres
and wars they have laid whole countries waste.   But we must not
confuse these travesties of Christ's teaching with the ideals that he
actually enjoined.   These are innocent as well as inspiring, and are,
therefore, altogether admirable—Sympathy for others, the self-
repression that manifests itself in Purity, Sobriety, Sincerity and

Humility, the magnanimity of Forgiveness, Mercy, Tolerance, Patience, Loyalty, and Generosity, and the harmony of Justice. We may be fanatic in their pursuit. But we shall injure no one.

8 Imaginative Activities

In the ordinary course of mental activity, we isolate the qualities of persons and things from their possessors, as when we think of the " sharpness " of the wind, or the " self-sacrifice " of a martyr. When the qualities are of the subjective kind and are strong, harmonious, or excellent, we may, as we have seen, idealistically admire and imitate them. Under the influence of imagination we go further : we " emotionalize " them—that is to say, vivify them ; and since life seems to involve personality, we also personify them. So the " wickedness " of evil is personified as Satan, and the " golden-hairedness " of the dawn as Aurora. That ideas of qualities should be emotionalized in this fashion is explicable in some degree if we realize that, as a spontaneous process, imagination is the consequence of a flow of emotion into the mind. It may be exercised as a voluntary faculty, because the will can energize any of our natural processes of movement and thought. But spontaneous imagining is always the result of emotional excitement. The emotion may be that of admiration which is aroused by a quality. In this case imagination resembles idealism in its origin. But, whereas idealism admires and imitates a subjective quality, as such and in itself, imagination transfigures a quality—which may be objective as well as subjective—into an animated existence. And since animated beings are perceivable by the senses, the transfiguration has the effect of giving a " sensory ", or concrete, existence to mental abstracts. It invests them with " individuality ". This is possible because in ordinary life the perception of things as individuals is a subjective, not an objective, process. The senses merely reveal to us *qualities*—" appearances " of colour, shape, and movement and nothing more—and (as we shall see at a later stage) we endow these with individuality because they are detachable from their surroundings, and, so far, resemble ourselves. There is, accordingly, individualization in perceiving as well as imagining. In the one case it is reflective, in the other emotionally " deflective." The imagination is a development of thought, and can more appropriately be discussed in connection with thought than with motives. But it influences conduct, and is, so far, a motive. It is the origin of the artistic activities that play a part of such immense importance in our lives, and we must, therefore, make some reference in this Section to its peculiarities.

Our imaginative aptitudes obscure their origin by flowing from three different although connected sources. They may originate spontaneously from emotional excitement of any kind: one is strongly imaginative under the influence of fear or love. They may be inspired by the admiration of a quality—as, for instance, by the glow of a sunset—or by pity for a condition, as for that of death. And, thirdly, they may be prompted deliberately by the will. We may distinguish these phases as the spontaneous, the inspired, and the ingenious.

Spontaneous imaginings.—The effect of emotion upon thought is displayed to us by a change in the manner of speech. Under the stress of emotion language becomes more forcible and picturesque, and this signifies that a similar change has occurred in the character of the thoughts that prompt it. They revert to their sensory origin, and become "images" or "visions". Fear presents its possibilities as ghostly phantoms. Love transfigures what it adores. A passionate admiration can present hallucinating appearances of its object so clear and distinct as to be undistinguishable from sensations. Intrusive and uncontrolled currents of expansive or contractive excitement appear to be the origin of our good and bad dreams. In all these transfigurations we can perceive a law. Through analogies, a quality of sensory, or "objective", experience, is animated with life and feeling, a "subjective" quality of feeling is materialized with an appearance. The impression of a sound becomes a "voice": a fear becomes a "bogey". It is a curious fact that our facial expressions of emotion follow the same lines. They *animate* the external appearance—for an expressionless face lacks the charm of vivacity. And, at the same time, they materialize feeling by manifesting it.

Inspired imaginings.—These are stimulated, not by a passing flush of emotion, but by the enthusiasm of admiration or pity for a quality or condition. This is imaginatively individualized. If it is a quality that is perceived by sensation, it is given an *animated* existence: so Shelley personifies the dead leaves of autumn as "pestilence-stricken multitudes", and Browning vivifies Nature's kindliness in his "good gigantic smile of the brown old earth". If it is a quality of feeling, it is *materialized*, as in Wordsworth's apostrophe of Duty, as " Stern daughter of the voice of God." The effect of these individualizations of the admired is to impel us to imitate them objectively in expressive action by dramatizing them, delineating them or describing them. Art, in these forms, may be dignified as " inspired imitation ". But its imitativeness differs from that of idealism in being objective.

Ingenious imaginings.—The imitative expression of an imaginative thought involves muscular movement or utterance, and, since all controlled movement or utterance is willed, imaginative expression becomes deliberate. The artist can hesitate over his work and choose his lines. This development reacts upon imaginative *thought*, and brings it under the influence of the will. He can make use of the faculty in cold blood, consciously summoning the analogies that occur spontaneously to emotional thought, and using them as our instruments. Indeed the word " imagine " is very commonly used in the sense of " deliberately suppose ". Much modern art and poetry is conceived in this practical fashion. And, coming under the influence of the will, imaginative talents can be used for practical purposes, such as the earning of a livelihood, or the winning of fame. But these voluntary imaginings lack the fire of emotional art. The poet who is emotionally imaginative is impelled to create by such an enthusiasm as inspires the song of a skylark—and, like the bird, is set a-tremble by it.

Religion.—In the generation of religious beliefs the appreciative and the imaginative faculties combine. Wonderful qualities of ourselves and of the nature that surrounds us are carried back to their unknown *causes*. These are imaginatively individualized as divine powers. Their personifications excite feelings of admiration, respect and faith which impel us to imitate their supposed wishes, as far as is possible—sympathetically and obediently, to adore them and glorify them.

There are marvels within us as well as outside us, in the varied and forceful changes that occur in our subjective feelings. They are referred to their causes in the creation of such divinities as Mars, the god of anger, Venus, the goddess of love, Minerva, the goddess of prudence. How wonderful are the phases of objective Nature— the heavens, the mysteries of birth, growth and death, her power for good or evil, shown in the various dangers with which she threatens us, in the mysterious alternations of sunshine and storm, plenty and famine, peace and war, health and sickness, riches and poverty, good and bad luck. These changes must have causes of immense power. They excite the imaginative emotion which is humanity's most distinctive ornament, and are consequently deified. If such a Cause become incarnate in human form, the objective and the subjective would be combined ; and this union of God and Man has suggested itself in various forms and in many religions.

The practical side of our nature shows itself in the desire to derive some benefit from these transcendental forces, to win their favour by propitiatory ceremonies and prayers, and even to exact it by magic incantations that can bring the deity within the influence of man's wishes.

We need not insist upon the power of religion as a motive of thought and conduct. It gives confidence and comfort. It strengthens moral rules and obligations by crediting them with inspiration. But it undeniably narrows the scope of intelligence. And differences of creed have caused so much misery to mankind as to lead some philosophers to wonder whether religious enthusiasm has not been more of a curse than a blessing.

9 Emotional Expression

Many of the most active hours of our lives are spent in simply expressing our feelings, with no object except to express them. Yet, by an extraordinary misconception, we expect to find a *practical* purpose in all the workings of Nature. We imagine that animals and plants owe their shape, colours and habits solely to the utility of these qualities, whereas, judging from ourselves, it is probable that very many of them are the manifestations of nervous energy that must free itself ; and frees itself in methods that are infinitely more striking than those which serve the material purposes of the struggle for life.

Emotion may vent itself instinctively—or naturally—in gestures, ejaculations, laughter, tears and facial movements of which we are hardly conscious. It may use, as its " escapes ", acquired methods of behaviour, as in applause, cheering, and the play of children. Nothing gives one a better idea of the *pressure* of a surge of emotion than the frantic manifestations which greet a popular politician, actor or football-player. And the insistence of this pressure is brought home to us by the relief which expletives or muscular movements afford us on occasions of emotional excitement. When angry, nervous or delighted, it is almost impossible to remain still.

Under the stress of emotion, the most self-contained of men may feel that he must " walk it off ".

Children's play may simply be an instrument of amusement, as in Blindman's Buff, for example. But in its dramatic forms it is plainly an imitative unpractical expression of admiration for that which is dramatized, whether it be paying calls, going shopping, or the wonders of horses or steam engines.

In its higher phases, emotional expression includes dancing, music, the various branches of Art, and the ceremonies of religion. These are phases of behaviour and will be considered in Part IV. But we may emphasise at once a point of much importance. All these manifestations are expressive in those who originate them, stimulative—that is to say, *impressive*—to those who are influenced by them. Dancing originated in such rhythmic steps as might suggest themselves to excited children : singing as an artless expression of mood : acting and delineating as spontaneous imitations : rhetorical description as impassioned utterance. Their origination becomes more and more deliberate, as the value of skill is appreciated : it may become a purposeful means of earning money. But it remains fundamentally expressive. To those, however, who submit themselves to their influence, these expressions are instruments for the stimulation of emotion. By deliberately dancing, or playing music, one " infects " himself with excitement—also by watching a drama, listening to music, visiting a picture gallery, reading poetry and fiction or attending a divine service. An actor is emotionalized by the part he is playing. This curious reversal of properties is obviously due to the action of auto-suggestion—that is to say, of associative re-stimulation. Unless they have become purely formal, expressions of emotion, however much elaborated, retain their instinctive association with emotion, and can, therefore, re-stimulate the excitement of which they are the manifestations. This restimulated emotion is enhanced by admiration for the skill with which the artist elaborates his expressions—a feeling that lends some attraction to Art that has become quite lifeless and uninspiring.

10 Individual and Racial Peculiarities of Character

Education and habit count for infinitely more than is ordinarily realized. But infants differ very greatly from one another at birth, possessing peculiarities of character which seem at first sight to be too anomalous to be assignable to definite causes. Our examination of origins and motives indicate, however, that most of them may be ascribed to strength or weakness in one or other of nine capacities—sensory impressionability (including the appreciation of harmony and discord), self-conscious sensibility, retentiveness of memory, acuteness of intelligence, inclinational impulse as contrasted with emotional excitability, emotional reaction to shock, effortful reaction to discord and power of resistent endurance. Of these capacities the four last are typically masculine, being emotional reactions to the harmonious and discordant.

I. " Psychometric " tests have proved that individuals differ very markedly in the delicacy of their sense-receptiveness. We have familiar illustrations of sensory obtuseness in those who are colour-blind, or deaf to the charms of music. It is evident that some persons are less sensitive to harmony (including that of justice) than others, and that sensibility to smells and tastes varies greatly. Since pleasure and displeasure are evolutionary stimuli of likes and dislikes, these differences in impressionability must produce differences in the strength of inclinations, and of the desires and aversions that spring from them. One whose sense of taste lacks acuteness is not likely to become a *gourmet*.

II. By " self-conscious sensibility " is meant the capacity of subjective perception—of realizing one's own motives and emotional conditions. There can be little doubt that this capacity is stronger in some men than in others. Dullness of subjective sensibility may have a momentous effect upon character. It may blunt a man's apprehension of the revulsion of shame as a subjective condition. He may retain a very lively appreciation of " objective " shame— that is to say, of the disgrace of reprobation, of being " found out ". But when his failure, or his fault, is known to no one but himself, he may escape the misery of one who is keenly self-conscious. In this case he will be uncontrolled by the voice of conscience. He will, moreover, be unimpressed by that which is the ultimate origin of our ideas of justice—the harmony between virtue and its reward in pride, vice and its punishment in shame.

III. We are well aware that in some children mental memory is more retentive than in others. There are great differences, for instance, in the facility with which poetry can be learnt by heart. But memory is not merely mental. It is the foundation of habit. Strong memorial aptitudes conduce, therefore, to the tenacity of habits of mind, prejudice and beliefs, and also of affections. It is the memory of a *physical* kind that gives us our muscular dexterities. One is skilful at golf when, having made a good stroke, he can repeat it. Memorial capacities can, then, be distinguished as mental, inclinational and muscular, and strength in one of these directions may be accompanied with weakness in others. That is to say, the capacity for associative re-stimulation may vary with the kinds of nerves that it affects.

IV. Acuteness of intelligence displays itself in the appreciations of samenesses between things that are different—in the perception of analogies. It varies with the kinds of analogies to be detected. There are great differences between individuals in the rapidity with which they see the analogies that underlie jokes. Some persons are abnormally quick in recalling words that are analogous to other words in sound—that is to say, that rhyme, or are in alliteration with them—a talent that is essential for a poet. Others are peculiarly appreciative of the analogies between numerical and quantitative relationships upon which rests the framework of mathematics. Others, again, are readily struck by the samenesses that call to mind parallel cases which confirm or discredit first impressions or decisions. They are consequently " broad-minded ". For the effect of these parallels is generally disillusioning : it contradicts beliefs that rest upon the narrow base of personal like or dislike, prejudice or habit.

V and VI. Inclinational impulse and emotional excitement are, respectively, the typical products of feminine and masculine influence. From them arise the dispositions which we contrast as the practical (or " matter-of-fact ") and the emotional : and character is obviously affected very greatly by any variations in the relative strength of one to the other. It is a fact that this differs in different individuals from earliest infancy—that some babies are more " grasping ", some more excitable than others ; and it is, then, clear that personal peculiarities in this respect are due to nature, not to nurture, although the latter may certainly accentuate them. Those in whom inclinational impulse is relatively strong have a " practical " bent : life is for them an occasion for seeking and acquiring objective means of enjoyment. The pleasure may be simply that of the senses. But it may also be the gratification of æsthetic tastes, or of amusement, or that which is given by success—in its most material form the acquisition of riches. These inclinations may become obsessions. So are enslaved the sensualist, the drunkard, the gambler and the miser. Emotional excitability, on the other hand, inspires rather than inclines : it gives rise to enthusiasm which grows into admiration, loyalty and faith, and flowers in imagination. Inspiration, like inclination, may become obsessing, as in ecstasy and mysticism. These two types of character are freely recognized in common speech : we contrast the realist with the idealist, the prosaic with the romantic, the " business-man " with the enthusiast, the bourgeois with the Bohemian, the profiteer with the " gentleman ". As man grows up emotional enthusiasm gives way to prudence : it is at its strongest during childhood. A precisely contrary tendency is illustrated by the caterpillar and the butterfly.

VII. Reaction to a shock commonly manifests itself in laughter. when it is emotional, not effortful ; and there is no question that some babies are more disposed to laugh than others. To some children tickling is a mixture of pleasure and pain : to others a pain : others, again, are indifferent to it. The capacity for being amused varies between different individuals from infancy. To appreciate the humorous or witty, intelligence is required as well as nervous elasticity : the stupid cannot " see a joke ", and cannot, therefore, be relieved from its shock by realizing that this is really causeless. But intelligence is of no avail if nervous elasticity is wanting. If this has run down, through grief or illness, the brightest of men will be disgusted by the comic and scandalized by mere flippancy of speech. The sense of humour testifies, then, to the possession of a nervous susceptibility which may be cultivated, but is, without doubt, inborn. It is one of the choicest of man's heritages, and its influence upon character is incalculably great.

VIII. *Effortful* reaction to discord is involved in anger, indignation, and jealousy ; and also in the very different motives of curiosity, courage and hopefulness. Acute neurasthenia, therefore experiences none of these feelings ; and there are individuals of the " mollusc " type, whose ordinary state is almost as apathetic. From earliest infancy children differ in irritability and quickness of temper, inquisitiveness and courage, and their peculiarities in this respect must accordingly be innate. These reactions all require elasticity of nervous tension. But this is not the only factor involved. Were it so, quickness of temper, curiosity and courage would always go together, and this is contradicted by experience, although courage is certainly assisted by anger. Two other factors come into play, sensibility to discord, and imaginative vivacity. It is obvious that reaction to discord must vary in degree with sensibility to discord. Anger, jealousy and indignation are reactions against the discordant effects of injury, humiliation and " unworthiness ", and their occurrence and strength naturally depends upon the intensity with which these effects are felt. Keenness of sensibility increases quickness and frequency of resentment, and may bring about a condition of almost persistent ill-temper. Curiosity, again, is resistance to the confusing effect of the strange. But this must be felt in order to be resisted. Some children are so phlegmatic as to be almost incapable of being " surprised ", and others quickly lose curiosity as their wonderment is blunted by the constant succession of unfamiliar experiences, or by the misleading, but satisfying, explanations that they receive from their elders.

To the birth of courage and hopefulness there contributes a third element—that of imaginative vivacity. The emotion of fear which is conquered by courage is caused, not by an *actual* discordant experience, but by the idea of one that is called " danger ", and to an individual of imaginative temperament an idea may be more disconcerting than an actuality, since it is exaggerated into a menace that he cannot resist. There is truth in the saying that spontaneous courage is unimaginative. Accordingly one who reacts violently to injury or slight may still be of a timid disposition. But he may be hopeful nevertheless. For his imagination exaggerates the favourable as well as the unfavourable. Hence it comes that optimism may be allied with nervousness, and pessimism with unthinking courage.

Spontaneous resistance, as we have seen, is the ultimate origin of volition, or will power. But this is a faculty which is developed by experience and education, not inherited at birth.

IX. A reaction is merely a " flash in the pan " unless its resistence is enduring. Nervous tenacity is a quality that shows itself in infancy as obstinacy. It can harden courage in the face of difficulty, and even of defeat : it renders curiosity pertinaceous, and angry feelings implacable and revengeful. The mental reactions of efforts of will become " resolute ", and give a " decisive " or " determinative " tone to character. Industry is imbued with perseverance, self-repression grows into discipline, and ambition can only sleep with open eyes.

Racial peculiarities.—It has become fashionable to regard inherited peculiarities of character as in great measure " racial "—as more generally innate in some races than in others. Such a generalization must be accepted with caution. So extensive has been the admixture of blood through wars, immigration and commerce that races with any pretensions to purity have ceased to exist—in Europe at all events—except in very sequestered corners. The educative effect of environal influences—especially in the development of idealism and will power—accounts for much more local distinctiveness than may be supposed. The character of a people may apparently be entirely changed by a new idea : the Arabs were transformed by the ideas of Muhammed. Nevertheless it must be admitted that mankind can be broadly classified into racial strains, such as the negro, the Mongolian, the aquiline brunette and the aquiline blond, which are distinguished by peculiarities of feature that are clearly innate, and are accompanied as a general rule by certain peculiarities of character. There is certainly a contrast between the people of Northern Europe and those of the Mediterranean, which seems to result from innate differences in their endowment with emotional susceptibility and resistant energy. The " Nordic " peoples, as they are called—and especially the Scandinavian tribes—possess less of the former and more of the latter—very possibly because energy is developed by recurring periods of cold. We all know the bracing effect of cold upon the spirits. Once acquired, this peculiarity can withstand for a few generations the effects of migration to a uniformly warm climate. Nordic people are less impulsive, less obedient and less artistic than those of the Mediterranean. But their resistant energy endows them with an enduring courage that has enabled them throughout the whole period of recorded history to over-run the South and subdue it, and at the same time to leaven the Southern peoples for a period with their characteristics. Their powers of self-control render them prudent, calculating and orderly. These are qualities that are essential for the success of democratic government ; and history seems to show that, when they are lacking, democracy can never realize the meaning of its name.

PART III

SENSATION AND THOUGHT

1 Sensation

Sensations, we have seen, may be either objective or subjective. In the former case they have a sensory basis : they arise from impressions upon the sense-organs—roots upon which the mind builds up the flowers of conscious ideas. They are, in fact, " sensori-mental ". Subjective sensations, on the other hand—those of our motives and emotions—have no such foundation. They are purely mental. We commonly distinguish them as " feelings ". But this term is ambiguous and confusing, since it is also used for objective sensations of our bodily conditions and movements.

Objective stimulation.—Communication with our environment through the sense-organs would be explained if these contained nerve-cells that were " tuned " to respond to certain kinds of vibratory conditions and chemical changes. Sound is demonstrably a vibration ; the vibratory nature of light can be inferred ; and science believes that what sensation presents to us as quiescent matter is in reality agitated by vibrations which could be received by the tactile nerves. Smell, on the other hand, is believed to be the conscious presentment of chemical charges. To affect the nervous system a sensory stimulus must be outside it. But this does not mean that it should be outside the body. The movements of our muscles impress us as a rapid series of touches. Injuries make themselves known as pain. And we are stimulated internally by the chemical action of a number of secretions—the *hormones* and *chalones* of the endocrine glands.

Touch is the most archaic, and by far the most important of our senses. We may infer from the behaviour of the simplest living organisms that they are sensible to touches if to nothing else. Touches may be external or internal. By the former we are sensible of external resistance (which consciousness represents as solidity), of surface and of its texture. Two or more simultaneous touches reveal to us separateness, and plurality. Through this sense we become acquainted with the conditions of heat and cold, and are therefore introduced to ethereal forces. And we become aware of movements in objects with which we are in contact, which, if not felt as abrupt shocks, impress us as a running succession of touches. Internal touches and pressures reveal to us our own movements in a similar form. So our smiles and frowns, as well as our gestures and movements of the mouth, become known to us. The muscles are abundantly supplied with sensory nerves. It seems also that it is through internal touch that we are sensible of the injuries and ailments of which we are conscious as pain. It has been demonstrated that the pangs of hunger are caused by a cramped or constricted condition of the stomach, and there is nothing against the view that a toothache is caused by pressure. It can certainly be increased by it ; and there is not much difference in quality between the agony of gout and that caused by ill-fitting boots.

Touch that is combined with movement—as in actively " feeling " a thing—is of such momentous importance to us that it may almost be treated as a sense apart. It is the source of our ideas of shape, or form. This is a relationship between different points on a surface which can only be detected by touch that is accompanied by movement. To one who could not " feel " things by passing the fingers over them, the environment as shown by touch would be simply a collection of shapeless obstacles. It seems, then, that " feeling " is the most instructive of all our sensory processes. It is the infant's instrument for exploring the world—shared by it with the octopus and the sea-anemone.

Smell is believed to be the conscious presentment of chemical action. Touch and smell, therefore, typically represent the two stimulating activities, mechanical and chemical, by which electricity is generated. It is, as has been noted, through chemical action that we are stimulated by our internal glandular secretions ; and it is not improbable that the distresses of hunger (apart from its pain), of thirst, and of lust, are of chemical origin. Taste is a combination of touch and smell. The tongue is the most delicate of our tactile organs, and its impressions are blended with those of the chemical effects of things received by the mouth.

In hearing we are impressed by vibrations of different rapidities, each of which is apparently taken up by a sensory nerve-cell that is " tuned " to it. Whether they occur in substances or in the atmosphere, they are *material*. The eyes extend our introduction to another world—that of the æther—for the vibrations to which their nerve-endings are " tuned " are ethereal. Sight presents us with colours, and with outlines that are constantly varying as we change our position. By our experience of perspective we interpret these outlines as the surfaces of objects that are at different positions and distances. But we make this interpretation by associating recollections of touch and movement with our visual sensations. We cannot distinguish the two apart because they occur simultaneously—having been associated by simultaneous experiences that come to us every moment of our lives. We may watch an infant initiating these associations by carefully touching what it sees. Unassisted by memory sight is, in fact, very uninforming. It merely gives us[1] clues which develop recollections.

It may be observed, however, that our memorial appreciation of solidity in what we see is justified by our double vision. For this invests an object with two outlines that are not precisely co-incident with one another ; and since each eye sees through the " outlap " of the image received by the other, and the two images are, nevertheless, combined, we seem to see *round* the object and *behind* it.

By the evolution of smell, hearing and sight, life has progressively extended the radius of its sensibilities. Touch, generally, requires contact ; and if some animals, such as bats, can detect obstacles in their path before they come into collision with them, (possibly through increases in air pressure) they must approach them very nearly before this is possible. Through smell the range of sensibility is extended to furlongs ; through sound to miles ; and sight puts us into connection with stars that are millions of miles distant. It is a noticeable fact that, as each of these progressive senses is refined by practice, those of shorter radius become less acute. When sight is lost, tactile sensibility gains immensely in delicacy.

Sense-impressions become conscious " sensations " when they are transformed into mental presentments by a process which, we have inferred, involves interaction between the sensory faculties of the brain and masculine emotion. In this form they lose all resemblance to the roots from which they spring, and can be connected with them only by inference. So we have learnt, for instance, that what we mentally conceive to be sound is in reality the activity of vibration.

---

[1] If there are dormant visual sensibilities in the skin (as is maintained in M. Jules Romain's *Eyeless Sight*) they might by practice be developed so as to give clues that might be expanded through associated recollections into seeming visual impressions.

Subjective sensation.—This affects the mind only, and leaves behind it far less definite traces than stimulation through the senses. There is a convincing proof of this. We cannot recollect a particular motive or emotion—a fit of anger for instance—apart from its objective cause, whereas sensory experiences can be recalled in themselves. We have vivid recollections of a friend—or of a toothache —but none of an affection except through the memory of the person who inspired it. The recollection of an objective experience is simply an idea of it ; that of a subjective experience must be associated with an idea of its cause. Subjective sensations are, therefore, far less *impressive* than objective, and are consequently held in less account.

Our subjective sensations, or " feelings ", present to us our motives and emotions. We are well aware of our likes and dislikes and the various motives into which they enter ; our emotional crises and changes are, indeed, the most poignant of our conscious experiences, although they leave fainter traces behind them than our sensations of sight and touch. Our awareness of them includes some objective elements, as of muscular bracings, relaxings and tremblings, and changes in breathing, circulation and secretion ; we are in fact conscious, not only of animative conditions, but of their physical accompaniments. From these material elements arose the old-fashioned notion that certain emotional crises were connected with particular organs of the body, as love with the heart, courage with the liver, jealousy with the spleen, and compassion with the bowels. But these objective feelings are merely incidental. Our consciousness of a motive or emotion is one of a condition in itself, and not merely of its objective consequences. For we know that these are in themselves unable to produce a " feeling ". The force of habit, for instance, produces objective consequences which enable us to infer its existence. But, being unemotional, we are quite unaware of its power and persuasiveness, and do not realize that we owe to it the great mass of the beliefs and convictions upon which we pride ourselves.

2 Perception

Perception is again much more complicated than sensation. It involves the co-operation of the mind with the sensory organs in the three processes of individualization, memorial amplification, and comprehension.

Individualization.—Sensation in itself reveals to us nothing but *appearances*, as of hardness, roughness, colour and sound. We give these appearances a " substantive " existence, as individuals, by investing them with such individuality as we possess ourselves— that is to say, by a mental process which is distinct from sensation. They are endowed with solidity and distance by the re-stimulation of ideas of touch and movement. But their existence as independent and separate individuals is given them by inference. Were this not so, the images of the cinema—which are merely shapes and colours— would not appear to us to be life-like. We can assure ourselves of the fact that sensations that are not mentally individualized are simply immaterial appearances. For such is the nature of visual impressions which lie outside the circle of attentive vision. They are merely " phenomena " of shape and colour.

Memorial amplification.—We do not " perceive " unless the senses are assisted by memory. A sensation that attracts attention immediately re-stimulates recollections that connect it with previous experiences, identify it with a *kind*, and give it, so to speak, a history. A sensation which manifests any of the peculiarities of a kind recalls the idea of a kind, and we " see " it as a bird, for instance, although, as a matter of fact, it is only a moving speck against the sky. Qualities are thus called to mind which are not apparent to the senses, as, for instance, that the bird has feathers. If we see smoke we know that there is fire. A sensation which is not accompanied by ex- planatory recollections strikes us as strange or surprising.

Amongst the recollections so recalled by visual impressions are those which invest things seen with solidity and distance. They are recollections of experiences of touch and movement that have become intimately associated with certain visual perspectives. It is by their assistance that we " perceive " a table to be round, although we actually see it as an oval ; its real shape is a series of relationships between one portion of its outline and another, which we have learnt by passing our fingers over it. There are some striking facts which prove that vision of itself deceives us. Those who have been operated upon for congenital cataract " perceive " nothing when the bandages are first removed. They have merely a confused impression of patterns in the eyes. Gradually as they touch, or move to, the things which present themselves in this indefinite fashion, the images gain shape, solidity and distance. There have been cases of violent concussion of the brain when, owing to the interruption of re-stimulating activity, the sufferers have been reduced to a like condition : until they have re-established memorial associations between visual impressions and recollections of touch, their sensations of sight have been merely kaleidoscopic. Such are, indeed, our visual impressions when we are absorbed in thought. They are merely schemes of flat colours.

Visual sensations of another's facial expressions and manners similarly recall ideas of feelings that are associated with these manifestations in ourselves. The sight of one who is frowning, for instance, enables us to " perceive " that he is out of temper. Our perception is, in fact, the recall of ideas concerning ourselves, that are re-stimulated by impressions of appearances with which they have been associated. It is through these memorial amplifications that we invest the moving images of the cinema with living motives. We ascribe internal (or subjective) conditions to other persons by " projecting " conditions of our own into them—a process which has been given the misleading name of " empathy ". Sensation only impresses us with their *appearance*. When we see that a man is running, our senses merely tell us that he is rapidly changing his place : we ascribe to him the active condition of running by assimilating his appearance to our own when running, and investing him with the condition that goes with this appearance in ourselves. When we see that the sun is " rising " we are ascribing to it an activity of our own. It is almost impossible to realize that our perceptions of the conditions of persons and things are, in fact, transfers to them of ideas of our own conditions. Yet proofs of this abound. The most striking of them is, perhaps, that, arguing from ourselves, we think of an object as " having " or " possessing " a quality, such as a colour. The relationship between it and its quality is clearly one of simple combination. Yet we ascribe to the object *power* over its quality, because in our own case association is generally possessive, and possession implies power.

In like fashion the sensation of an object recalls its name. Recollections of things and recollections of their names are, of course, separate mental existences. But they become so intimately associated by the familiarity of everyday experience that one immediately brings the other before us. So a word instantaneously recalls the idea for which it stands. For words are sensory impressions of hearing, sight or feeling. We are impressed by hearing or seeing the word " motor-car " exactly as we are impressed by the sound or sight of a motor-car. And, since the utterance of a word involves movement, we *feel* its utterance as we do the movement of a finger, although our consciousness of the feeling is deadened by habit.

The amplifying recollections, to which we have referred so far, present themselves simultaneously with the recalling impression because they have been simultaneously associated with similar impressions in the past. We can see a thing and handle it simultaneously. If, on the other hand, the two impressions have occurred successively, the recurrence of one of them will recall a recollection of the other in succession. So every action recalls an idea of its consequence : if we grasp a door handle, we immediately think of the future opening of the door : if we see umbrellas go up in the street, we perceive that it has begun to rain, because in experience rain has always preceded their use. These memorial flashes into the future or the past are the beginnings of the process of inference.

Comprehension.—By this is meant the grasping of the relationships that connect things with their environment and link them with the past and the present—as, for instance, that a bird is *in* the sky, is *like* a skylark, and *has been singing*. These various relationships have been touched upon already, and will be described in detail when we deal with ideas and their formation. But it is necessary to make some reference to them here.

Experience—that is to say perception assisted by recollection—presents life to us as a series of scenes, each of which is composed of a number of things that are in coincidence with one another, but in a coincidence that is constantly interrupted by change, movement, growth and development. Accordingly, one thing is linked to another, either because it coincides with it, or because it precedes or follows it—that is to say in sequence or succession with it. A man whom we see is coincident with his qualities of appearance, emotion and action, with his name, with a place in space and a point of time. But, in time, his conditions follow those of yesterday and precede those of to-morrow. If he moves, there is a sequence between the beginning and the end of his movement. These relationships that are impressed upon us by experience may all be described as phases of inter-dependence through *combination* (or association) in coincidence or sequence.

Intelligence, on the other hand, discloses to us relationships of quite a different kind—that a thing may be the same as (or identified with) another thing, may resemble it, or be different from it. These relationships are obviously the result of *comparing* the two. They may be distinguished as relationships of *comparison*.

Our understanding of relationships is confused by the fact that sequences, or successions, of experience are represented in thought by a string of coincidences. There is a succession in going from one place to another. Yet in the thought " I motored from London to

Bath ", the journey presents itself " statically " as a single event. It might indeed conceivably be expressed by a single word, since the sequence of movement is expressed by an idea of *direction*. And, since successions are figured in thought as coincidences, they can be expressed backwards as well as forwards : an outcome can be placed before its origin, a consequence before its cause. We can say " from London to Bath ", or " to Bath from London ", the " son of his father ", as well as the " father of his son ".

Relationship of combination, or association.—These, as coincidences, include the *liaison* between a quality, condition or activity and the individual to which it belongs—which possesses or " has " it. A thing is in coincident relationship to its colour and form. Of this class are also the relationships between an individual and a place or point of time, between a movement and its direction, between a distance or condition and its length or duration. Relationships of combination in sequence or succession include not only the *liaisons* between an origin and its outcome, a beginning and its development, a cause and its effect, but all movements that occur in space and changes that occur in time. In every movement there is a relationship between its start and its finish. All changes are relative to that which preceded them. Their existence depends upon the existence of a predecessor.

Relationships in comparison.—These all arise from the fact that an element or trait that is common to two recollections or ideas enables one of them to originate the re-assemblage of the other, and is therefore a link between them which brings them into comparison. There are resemblances between feelings as well as between sensory impressions : courage and self-control are obviously connected. Similarity may be in function, or circumstances, as well as in character : a butterfly resembles a bird in flying : choice resembles the process of weighing in that they both involve *balancing*. Metaphor, which assists us so greatly in devising words to express ideas, is suggested by relationships of resemblance. When we speak of a " melancholy day ", we liken it to ourselves.

It is through comparison that things are *measured*. Relationships of quantity or intensity are those between a quality and a unit of the same quality whereby the first is measured in comparison, as when we say that the electric light is brighter than gas. But all qualities that vary in degree or in intensity, such as length, size, weight and velocity, involve comparison with a unit, although the comparison is not expressed. When we speak of a " large " tree or a " fast " horse we are comparing them with a unit of *average* size or speed that is in our mind. For these average mental units, material units are substituted. This is the origin of *measurement*.

The reality of relationships.—Between our consciousness of things or qualities and our consciousness of relationships there is a difference of vast importance. The former is deceptive : the latter is true. Our sensations and feelings are merely symbolic presentments of reality. The world, as known through the inferences of Science, is astonishingly different from our conscious ideas of it. But things may be symbolic in character without falsifying the relationships which connect them. A game of chess is symbolic of battle. Its pieces have no actual resemblance to combatants. But their relationships in time, place, function and power, are such as those to which combatants are subject. If the external changes of which we are conscious did not occur in succession—that is to say, in time—there would be no interval between sunrise and sunset. If things were not separated in space—that is to say, by distance—we should not have to move in order to shift our position from one room to another. When we put coal on the fire we certainly put something on to something else. When we recognize a similarity between a tree and an umbrella there must be a real resemblance between them—that of form. The sun and moon are actually round. The resemblance between a note of music and its octave exists between the rapidities of their vibrations, which, multiplication apart, are the same. And if the question be asked—why should our knowledge of relationships be true when our impressions of the character of things is demonstrably false, there is a convincing answer. This imperfect knowledge suffices for the requirements of life. So long as conduct conforms to the relationships of our environment, it is not prejudiced by errors of apprehension regarding the nature of things. Our lives are not endangered by ignorance of the real character of arsenic so long as we correctly realize its relationship to certain consequences. Life could not exist if it misinterpreted relationships.

3 The Process of Recollection

Recollection is clearly the beginning of thought. It involves the revival of a sensation as a kind of " echo " or " shadow " of itself. Recollections may be classed as objective, subjective, or " relative " —that is to say, recollections, not of things, but of relationships

between things.   It will be convenient to take subjective recollections first.   They are mental " echoes " of motives and emotions,
and must be sharply distinguished from actual re-stimulations of
these subjective energies.   By a thought of its object (or cause),
a motive or emotion can be easily revived in actuality ; and, since
words recall thoughts, they may be equally effective.   Subjective
recollections are not to be confused with these resuscitations of
feeling : they are merely " ideas " of feeling—notions of qualities
rather than occurrences.   They differ markedly from re-stimulations
in that they can be recalled directly by words that signify them—
" courage ", for instance—whereas to re-stimulate a feeling in
actuality a thought of its *cause* is required.

Objective recollections are of a much more definite character since
they are based upon sensory impressions.   But here again we must
distinguish memorial from actual re-stimulation.   Under the
abnormal emotional conditions of hallucination, objective sensory
experiences may be re-stimulated in actuality, so that a sensation
repeats itself, in the absence of any external stimulus.   A sensory
hallucination is, then, comparable with an emotion that is re-
stimulated by an idea of its cause.   Objective recollections are of a
much less vivid quality.   They apparently involve some re-stimulation of sensory conditions, but of conditions that are derived from
sensory impressions, not of the impressions in themselves.   They
are popularly supposed to be located in the brain.   But it is really
inconceivable that the brain should present them without the co-
operation of the sensory organs.   The recollection of a tune, for
instance, must involve repetitive activity in the nerves of the ear.
When we recall a particular touch or taste, the nerves of the place
touched, or of the tongue, must contribute to the recall.   And it
seems unquestionable that the recollection of a movement must
include assistance from the nerves of the muscles that were moved.
If, for instance, we move a foot and then recollect the movement,
we can detect that something in the foot contributes to the remembrance.   We may, then, conclude, it seems, that a recollection of a
sensory impression is to some extent localized in the nerves which
received it.   There is, it must be admitted, an argument against this
view.   One who has lost a limb can, nevertheless, for some time
afterwards, recollect, or think, of moving it.   His recollection is
perhaps a general idea of movement which is, through the force of
association, erroneously located in the missing limb.   But, however
this may be, it is impossible to account for a recollection of movement unless it arises from an echo of the sensation of movement,

or for a recollection of hunger unless it is connected with the nerves of the stomach.

Relationships are recollected as part and parcel of the stream of re-stimulations that constitutes " remembering ". If we remember a book, we may at the same time recall the person to whom it belonged, the time and place at which we saw it, and the purpose that was in mind at the time. A recollection of an amount, or intensity, as of a " large " book, or a " half-stroke " at golf, involves an idea of a normal with which a comparison is made : if it is *definite*, it includes the idea of a unit of measurement. The recall of such standards of intensity would be wholly inexplicable if recollections were, as popularly supposed, " stored " in the brain. But, if they are sub-repetitions of conditions of the past, the recall of an idea of an intensity is less mysterious : in our illustration from the golf-links, the intensity of a full stroke is recalled as the echo of a feeling and forms the basis of a relative muscular effort. Of the same kind are our recollections of the normal duration of certain kinds of periods, such as that which enables us to think that a particular period is unusually long or short. If by habit a normal or average duration has been established for any particular course of activity, on the completion of the normal, the memory suggests an idea of its completion. So we come to feel that a meal, or a game, has lasted " longer than usual ". We clearly owe to these automatic reminders our capacity for estimating the intervals of a series as of equal or unequal length—and our ability to " beat time " correctly.

Subconscious memory.—It is difficult to think of recollections as being other than *conscious* experiences. Yet it seems quite clear that the memory can act unconsciously, and in this case a recollection must exist apart from its presentment in consciousness. We can, beyond doubt, receive sensory impressions during a period of unconsciousness : we could not otherwise be awakened from sleep. One who is under hypnotic influence not uncommonly shows a knowledge of facts of which he was consciously unaware, and must, therefore, have struck him unconsciously. A recollection, which suddenly presents itself after an interval of forgetfulness, must be called up by an unconscious re-stimulation. And it seems clear that thought may proceed without consciousness. It is within the experience of many men that a problem which was insoluble over night has presented itself solved in the morning. These facts provide a definition for the term " subconscious "—a word which is often used very vaguely indeed. " Subconsciousness " is a phase of unconsciousness which permits of the re-stimulating action of memory and intelligence.

Recollection and the brain.—It is a peculiar feature of recollections that they grow in detail as we think about them. Our recollection of a train, for instance, is at first little more than symbolic. But as it is dwelt upon, it grows—like a plant from seed—into a complicated presentment of form, colour, energies and sounds. The co-operation of the sensory organs is, in fact, initiated and controlled by the action of the brain. The anatomy of this organ is extraordinarily intricate, and in regard to the functions of its various parts physiology has hardly crossed the threshold of knowledge. But one definite fact is known. A study of the *post mortem* conditions of those who have suffered from paralysis in its various forms has established that each phase of this affliction is associated with disease or injury in a particular area of the cortex of the cerebral hemispheres. If the surface of the occipital lobe is affected, the sufferer loses the intelligent use of his eyes : he may " see " things but does not recognize them. While continuing to receive visual impressions, he is unable to summon the recollections that are required in order to complete them and endow them with meaning. The process of hearing is similarly sterilized by injuries in the temporal lobe. When an injury affects the parietal lobe, the process of voluntary movement is interrupted. The sufferer may be able to move his limbs involuntarily under the action of an outside stimulus, but cannot use them deliberately—that is to say, cannot initiate movements by ideas of them, although such ideas may present themselves. He may, for instance, be able to think of moving a finger, but the thought will have no effect. And it has been established that the particular limb-muscles which are isolated in this fashion depend upon the position of the injury in the parietal lobe : they are those of the feet if the lobe is injured at its summit, and they lie higher and higher up the body as the injury is lower and lower in the brain. In fact, areas of the parietal cortex correspond with areas of the body in reverse order. In the injury affects a patch in the parietal lobe of the size of a hazel-nut (Broca's convolution) the sufferer loses the power of uttering words voluntarily. It seems clear, then, that upon the parietal nerve-cells depends the power of re-stimulating motor conditions by thoughts of movements, whereas the occipital and temporal nerve-cells are concerned with the re-stimulation of sensory conditions. Paralysis is an affliction of the same kind as loss of memory.

These facts give support to the view that each recollection (or sub-repetition of sensory conditions) is initiated in the cortex of the brain by what may be termed a " symbol-key ", which is at once its representative in symbolic miniature, and a centre from which it can be re-stimulated in full. The word that " names " a recollection is intimately associated with its symbol-key, and can, therefore, bring it into action. If, for instance, in conversation we are " reminded " of a particular friend, we at first call him to mind symbolically—in " short-hand ", so to speak—through the expression of his features. But, if we allow ourselves to dwell upon him, this symbolic recollection develops into a more or less definite recall of his various attributes and possessions. What was primarily merely a brain-sign becomes a sub-repetition of various sensory conditions in detail. The brain-cell is, then, not merely a symbol. It is a " key " through which a complete recollection can be revived, just as a piano-key is the instrument through which a note is sounded.

These symbol-keys would be drawn into association by simultaneous or successive occurrences of the sensations of which they are the brain-signs. They would, therefore, re-stimulate one another in ordinary course, and each on being re-stimulated would evoke the recollection for which it is the " key ".

This hypothesis is by no means out of accord with the constitution of the brain as a whole. Its basal portion is intimately connected with the sense-organs, the spinal cord, and the sympathetic chain. It may be likened to a knot to which nerve-strands of various kinds contribute, and in which the physical and animative elements of our nature are both represented. The hemispheres which overlie the basal " knot " consist of myriads of nerve-fibrils in a compact mass that lie between various aggregates of nerve-cells below, and a layer of nerve-cells that is spread over the upper surface and constitutes the " cortex ". The fibrils would provide a means of inter-association between the nerve-cells below and those of the cortex, and between the nerve-cells that compose each of these aggregates. There are almost infinite possibilities for the re-stimulation of one nerve-cell by another ; and it may be argued that the constitution of the brain reflects very strikingly the vast importance of the process of nervous re-stimulation in physical and mental life.

4 The Development of Thought

There are some curious analogies between thought and movement. Both are under the control of the will—that is to say both can be deflected in course by an effort. It has consequently been held by some psychologists that thought has evolved from movement. But this strains the analogy too far. For the materials of thought are recollections, and ideas which (as we shall see) are derived from recollections. The evolutionary origin of thought must therefore be sensation that is accompanied by memorial re-stimulation. There is, however, one phase of sensation—perhaps the most fundamental —to which movement is essential. This is sensation by tactile " feeling ". There are some striking resemblances between this process and thought. The movements of feeling are a succession of trials ending in a grasp. This is illustrated very clearly by the behaviour of animals which rely upon tentacles for their food, and by ourselves when, for example, we search for a box of matches in the dark. We pass our fingers tentatively over a number of objects and grasp the box when we come across it. This closely resembles the process of thought. It passes ideas in review until one presents itself that enables it to grasp the clue to a difficulty. It then, by an effort, forms a decision or conclusion, which, when it affects behaviour or speech, is called a " choice ".

There is another connection between thought and movement. The one takes the place of the other. The primary effect of a like, or inclination, is a movement of approach. We can, however, satisfy this impulse by " thinking about " our object. We should otherwise be as impulsive as a little child. Those are most impulsive who think the least.

The reception of sense-impressions may, as we have seen, be unconscious. And it seems clear that " thought " may also progress in unconsciousness, although we have no means of ascertaining what forms its " ideas " then assume. It is only on this assumption that the fact can be explained that one may awake with a definite conclusion on a point which had been quite baffling over night.

It is impossible to discuss the process of thinking until we have arrived at some definite conclusions as to the nature and origin of the ideas which are its materials. But one point may be emphasized at once. We think about a thing by ascribing to it something which is in relationship with it, as a quality of appearance, feeling or conduct, a position in place or time, an identity, a resemblance, a difference or an intensity. Whatever be the drift or purpose of our thought, this ascription may be made under one of three very different influences. It may be made rationally, inclinationally, or emotionally. A *rational* ascription is based upon a general rule or law that is deduced from experience, or is dictated by intelligence. We argue from experience when we ascribe truthfulness to another's statement because it is to his discredit, and experience shows that men never deceive when it is against their interests to do so. The law is brought into thought by the intelligent grip of an analogy : there is a sameness between the statement we are considering and statements generally. We argue by intelligence when we conclude that since *a* equals *b*, and *b* equals *c*, *a* must be equal to *c*. An ascription is *inclinational* (or " tendencious ") when it is urged by habit, or by a like or dislike : we may accept another's words because we ordinarily do so, or because we like either him, or the information that he gives us. We ascribe *emotionally* when actuated by such feelings as love, admiration or faith, or when we are thinking imaginatively. And we must refer to a further complication. Whether an ascription is rational, inclinational or emotional, it may be made either spontaneously, or by the effort of will that is evoked by a difficulty or discord. We are spontaneously rational in ordinary thought : one ascription follows another by inferences from experience, or intelligently appreciated samenesses, which are drawn so smoothly and rapidly as to escape our consciousness. But if no law is forthcoming, we exercise the will in seeking a clue to one. The habits or prejudices that sway inclinational ascriptions may similarly affect us automatically, or urge us to an effort. Emotional ascriptions are spontaneous when enthusiastic, willed when ingenious.

It is certain that ascriptions of the rational kind are those which are normally made when thought is free from outside influences. For they run from the particular to the general and back to the particular, and this is the order of perception. We see a thing, refer it to its kind, and deduce its qualities from its kind. Thought, as a development of sensory susceptibility, *naturally* follows the lines on which the process of perception has evolved. But it can be swayed by influences from either the feminine or masculine side. In the first case it is deflected by like or dislike, or by habit—the attraction of familiarity. In the second it is up-lifted, and may be imaginatively transfigured, by emotion. In both cases " reason " is submerged. And it is not an uncommon experience that perception is similarly deranged by prejudice, habit or enthusiasm.

5 The Formation of Ideas

We have, so far, been considering recollections as the materials of thought. But actually we most commonly think in " ideas " that are derived from sensations and recollections, although greatly differing from them ; and before commencing to discuss the various processes and phases of thought we must attempt to trace our ideas to their origins. This will involve a difficult and laborious process of analysis. But it is worth an effort if by making it we can dissipate some of the mist that obscures from us the wonderful ingenuity of our mental faculties.

In ideas sensorial impressions appear to be sublimated into extreme tenuity. For an idea is, typically, the notion of a *quality* or group of qualities, that is isolated from substantial existence. The quality may be a trait of external appearance, a trait of internal feeling, or a relationship linking two things together, as, for instance, that of being connected together as cause and effect. It is an attribute to one who runs that he is energetic, of one who is energetic, that he is hot. The energy and the heat, as mentally isolated, become free of all particular attachments, so that they can be ascribed to very dissimilar objects. Energy can be attributed to a steam engine or a thunder storm : heat to a cup of tea, or the weather.

Words and ideas.—It has been held that the most abstruse of our ideas could not exist unless there were words to express them—that in fact words came into existence before the ideas that they signify. This is tantamount to holding that the sounds of a telephone receiver cause the current that agitate it. For utterances being *manifestations* of ideas, an idea must exist before there can be a word to express it. There is, moreover, a fact which demonstrates that highly complicated ideas exist in the mind independently of the words that signify them. For we may hesitate over the use of particular words to express an idea that is in mind, and choose between alternatives, as between " involve " and " entail " for instance. Words may, however, exist without ideas (as in a language we do not understand), and may be used—and, indeed, are very frequently used—without clear ideas of their meaning.

Ideas and " things ".—Our only knowledge of our environment consists in our ideas of it, and we unconsciously recognize this fact in using the word " thing " for ideas as well as for material objects or conditions. We speak, for instance, of a " thing " which we have in mind. And it is noteworthy that, having regard to the origin of the word, its primary meaning is that of a *phenomenon* or " appearance ". For it is derived from the O.E. *thenken*, " to appear ", a vestige of which remains in " methinks ". We shall, from time to time, use it as the equivalent of " idea ". It is convenient, since it expresses the objective through the subjective, and it is of such indefinite application that it can include the animate as well as the inanimate.

The sources of ideas.—It can be shown that ideas—however ethereal they may appear—all spring from our objective and subjective experiences of sensation and recollection, including the relationships to which these introduce us. Under the operation of certain mental processes that are in fact developments of associative re-stimulation, these experiences become, as it were, germs that can produce, not merely such simple leaves as are a plant's first essays in life, but a branched structure of ideas, the most highly elaborated of which may not inaptly be likened to flowers. These mental processes may be distinguished as individualization, combination, comparison and deduction. By *individualization* we give a separate existence to the appearances that are presented to us by sensation and feeling. By *combination* we blend together ideas of them. In the process of *comparing* two things, the elements or traits that are common to both are separated from those that are peculiar to each of them : the former are therefore isolated by *assimilation* the latter are isolated by *differentiation*. Thus, for instance, all roses are assimilated through their generic similarities to form the general idea of " rose ", as a quality of *kind* : their various colours are differentiated as their peculiar qualities. Comparison, moreover, gives rise to new ideas in the relative conditions that it brings about—those of resemblance and intensity, for example. The process of *deduction* is also creative. Our experience of life's successions convince us that everything must have a cause or origin. Accordingly, when no origin is evident, we deduce one in the form of an abstract continuity, such as Space, Time and Virtue. By deduction an idea may also be formed as the *contrary* of one that has been established by experience. We know of the relative : we deduce the existence of an Absolute.

These processes can all be traced to the law of associative re-stimulation. Under this law an idea of one quality will re-stimulate the idea of another—and be *combined* with it—if the two have been associated together in sensation. It is obvious that two ideas are *compared* when one re-stimulates the other through a sameness. And abstract ideas are *deduced* as origins of immaterial conditions, because the process of re-stimulation ordinarily presents to us the antecedents of our experiences, and, when no antecedent is known, we are urged to supply one.

The growth of ideas.—We can no more expect to watch the evolution of ideas than the evolution of plants and animals. It has slowly pursued its course during uncounted ages ; and, from the very slowness of its march, is the greatest of human accomplishments. It is infinitely easier to learn than to invent, so that, when an idea has been " caught " and labelled, it is readily appropriated by the rising generation. On the other hand, the process has been thrown back—often nearly to its beginnings—by the destructiveness of war. But it is not necessary to watch the action of a process in order to understand it. We can infer its course from its results. If, for example, we examine a classified collection of flowers, we can infer the principles that have guided its arrangement. Similarly, by analyzing our ideas, we can discover the methods of their elaboration. It is, of course, by analyzing plants and animals that we have formed the conclusion that they have come into existence through a process of evolution.

Individualization.—Our sensations and feelings are in themselves merely impressions which appear to us in consciousness. Some of them—hunger and anger, for instance—are within us, while others, such as feelings of solidity, smell, taste, colours and sounds, affect us on the outside. Actually, both are alike in being part of ourselves : a sensation of sound is as much ourselves as is a headache. In itself it is " subjective ", and is objective in that it is *caused* by something that affects us externally. The indications that our eyes afford us of the nature of these external stimuli vary with every alteration in the position of the body and the eyes : a thing rarely presents exactly the same appearance twice running, and we need not wonder that a baby regards this meaningless kaleidoscopic entertainment with round-eyed astonishment.

Amidst these bewildering changes one thing remains constant— ourselves. Our feelings alter from time to time. But they are continuously linked in relationship with one another so as to form an individual unity. This continuity becomes our " personality " when combined with a notion of external appearance. Arguing analogically from ourselves, we individualize everything that can be separated from its surroundings—that is to say we " form an idea of it " as a separate *thing*. This process is at its simplest when it deals with tangible or " substantial " objects, since these can be separated from their environment by being moved—as a cloth from a table or the limbs from the body. It is extended analogically to everything which possesses a separable existence—to manifestations of activity, such as movements and sounds, to our own states of feeling and to conditions of relationship, such as *position* and *resemblance.* For all these " come and go " and present therefore an appearance of independence. The picture-stream of sensation and feeling is thus crystallized into *things.*

Combination.—Ideas combine with one another when they are derived from repeated simultaneous or successive experiences. For in this case one immediately re-stimulates the other, so that they present themselves together. Combination may be either *intrinsic* or *extrinsic.* In the first of these phases it creates single ideas out of a multiplicity of elements by compacting them together. The vast majority of our ideas are highly complex " combines ". A multitude of qualities enters into our notion of a motor-car, for instance. The active and passive conditions which are signified by verbs may be compounds of activities, instruments and objects ; *sewing* involves the idea of a needle, *drinking* that of a liquid. Ideas of instruments include implications of purpose ; apart from its purpose a pencil is simply a pointed cylinder of wood. In our idea of an emotion is combined an idea of a like or dislike with one of an emotional state of expansion, contraction, or discord. It is by this process of combination that our visual impressions of objects immediately recall ideas of solidity, position and distance, and the sights and sounds of another's behaviour and utterances present to us ideas of his feelings and thoughts.

By *extrinsic* combination ideas are connected together in a series. This is the process of thought, which is for separate discussion hereafter. We are now concerned with the formation of ideas. But it must be mentioned here that the linkings of thought are rendered possible by the extrinsic combination, with particular ideas, of " blank " ideas, or " somethings ", that serve as connecting links or " catches ". We call these *somethings* " implications ". An adjective implies a possessor ; a verb, a subject, and, if active, an object : the demonstrative " this " implies the existence of an indefinite something that is combined with the idea of *nearness.* These combinations with blanks are formed by a series of comparisons which, as we shall see, can eliminate the *particular* element of a combination. So a quality can be isolated from any particular possessor. But there remains an implication of being possessed— of an indefinite possessorship—a blank into which a particular can be fitted.

Comparison.—The process of comparison leads to the formation of new ideas through its consequences in assimilation and different-iation. Traits or qualities that are possessed by both the things that are compared are isolated because they are assimilated to one another, whereas qualities that are possessed by only one of them—and are *peculiar* to it—are isolated because they are differences. A baby sees the dog of the family in dozens of different positions, recollections of which will be recalled by each sight of it. Certain traits will be included in all of them—that is to say, will be assimi-lated to one another as essential, whereas those that vary are accidental. These essential traits, coupled with a particular name, will constitute its idea of the " concrete " particular dog. It is, then, clear that our ideas of particular things are generalized from a number of different impressions through the assimilation of essentials.

It may be objected that comparison involves something more than the mere bringing together of two ideas through the process of associative re-stimulation—that it entails an active capacity of *appreciating* sameness and differences. We possess such a capacity in our acute sensibility to harmony and discord. Sameness is harmony in its completest degree—the harmony of unison. Differ-ence is a form of discord.

It must also be realized that comparison may be spontaneous as well as " willed ", and that we are now referring to the former kind. We are so accustomed to the voluntary, effortful, use of our faculties, that we hardly realize that willing is a capacity which has evolved through the infusion of effort into processes that are primitively spontaneous.

Generalized ideas of qualities of kind.—By comparing and generaliz-ing concrete things we also form ideas of qualities of kind—that is to say, of the qualities that are common to a class of individuals. If we compare a green-finch with a linnet, the traits that are common to both are isolated by assimilation as those of the finch kind. In the same fashion we form ideas of the qualities that unite social classes, fellowships, and nations. Comparison then not only frees ideas of individuals from qualities that are varying or accidental, but classifies individuals by assimilating traits that are common to all of them.

It is obvious that by successive processes of comparison and elimination all the qualities of an object can be divorced from it except that of simple concrete existence. If two very different objects are drawn into comparison simply because they both are tangible, there is nothing to be assimilated but mere substance, and this is eliminated by such a comparison as that between a flower and a note of music. There remains only the idea of bare existence— which we express by the word " thing "—" something " if an idea of a *kind* persists, " anything " if this is also eliminated. This vague idea of undefined individuality plays an essential part in thought. When we ask : What is it ? we recognize the existence of something of whose precise kind we are unaware.

The essential traits of individuals and kinds, being isolated by assimilation, not by differentiation, are by no means clearly marked. It would puzzle one to define precisely the characteristic traits of a particular person, or of a dog. They seem to be traits of movement and expression rather than of form and colour. It is the *expression* that marks the friend, and also, it appears, distinguishes the dog kind.

We think, for the most part, in " generals "—that is to say, in ideas of individuals that are characterized by possessing the qualities of a kind. If we wish to specify a particular individual we attach a proper name, or define a general idea, by giving it a special relation to a place or person (*this, that, mine*), or by indicating, through the definite article, that it is a " particular ". General ideas may be broadened by the amalgamation of two or more kinds : dogs may be grouped with horses as *quadrupeds :* various kinds of self-repression are grouped together as *virtues : colour* is a group of numerous different tints which are alike in their effect upon sight. And kinds can be narrowed by subdivision, as, for instance, by the distinction between dogs of different breeds.

Differentiated qualities.—As ideas of objects and kind-qualities are formed by *assimilating* properties that are common to various impressions, so ideas of particular qualities are formed by *differentiating* properties that are peculiar to individuals and kinds. Such are the colours of the two finches—green and brown, and their song-notes. The process of evolution then reverts to assimilation. The qualities that have been isolated are themselves generalized by being assimilated with similar qualities that are possessed by other things—the green of the green-finch, for instance, with the green of a leaf.

A quality as thus isolated is an attribute, such as " red ", which is meaningless in itself. But it can be individualized with an implication of being possessed : we use " red " in this sense when we say that " red is startling ". And it can be further individualized as a condition of possessing it, as in " redness ". The quality " solid " is an attribute : it is individualized as " solidity " and can be further individualized as a condition of possessing it (solidness). " Solidity " as an individualized quality must be sharply distinguished from " solidity " as an abstract. The former implies something to which the quality is attached. " A solidity " cannot exist without something that is solid. But as an abstract, " solidity " is free from any such implication, and possesses an independent existence.

Subjective conditions, such as fear and pleasure, which come and go, can be regarded as qualities, since they *qualify* the persons that they affect. But their phase as a quality is derived from their phase as an individualized condition, as " virtuous " is from " virtue ". With some limitations, this also applies to conditions of relationship, such as *time*, which gives rise to *timely*, as a quality, and to *timeliness*.

Quantities.—These are ideas of intensity or amount. They also are isolated by comparison. The comparison is, however, not between two different things that are connected by a sameness, but between two things that are alike in possessing a quality but possess it in different degrees. The greens of the bird and of the leaf are alike. But one differs from the other in being *more* or *less*, and the excess or deficit can be estimated by using one shade as a unit of comparison and bringing the other into a relationship of proportion with it. An intensity, or amount, can also be estimated by comparison with a normal, or average—that is to say, with a generalized idea of it. Its accurate measurement is only possible when the unit of comparison is artificial and can be rhythmically subdivided.

Isolation of relationships.—So far of the effect of comparison in generalizing and differentiating ideas of individuals, qualities and quantities. It performs another function. By isolating the relationships which connect two things together it gives rise to the most abstruse of our concepts. Two things are related to one another when they are combined or compared. The word " Englishman ", for instance, expresses the combination of an individual with an attribute of kind : the word " likeness " expresses the consequence of comparing two things that possess a common trait. A relationship cannot exist apart from the two ideas which it connects. But it can, nevertheless, be partly, and even wholly, isolated by comparison, since for particular ideas, blank ideas of indefinite " somethings " can be substituted. We can illustrate the process by dismembering a word. " Englishman " connects a man with England by the relationship of " belonging to ". But other things may belong to England, and " English " may accordingly be isolated as an adjective, carrying a blank idea—or implication—of something that is English. It becomes an " idea related to a blank ". Such are adjectives, adverbs, the possessive, demonstrative and relative pronouns, and neuter verbs, each of which has an implication of " something " that is related to it as its subject. An active verb has two such implications—one of an indefinite object as well as of an indefinite subject. An adjective in the comparative is also related to two blanks—one of something that is compared, and the other of a standard of comparison. Reverting to our illustration, the syllable " ish ", which signifies the relationship of " belonging to ", may further be isolated by comparison, since this relationship exists between vast numbers of other things : " sheepish ", for instance, means something that appertains to a sheep. So isolated, it represents a condition of relationship that connects two blank ideas. Such are the prepositions (in most of their uses) and the conjunctions. " In " expresses a link of " inclusion " that is related to two blank ideas, " and " a relative condition of conjunction. These ideas can be isolated because a number of different things are connected by one being in the other, or by one being joined to the other. The comparative relationship of " likeness " between a horse and a pony can similarly be isolated, since there is likeness between a vast number of different things.

These blank ideas are the attachments by which thoughts connect themselves into a series. They are, so to speak, receptacles which can be filled by the attachment of particular ideas. It follows that thought and grammar have evolved through the isolation of relationships. Traces of this process survive. In Latin certain relationships in quality, space and time are signified by case-endings which have the effect of converting their nouns into ideas related to a blank. In English these links are expressed by prepositions, signifying conditions of relationship that connect two blank ideas—leaving, however, an evolutionary trace in the possessive case. The Latin verb expresses the person to whom its condition was linked, or ascribed. " Cogito " is a sentence in itself. In English the verb is isolated from particular personality, and is reduced to an idea related in blank.

Blank relationships, when thus isolated, are individualized as conditions, with implications of the two " somethings " which they connect. Precedence, for instance, is a relationship of being " before " another, and implies the existence of two persons or things, one preceding, the other following. Individualized relationships of this kind are amongst the most abstruse of our concepts, including such ideas as those of time, space, causality, energy and

K

thought. But although we describe them as " isolated ", they all carry implications of two somethings that they connect. A *space* is meaningless apart from ideas of two things or places that are linked by it, a *causality* unless there are ideas of a cause and a consequence, an *energy* unless there are ideas of something that acts and something that is acted upon. This fact is obscured by the use of these words in an entirely different sense—with an " abstract " signification. But with this meaning they represent, not actualities of experience, but transcendental continuities.

The process of comparison, therefore, simplifies things by separating from them traits and relationships that can be isolated by differentiation. We may liken combination to *mixing*, and comparison to *distilling*. It is an evolutionary instrument of refinement that acts gradually ; and, consequently, amongst backward peoples general ideas, that appear obvious to us, may be completely lacking. The Mohicans have words for cutting various objects, but none to convey *cutting* simply. The Zulus have such words as " red cow ", " white cow ", but none for cow generally. In Cherokee, instead of word for " washing ", we find different words according to what is washed—I wash myself—my head—my clothes, etc. In old English there were two separate words for washing animate and inanimate objects.[1]

Deduction.—By this process we deduce the existence of an idea from the existence of another. We are impelled to do this by the influence upon us of our capacity of associative re-stimulation. For this process cannot complete itself unless an experience has an antecedent which can be recalled. If such predecessor is not revealed to us by sensation or feeling we bring it into mental existence by deduction, as a transcendental as opposed to an empirical concept.

So it is that we form our " abstract " ideas. They are concepts of continuities that serve as origins ; for the origin of a thing is explained if it exist from all time. We have no knowledge of " substance " apart from our tactile experiences. We deduce an abstract idea of " substance " as a continuity which underlies the material, precisely as the existence of gravity was deduced from the falling of an apple. The immaterial must also have an origin— the transient conditions, or " feelings ", of our subjective life, and the conditions of relationship which bind our experiences and thoughts into a *continuum*. It seems that no one could be virtuous or just unless these qualities were pre-existing energies. There

---

[1] Jesperson. *Growth and Structure of the English Language*, §51.

could be no velocity unless velocity had a continuing existence, such as that with which we invest the force of gravity. So again, space, time, energy and harmony must exist as continuities in order that there may be points and periods of time, place and distance in space, energetic conditions and such harmonies as those of truth and justice. Things that possess a material or sensory existence need not be so abstracted. For their " substance " is their origin. But Plato could think, nevertheless, that an abstract " tree " was the origin of all our ideas of trees.

Abstract ideas of conditions are liable to be confused with general ideas of them, since we employ the same words to express the two. But we can easily appreciate the difference of meaning between Virtue in the abstract, and " a virtue ", between Space and " a space ", between Time and " a time "—that is to say between abstract ideas and such generalized concepts of virtue, space and time, as are before us in such phrases as a " man of virtue ", a " point in space ", or a " period of time ".

An individualized *quality* is shadowed by the idea of something to which it appertains, since this cannot be altogether eliminated by the isolating comparisons. But an abstract is free from this implication since it is not drawn from experience but is imposed upon it.

Abstracts are of immense importance, since they affect our outlook upon life. They are " metaphysical " ideas, *following* " physical " ideas in the sense of being deduced from them. " Mind " in the abstract, seems to be a directing force which exists independently of the mind of man. As a kind of relationship, " truth " is accord between a conclusion and experience or intelligence : in the abstract it presents itself as an eternal influence which is the origin of truth in man. The difference between the individual (or " concrete ") and the abstract is that which distinguishes History and Science from Metaphysics, Theology and Logic. But Science trespasses across the border line, using concepts that are purely metaphysical. Such is its idea of Energy as a continuously self-conserving force. All that experiment tells us is that an energetic condition of one kind may expend itself in giving rise to an energetic condition of another kind (as a motive stimulates a movement), and that the intensity of the second will be proportionate to that of the first.

6 The Various Kinds of Ideas

The classification of ideas is exceedingly difficult because it can be effected from two points of view which cross one another. We can distinguish ideas according to their *uses*, or according to their *kinds*. The former is the grammatical classification to which we are accustomed : the latter is more fundamental, since it traces them back to their origins. Grammar arranges ideas (through the words that express them) into " parts of speech ", which may be distinguished as either nominative, ascriptive or descriptive. A *nominative* (or noun) is the subject of a thought, an *ascriptive* (or verb) connects the subject with a personality, condition, or quality of some kind, a *descriptive* defines or amplifies the subject or the ascription. Nominatives are commonly known as " substantives ". But it must be observed here that this term is misleading. For it implies that they are not " relatives ", and as a matter of fact all our ideas are relative, with the exception of abstracts. An idea is relative if its nature is dependent upon another idea so that its character is changed if this is withdrawn. This dependence is most conspicuous in the case of the contraries styled " correlatives ". For if one of these ceases to exist, the other vanishes with it. There is correlation between origin and outcome, in direction of movement, in change, and between active and passive conditions. There can be no son without a father, or cause without a consequence, no motion towards one thing that is not also away from another, no change unless one thing is transformed into another, no power without a corresponding constraint. But interdependence may fall far short of this and still produce a condition of " relativity ". An idea of any object, for instance, is changed if an idea of one of its qualities is withdrawn. An idea of a quality implies an idea of something that possesses it. Abstracts are " absolute " because they are not adopted from experience but deduced from it. They are conditions or qualities that are mentally endowed with existence in themselves.

Grammatical distinctions cannot be considered apart from the process of thought. But, before discussing thought, we wish to group ideas according to their *kinds*, or origins, irrespective of grammatical specializations. For this purpose we should view them all as nominatives, or nouns. But it is really impossible to carry this limitation rigidly into effect, and at least two grammatical distinctions—those of the adjective and the verb—insist upon intruding themselves into a fundamental survey of origins.

The difficulty of our task will be lessened if we attempt it on evolutionary lines—that is to say, if we endeavour to put ourselves in the place of an infant, and follow the earliest of its experiences in feeling and sensation. With the very beginning of consciousness, it would become aware of its own existence, as a *continuity*—that is to say, of its personality. Amongst its first objective ideas would be that of resistance to touch. This is in fact one of *substance*, to be broken up by individualization into *objects* possessing various qualities. It would at the same time be impressed by activities of movement and sound—whether its own or in the world outside it. Its subjective existence would appear to be a procession of transient conditions such as those of hunger, pleasure, pain, joy and fear. It would gradually isolate the *qualities* of things—and amongst them its subjective feelings as qualifying itself—and would arrive at ideas of *quantity* by comparing different things in size. The passage of its feelings, and the movements and sounds that are perceived through its senses, are *changes* which present *time* as a succession of intervals between them. Its movements of exploration would reveal to it *spaces* between things and their relative positions. Time and space are both conditions of relationship, since they do not exist except as intervals between two points. Other simple conditions of relationship, such as *likeness*, would present themselves. And throughout this process of mental growth, it would be constantly making new connections between itself and conditions of activity, of feeling, of relationship, of quality and of quantity by *ascribing* them to itself ; and would make like connections between these conditions and the things that were the subject of its observation and thought.

These primitive experiences enable us to classify our ideas as those (1) of personality ; (2) of objects ; (3) of objective activities ; (4) of conditions of subjective existence ; (5) of qualities ; (6) of quantities ; (7) of conditions of relationship ; and (8) of ascriptions. To these we must add a ninth class—of abstract ideas—a later and more refined development. The origin and character of abstract ideas have already been traced. We will now pass in review the other eight classes.

(1) *Personality.*—This is expressed by the personal pronouns. The first and third of them express self and particular personalities which are not self but are created by associatively investing others

with conditions such as our own. The second expresses a person-ality which is in communication with us as we are with our " other self "—which is, in fact, substituted for our other self. In moments of self-admiration or self-reproach we commonly think of ourselves as " you ". But the personality of one who is in communication with self can always be expressed by a title—" Your Excellency " for instance, and, since this is more respectful than direct address, mankind has devoted an immense amount of ingenuity to the elaboration of indirect means of indicating the second person.

(2) *Objects.*—In this class are included ideas of things which possess substance, or qualities of shape that are associated with substance. These ideas differ from recollections only in that they are generalized —that they are ideas of kind, not of particulars. All of them are complexes or " idea-combines ", for there must always be an idea of some quality that has been combined with that of substance by sensory experiences. The quality may be of origin and outcome, purpose or function, as well as a possession. " Father " is mean-ingless without the idea of a son, and *vice versa*. The idea of a piano involves one of its use. Emblems and symbols have a meaning because of their " implications ". In the emblem this is connected with the object by an analogy : an anchor *resembles* hope in that they both " hold fast ". In the symbol—the national flag, for instance—the connection between the two is artificial. But, quite apart from these implications, ideas of objects include a vast number of sensory qualities that are combined in relationship to form their character. Our idea of a motor-car, for example, is a combine of extreme complexity. Places are conceived as objects because they are marked by objects. A town, for instance, is marked by its houses.

Creations of the imagination are objects, because, although they only exist in the mind, they are fabricated out of sensory ideas and possess shape. Hence a fairy, although actually unsubstantial, is still " objective ".

(3) *Objective activities.*—Our movements and utterances are sharply distinguished from our feelings. For they are perceived through the senses—not directly by consciousness. This is also the case with the movements and utterances of others. But these differ in character from our own in that they are *manifestative,* whereas our own movements and utterances are *expressive.* But both are objective as opposed to subjective. They are individualized as activities and expressed by such substantives as *step, blow, deed, sound, voice, word.* Activities may be exceedingly complicated. They include a football match, a compliment, poetry and music.

They pass into the class of objects, if they are given a material form —if they are acted, painted or printed. But they remain peculiar in that, as manifestations, they convey the meanings of what they express. It is by this association that the behaviour and speech of others are *significant*. In themselves they are merely sights and sounds. But they are identified with similar activities of our own, and re-stimulate ideas of the bodily and mental conditions which accompany them in ourselves.

In this class also fall all our ideas of *manifestations* of natural forces—of the movements of things, of growth and development, weather changes, thunder and lightning, rainbows and sunsets, and the varied manifestations—as of gravity, chemistry and electricity— that constitute objective science. They are all that we can actually perceive of the forces that surround us ; and we construe them, exactly as we construe the words of another, by " reading into them " forces that are in fact derived from our own—as, for instance, the " pull " of gravity, the " force " of explosion, the " energy " of movement, and the " attractions " and " repulsions " of electricity. Objectively, the movement of a thing presents itself as a succession of changes of position, whether we are ourselves carried along by it or observe it from outside. We perceive nothing of the energy that lies behind it.

(4) *Conditions of subjective existence.*—Our subjective life' is a drama of inclinations, antagonisms, efforts and emotions, which are individualized as *conditions*, and are expressed as substantives by such words as love, pride, pleasure, harmony and power. They are the *causes* of our activities. We invest others with them by asso- ciating ideas of them with our impressions of the behaviour and speech of others. We " understand " the natural world around us in precisely the same fashion—by attributing to it conditions such as we ourselves possess. Indeed, we speak of the weather in the same terms as of our feelings. Our idea of movement as the ener- getic overcoming of *inertia*, not as a mere changing of place, is drawn, subjectively, from ourselves. Our views of Nature are then, and must be, fundamentally anthropomorphic, although the results of scientific experiments are constantly limiting and correcting the application of our own feelings to the inanimate world.

Our personality is a combination or succession of these subjective conditions and they may consequently be figured as *qualities* of personality. Anger, for instance, *qualifies* for the time one who is affected by it, and can, therefore, be given an attributive form in *angry*, and its possession can be individualized as *angriness*. So again with such conditions as those of *beauty* and *use*, which are subjective in that they involve harmony. They assume an attributive implication in *beautiful* and *useful*, and are individualized as possessionships in *beautifulness* and *usefulness*.

(5) *Qualities.*—We ordinarily think of a " quality " as an attribute that is apprehended objectively by the senses. The isolation of a quality from the thing that posesses it is a mental process, and has of course no foundation in reality. Accordingly, ideas of qualities always include an implication of *attachment*, save in the cases when they are etherealized into abstracts. The primary idea of an objective quality is that of an attributive (or adjective). From this are developed ideas of individual existence—with an implication of possession—and of the condition of possessing the quality, as in *solid, solidity, solidness*. The course of development differs, then, from that of ideas of subjective qualities, in which, owing to their emotional influence, conceptions of individual existence force themselves to the front, so that an idea of individuality is formed before that of an attributive, as in *courage, courageous*. But in the case of qualities which involve harmony as well as sensory apprehension, the objective and the subjective may be confused. The idea of *use* takes its primary form as a noun, that of *justice* as an adjective.

Qualities apprehended by the senses may be distinguished as actual, consequential, potential or proportional. Of the first kind are such attributes as *rough, yellow, shrill :* of the second kind those that are the consequences of sensation, such as the *good*, the *just*, the *decent*. The third class comprises qualities that are expressed by adjectives ending in *able* or *ible*, signifying potential attributes. The fourth includes the qualities which vary in intensity, such as those of size, length, value, rapidity and age. An idea of these involves comparison with a normal. A " large " dog is one that is " large for a dog ". To each idea of kind is attached an idea of a normal amount of intensity with which the amount or intensity of a particular object or action is compared.

(6) *Quantities.*—An amount or an intensity can be *estimated* by comparison either with another amount or intensity, or with a normal. Arithmetical *measurement* commences when the standard of comparison is an artificial unit of amount or intensity, that is to say, of quantity. A new kind of individuality comes into existence, that of quantity as a unit, or units, of quality. A pound of bread is a pound's *weight* of bread.

The unit standards by which we compute quantities are conceived by accepting the intensities of amounts of certain definite objects as formal bases of comparison—as the pace, the foot, or the first joint of the thumb for the measurement of length, the weight or capacity of some well-known object or utensil for the measurement of weight and volume.   This could easily be multiplied by repetition. It was subdivided by being cut up into equal portions, which, being equal, could be added together by counting.   They are counted by being assembled progressively into groups, each of which contains one more unit than its predecessor—a process that is suggested by various groupings of the fingers.   The number V signifies a group of five represented by the fingers of one hand.   The Roman numerals were based upon this idea.   But a number may also represent an *interval* in numerical sequence, and in this case " five " is the name of the fifth interval in a series.   Used in this sense " five miles " is five *times* a mile.   This interpretation of number was impossible until the cypher, or zero (from the Arabic *sifr*) was introduced to represent the beginning of the first interval.   The two methods of counting are often confused, and we think of two intervals as including three numbers.

Arithmetical measurement and computation rest, therefore, upon the *equality* of subdivisions—that is to say, upon their rhythmic character, for rhythm is a procession of equal intervals.   We could hardly have obtained an idea of rhythm from the world outside us. Science holds that the ultimate conditions of our environment are probably rhythmic.   But their rhythm is imperceptible, except in the case of very deep sounds.   There is rhythm in the alternation of day and night, in the tides and in the procession of the seasons, but the intervals are not precisely equal, and are too long to have suggested the graduation of a measure.   There is rhythm within us in the beating of the heart.   But this is hardly arresting enough to have been the origin of our idea of rhythmic intervals.   We are, however, obviously rhythmic in our method of progressing by steps, and it seems that we owe our strong appreciation of rhythm to this instinctive aptitude.   The most primitive of our measuring units— the foot and the pace—are obviously derived from it, and we still apply the word " foot " to the measurement of rhythmic speech. Rhythm is harmony in movement or in utterance—the harmony of a succession of intervals which are of equal length, or are sub-divisions of the same unit.   It is a remarkable fact that, in slow or " processional " marching, the number of paces which is taken is approximately 60 to the minute ; and it is more than likely that the subdivision of the hour into minutes and seconds (which we owe to the Babylonians)—starting with the idea that one-twelfth of the day at the equinox was a convenient unit of time—was suggested by the fact that during this interval progress at a slow march includes about 3,600 paces. The division of this number by its square root gives 60 minutes each of 60 seconds. That our measures of time are derived from stepping is all the more probable in that movement is the most obvious and the most satisfactory instrument for time-keeping. The duration of an interval can be estimated through a physical change : in the East the withering of a leaf or the burning of a cigar is sometimes used as a measure. But all modern time-keepers rest upon movement—that is to say, upon changes, not of physical character, but of position in space.

It may be observed that stepping offers a simple origin for the processes of multiplication and division. Five steps are multiplied by repeating the series over and over again : hence 25 is five times 5. Division is the contrary process : the series is " cut up " into equal portions. Having once realized the essential points that units of measurement must be equal, or rhythmic, " calculation " could be carried further by the manipulation of pebbles, each of which symbolized an equal unit. This method of computation survives in the *abacus*.

(7) *Conditions of relationship.*—We have seen that a relationship is a link between two ideas that have been combined (or associated) by experience, or drawn together through intelligence. Experience connects them in coincidence or in succession : intelligence connects them through sameness. Relationship in itself is, there-fore, simply the effect of coincidence, succession or sameness in mentally connecting two things—that is to say, in enabling an idea of one of them to re-stimulate an idea of the other. But there is good reason, as has been shown, to believe that these mental con-nections correspond with actual connections in the world outside us and within us. The consequence of a relationship is a condition, or phase, of relationship, in which the linking is combined with the ideas that are linked. But one or both of these things may be implied—that is to say, may be represented by a blank " something." Conditions of relationship can, therefore, be individualized in themselves, as in such ideas as those of *qualification, succession, causality, origin, position in place or time, identification, correlation* and *measurement*.

Accordingly, in reviewing our ideas of conditions of relationship we must sharply distinguish between (A) those of simple combination or succession in experience, and (B) those which are intelligently isolated through comparison. In each of these classes there are several sub-classes.

A. Conditions of combination (or association).—The relationships from which these conditions proceed may be intrinsic or extrinsic : they may have the effect of *compacting* a complex idea by binding its elements together, or of *amplifying* it by attaching elements from outside. It may be observed that, in assuming these intrinsic and extrinsic phases, the combining power of associative re-stimulation curiously resembles the force which shows itself as " coherence " in compacting matter, and as " gravity " in drawing one mass to another. The essential qualities which form an idea of " kind ", and enter into the ideas of an instrument or a symbol, are *compacted :* accidental qualities are *attached* to it. But the one process passes into the other, as is shown by changes of phraseology. A man " of gentle birth " becomes a " gentleman ".

The combinations with which we are now concerned are extrinsic, and the elements which they attach are signified by words or syllables. These additions affect the character of ideas by amplifying them, or by connecting them with ideas of origin or outcome, object, purpose, instrument or method, or position in place or time. The combination may be expressed by such descriptives as adjectives, participles, the possessive and demonstrative pronouns and adverbs, or by the use of prepositions. We can say " with red hair " or " in a rage " as well as " red-haired " or " enraged ".

Amplifying combinations.—An idea is amplified by the attachment to it of a quality in coincidence. This is signified by a descriptive attribute—*round* or *good*, for instance. But the amplification may also be effected by the intermediary influence of an idea of power, possession or " having ". That is to say, with our tendency to regard all activity as resulting from will-power, we invest things with this capacity and figure them as using it to hold their qualities together. So we speak of a tree as " having " brown foliage, and even of " having " a place on our lawn. Using possession as an intermediary, a man may be qualified by his possessions ; a rich man is qualified by his wealth as a tall man is by his height. And the thing possessed is also qualified by its owner ; so we use possessive pronouns to qualify things descriptively.

The relationship between a quality and its possessor may also be signified by the possessive case, or by the use of the preposition *of.* This signifies " off " one thing in the direction of another, and expresses very neatly the " two-faced " character of a link. It can consequently be used to express the connection between a dress and its colour, or between the colour and the dress.

Combination with origin or outcome.—A father is qualified by his

son, and a son by his father ; a consequence by its cause, a box by
its material, and all of them *vice versa*. These combinations differ
from those which we have been considering in that they originate
from consecutive, not coincident, experiences. They are connections in time. But since, as we shall see, thought is a succession
of coincidences, all relationships of succession present themselves
spatially and are expressed in terms of space. The preposition *of*
signifies a direction in space, and can, therefore, be used to express
combination in succession, as in a " man of good birth ", the " heat
of friction ". But succession may also be expressed by a descriptive,
as in " a well-born man ".

Combinations with object, purpose, instrument and manner.—An
action is qualified by its object. This is expressed by the accusative
(accausative) case, since the object of an action is also its cause.
It determines at the same time its *direction*, and hence the accusative
is used to express the objective of a movement, as in *Romam*. Purpose is combined with motive, in terms of spatial direction, by the
preposition *to*. Qualifications of instrument and manner are also
attached by spatial prepositions—*by* and *in*. But the latter are
most commonly signified by adverbs. These include terms of
space and time—such as *there* and *then*—because in certain circumstances connections in space and time become manners of action.

Combinations with space and time.—Our conceptions of space and
time are of such far-reaching importance as to require separate
consideration at a later stage, and we will limit attention at present
to the conditions of relationship in combination to which they give
rise.

We must, first of all, safeguard ourselves against a misconception.
We habitually think of space and time in terms of measurement.
But their measurement is an accomplishment of comparatively recent
date, and has no bearing upon their existence. A distance or a
period exists quite independently of miles or hours.

Our experiences of space are of places, directions and distances
which are marked by things ; our experiences of time are of points,
successions and periods which are marked by *changes*—that is to say,
by events or occurrences. Space is one, and its intervals, or distances, persist ; for we can go over them again and again. Time is
multiple and its intervals can never be recaptured. Growth and
movement are successions in time, as well as day and night, life
and death, and the revolution of a clock. Space is a series of coincidences ; time a series of successions. Space and time are then
of the nature of contraries. Yet we use spatial relationships to

signify relationships in time—such as *after*, *in* and *at*, for example. For thoughts (like sensations) present themselves as a series of coincidences which can be conveniently expressed in terms of space.

Combinations with elements of space.—We know of space through movement. This leads us to objects which mark *places ;* and it tells us that an object may lie in various *directions* from other objects and from ourselves, and that objects may be together or at different *distances* from one another. Coincidence with a place is expressed by " at " ; the conjunction of one thing and another by " with " ; direction by such prepositions as " above ", " under ", " before ". The preposition " by " is curious in its varied applications. It seems to mean " next in succession to," as in " by the way." Slightly changed in form, it enters into combination as *beside* and *between*, and is even used in *because*, to mark the antecedent of a succession. " Because he was ill " means " next in succession to his illness as a cause ". Direction is expressed by words, such as " to " and " from," which are also used to give spatial expression to successions in time. Distance is vaguely described as " near " and " far ". The demonstrative pronouns are ideas of distance related to blanks.

Spatial relationships include those of shape. This is fundamentally a series of relationships of direction and distance between different points on a surface, that are primarily detected by moving the fingers over it.

Combinations with elements of time.—As space is revealed to us by movement, so time is revealed to us by change. In conditions of absolute unchangeableness, time would not exist. For it is created by changes that occur in succession with intervals between them. Each change, considered in itself, is an occurrence or event. There are innumerable changes occurring in us and around us, each in a series of its own. Movement is a succession of changes and is, therefore, timed. It is, then, possible to compare one series with another, and *coincidence* in time is always between two events in different series of happenings—such as, for instance, between tea-time and 5 o'clock. *Succession* in time may be either between two events in the same series, or between two events in different series.

The relation of an event to a point, or a period of time, is generally expressed as a coincidence between it and a point or period in a different series of changes. It cannot be timed in this fashion unless the series with which the comparison is made is a fairly regular, or rhythmic, alternation of changes and intervals that can be used as a standard of measurement. Nature offers us such standards in the rising and setting of the sun and the procession of the seasons, and we use them when we speak of " rising at dawn," " resting during the afternoon," or " starting next spring." But these standards are inexact, and are insufficiently sub-divided, and man has been pressed to devise artificial sequences to serve as standards of measurements. Such are the grouping of days into weeks, months and years and the regular movements of a clock. There is measured coincidence between points of time when lunch is " on Monday next " or " at 1 o'clock "—between periods, when one lasts " half an hour ".

One event may succeed another in the same series of changes (as " from sunrise to sunset ") or in different series, as when an occurrence is timed as " before sunset " or " after 5 o'clock ". By the use of prepositions that indicate spatial direction, these successions are expressed as coincidences.

B. Conditions of comparison.—Ideas are drawn into comparison by a sameness between the two which causes one to restimulate the other. The comparison gives rise to conditions of comparison which vary of course with the nature of things that are compared. There is a radical difference between conditions of combination and those of comparison. The former present themselves as ideas in combination—" rainy weather," for instance. The latter are *consequential* conditions of identity and contrariety, of resemblance and difference, of harmony and discord, of correlation, and of intensity and degree.

Identity and contrariety.—It is a little difficult to realize that two ideas may be, in fact, the same. Yet it is obvious that a recollection contains the same elements as the sensation which it repeats, and that an idea does not lose its identity if it is restimulated several times over. The identification of two ideas eludes consciousness because one is merged in the other. But it can be detected by inference. The recognition of an object must involve the identification of the sensation of it with a recollection, since we should otherwise be unable to know that it possesses a number of its properties which do not impress the senses. And in our speech we admit that identification does occur. " Yes " means that a thought or motive in mind is identical with it as expressed in a question ; and the relative pronouns, adverbs and conjunctions have the effect of identifying something in particular with something indefinite in the preceding sentence. They are " ideas related in blank identificatively ". The interrogatives put things indefinitely to be identified definitely in the answer to them.

Identification is involved in the *substitution* of one thing for another. The former represents the latter as a Member of Parliament represents his constituency. It is through identification in purpose that most instruments were invented ; they are substitutes for manual processes. Musical instruments are substitutes for the voice. And it is by identification in birth, nationality or interests that we think of others as our fellows in kind.

A relationship of identity is involved in measurement. What we measure is not a thing but a quality which it possesses—as of length, size or value—with which the measure of the quality is identified. When we speak of a " yard of cloth " we mean a length of cloth which is identical with a yard.

The contrary of an idea is its *replica* reversed, and contraries tend, therefore, to recall one another in thought. The reversal is commonly signified by the prefix *dis*. " Dissatisfied " is the contrary of " satisfied ", as $-x$ is the contrary of $+x$. It differs from the negative " unsatisfied " as owing five pounds differs from lacking five pounds. The mental processes by which ideas are contrarified and ascriptions negatived will be touched upon hereafter. Voluntary contrarification is, of course, one of the principal instruments of Algebra.

Resemblance and difference.—Things that are compared are assimilated by their identities, differentiated by their peculiarities. They are " like " one another if assimilation outweighs differentiation : unlike one another in the contrary case. Analogy arises from a sameness that underlies a difference. It may draw two ideas together that are really very distinct—such as, for instance, the " running " of an animal and that of water. It is through a relationship of difference that a change is distinguished from—that is to say, contrasted with—that which preceded it.

Harmony and discord.—These are the effects upon consciousness of certain kinds of resemblances and differences between two sensations or feelings. We experience them sensorily when certain colours and sounds present themselves together and thus are compared. They are harmonious if they are similar in some fundamental respects—as for instance, in the rhythm of their vibrations. There is harmony in movement when it is rhythmic—that is to say when its major intervals are equal. But our most poignant experiences of harmony and discord are in our subjective feelings.

When two ideas, which are combined by experience, are in harmonious relationship with one another the condition of harmony between them takes mental form in some of the most important of our relative concepts. The attainment of success is harmony between intention and accomplishment; usefulness is harmony between an instrument and a purpose. The quality of justice is a harmony of goodness or badness between conduct and its consequences in reward and punishment, that of truth a harmony between words and experiences, that of freedom (in one of its senses) a harmony between desire and occasion. The right is a harmony between action and intention or obligation; that hand is called the " right " which is the most effective; a right angle is one which enables a thing to stand " upright ".

Correlation.—Contrariety acts like identity in drawing different things into comparison. Through comparison we appreciate the correlation between father and son, cause and consequence, origin and outcome. Each is the contrary of the other, and each accordingly suggests the other.

There is correlation between an active and a passive condition— between beating and being beaten. If one person overcomes another, the latter is overcome. Power implies subjection or constraint; superiority suggests inferiority, an implication which, as we have seen, most masterfully affects the course of our feelings. The value (valour) of a thing is its power of overcoming another thing. It is *measured* in terms of the things which it overcomes. But its existence is independent of its measurement.

Correlative conditions of great importance are those of obligation, duty, and necessity. An obligation is subjection to a claim that is enforced by a penalty of some sort, be it only that of self-reproach. It becomes a duty if it is in pursuance of a general rule of conduct. Necessity is a condition of being constrained by the force of circumstances. If the constraint is relaxed, necessity becomes potentiality or permissibility. These conditions are used to qualify the conditions that are expressed by verbs, in the form of the auxiliaries *ought, must, can* and *may.*

A ratio (or relationship of proportion) between two numbers or quantities is a correlative. For a fraction is the contrary of a multiple.

Intensity and degree.—These are comparative relationships of qualities. There is such a condition between two qualities when one is used to indicate the intensity of the other. This is the process called " comparison " in grammar. The excess or deficit of intensity, or amount, is expressed in terms of more or less, qualified by such adverbs as " much " and " very much ". A similar condition of relationship comes into play when a quality is appraised by comparison with a normal : a " slow " train is one which travels slower than usual. Appraisement gains immensely in accuracy when a graduated scale of measurement is employed as the basis of comparison. Each of its degrees represents a certain intensity or amount of a particular quality, which is identified with the quality under measurement. Degrees when computed in number gives definite *amounts*.

There is that between two quantities or numbers—the *proportion* of one to the other—which is unaffected by their multiplication or division and is therefore independent of magnitude. This is the comparative relationship of *ratio*, the principal instrument of mathematics. It is curious that it should be signified by a Latin word which means " reason ". We reason through relationships, and it may be that the word originally signified the condition of relationship in general. It has now been appropriated to a particular phase of relationship.

Conditions of comparative combination.—It will have been observed that relationships of combination and comparison may work together in the formation of ideas. The idea of justice, for instance, involves the combination in succession of ideas of conduct and of retribution, their comparsion, and the formation of an idea of a kind of harmony. But the most distinctive products of this dual process are our ideas of the comprehensiveness or generality of the possession of a particular quality or attribute, or of the regularity of a particular succession in time. Experience shows that the possession of a quality or condition may be more or less generally distributed ; its various distributions are compared, and ideas are formed of relative conditions of distribution. They are expressed by such words as " all ", " most ", " some ", " few ". The successions of experience are similarly compared with respect to their regularity, and from their comparison are deduced ideas of invariability, generality or rarity that are expressed by the adverbs " always ", " often ", " seldom ".

These deduced conditions of relationship play an essential part in the process of reasoning. For a conclusion is only certain when the law upon which it is based is universal, or invariable. As the law becomes less and less general in its application, the conclusion declines, through various shades of probability, into bare possibility.

(8) *Ascription.*—By an ascription a new relationship is established in the mind—a new associative, identificative or comparative connection between the subject of sensation or thought and a personality, a kind, an objective or subjective condition or quality,

L

a point of space or time, or a standard of comparison. This new relationship is a coincidence in present time. For thought, being evolved from sensation, resembles sensation in being a present experience of a series of coincidences. Whether we are thinking of the present, the past, or the future, our ascriptions, like sensations must be in present time. A recollection is, of course, a present experience although it relates to the past. In order to convert the past and the future from a consecutive to a coincident complexion we conceive of the past as something to which we look back, and of the future as something to which we look forward. That is to say, ascriptions assume past and future timings by presenting themselves as in backward or forward directions, whereas present ascriptions are " close-ups ".

Ascriptions need not be expressed in speech. They are commonly left to be understood in Arabic, and are unexpressed in such ungrammatical phrases of " pidgin " English as " he bad man ", " I going soon ". The grammatical instrument for their expression is the verb. " He was ill " means that he is connected in a backward direction with a condition of illness that is itself untimed ; " he ran " that he is connected, looking backwards, with a condition of running that is also untimed, for the ascription may take the form of " he was on the run ". It is, then, evident that the simple past tense (aorist) of a verb gives a backward signification, not to the condition that is ascribed, but to the ascription that it makes— a distinction which must be realized if we would understand the effect of using auxiliary verbs with participles to express past events. The expression of a forward, or future, ascription is more complicated. We use the " purposive " (commonly called the *infinitive*) form of the verb, omitting the preposition " to " and employing " shall " or " will ", since purpose is ordinarily the consequence of an obligation or of an effort of will. The condition of " going " may also be used to complete a future ascription, as in " I am going to speak ", since it indicates a forward intention. In the Romance languages a future ascription is indicated by the use of the condition of " having " with the verbal purposive, as in parler*ai*. But these methods of expressing the future are alike in that they time, not the conditions ascribed, but the ascription. A future event is ascribed as a present intention or purpose.

Our verbal tenses do not, then, time the conditions or qualities which their verbs signify, but indicate the direction in which their conditions are to be ascribed ; " spoke ", for instance, does not mean a past condition of speaking, but a condition of speaking that is ascribed backwards. In the verbal participles, however, conditions are themselves given backward, close-up, or forward aspects, and hence by the use of participles (or of verbal forms signifying *intention*), in association with auxiliary verbs, time can be thrown into the condition ascribed as well as into the ascription. " He has spoken " means that he is connected in the present with a " back " condition of speaking ; " he had spoken ", that he is connected in a backward direction with a " back " condition of speaking ; " he will have spoken " that he is connected in a forward direction with a " back " condition of speaking. We use the verb " having " as an ascriptive auxiliary with conditions that are in the past because the past can be figured as an experience that is " possessed " in recollection. And by the introduction of the auxiliaries *can, ought, must* and *may*, the ascription can be qualified as potential, obligatory, necessary, and permissible.

Accordingly, by the use of ideas of *direction*, thought contrives to express the changing successions of time in the guise of coincident happenings, that is to say, it represents time in terms of space, and this is one of the peculiarities which renders it so difficult to understand. It deals with ideas of movement in precisely the same fashion. When we think of another that " he is going to Paris " or " is going to make a mess of it ", we conceive him to be *in the direction* of these ends, and so give static expression to conditions that are in actual experience dynamic.

The substantive verb " to be " may be used to express the subjective condition of simple existence ; but it generally signifies the existence of an associative, identificative or comparative relationship between its subject and something, as in " I am unwell ", " I am in bed ", " I am he ", or " I am like him ". That is to say it signifies an ascription. Other verbs signify conditions, or qualities, which, being changeable, can be ascribed in past, present or future. These conditions or qualities are, for the most part, of the class which we have distinguished as objective activities and their passive contraries. But amongst them are conditions of mind, such as *thinking, hoping* and *feeling*—another illustration of the curious connection between thought and movement. Subjective conditions are represented by verbs when they are motives of practical activity, such as fearing, loving, admiring· But, when they are purely subjective, such as pleasure and displeasure, pride and shame or jealousy, verbs are not uncommonly lacking for them, and they are expressed as passive conditions of " being " or " feeling ", as " to be joyful ", " to feel proud ". To be expressed as a verb a condition must be transient. There is no verb for " being red ". But we can speak of " reddening ".

A transient condition is a *change*. It can hardly be individualized as an existence, and no such noun is developed from a verbal participle as *solidity* is from *solid*. A timed quality can only take an attributive or descriptive form. Verbal conditions may be individualized in themselves, (speaking) or as attached to a person (speaker). But in these cases they are untimed.

7 Time and Space

Amidst the doubts that arise as to the reality of our sensations, we may feel sure of the actuality of time and space, as, indeed, of all the links between things which we apprehend as relationships. Time is a succession of intervals between changes, space an extension of distances between places ; each is an " apartness " the one in succession, the other in coincidence. If changes were not separated by intervals, our sensations and feelings would not occur at different periods ; dinner would follow as nearly upon breakfast as lunch. If places were not separated by distances, we should touch the table immediately upon entering the room. Our ideas of the real character of our meals, of our houses and furniture may be misleading. But we must be right in feeling the apartness of changes in time, and of places in space. For these are relationships ; and unless we appreciated relationships correctly, life would be unliveable.

In analysing our concepts of time and space we must not understand them in their abstract meanings. For, as abstracts, they are hypothetical continuities that serve to complete ideas as to origins which experience leaves blank—not existences the actuality of which is demonstrated by experience. If we are to deal with them in a scientific, as opposed to a metaphysical, spirit, we must regard them as they are revealed by experience. Viewed in this light, time consists of points, marked by changes—in the present, the past, and the future—and of intervals between these points ; space consists of distances between places that are aligned in certain directions. Time is a series of successions ; space a series of coincidences. Time passes ; space persists. We cannot recover the past except in recollection. But we can traverse a particular distance over and over again, and find that it remains the same.

This reflection is not so fatuous as it may appear. For there is a tendency in modern thought to regard time as an element of space —that is to say, to regard succession as an element of coincidence. It is true that the succession of *movement* is involved in the *measurement* of space. But this is the only connection between them.

Time.—A point of time is a *happening*, that is to say, a change, which may, however, only be the occurrence of sound after silence (as in the ticking of a clock) or a change of place. A period of time is the interval between two particular changes—-a relationship of *transition* that connects one change with another. There could be neither points nor periods of time in conditions of changelessness and immobility. It may seem that, even so, time would continue to exist. But we are thinking, in this case, of *abstract* time, not of time as we know it. In the abstract, time presents itself as infinite. This is a purely metaphysical conception. But it gains some consistence from the fact that we cannot think of a rhythmic series to which a beat could not be added—or of a step which could not be repeated.

We are surrounded, so to speak, by the myriad-footed beat of a vast multitude of successions—some advancing in space, others " marking time "—stepping with even and uneven paces of varying length and rapidity. They are welded into a whole by the fact that those whose intervals are short, or whose pace is quick are periodically embraced by their longer or slower concurrents, as the events of a particular year are bracketted together by its completion. Time being the intervals that occur in a succession of changes (each of which is a point of time) it follows that each succession has a time of its own, and that there are as many kinds of time as there are kinds of changes. Changes may be subjective or objective—within us or outside us. Of the former class are those that occur in our motives and emotions, and render life a procession of various dispositions. Our movements are changes, and are, therefore, timed ; for every movement involves a change of place—that is to say, a change in space. Thought is the most changeful of all our subjective experiences ; but since its successions are chains of coincidences (and are therefore reversible) it gives us no idea of the passage of time. Indeed, when thinking or reading, one is almost isolated from time, and has very little consciousness of its current.

Objective changes are illustrated by successive sounds, and sounds and silences, by changes of light, as from day to darkness, by fluctuations in the weather and the tides, which impress us so greatly that in French the former, and in English the latter are identified with

" timing ". There is time in the growth and decay of plants and animals. And movement, as perceived in our environment, is timed, since it involves, like our own movements, a change of place. In the case of vibratory movement a change of place is immediately reversed. But it occurs nevertheless.

The estimation of time.—The duration of a period of time may be vaguely estimated by comparison with a normal, or by the number of changes that occur during its currency. We obviously use normals in judging durations, as when we think that a meal has lasted longer *than usual.* We can trace the origin of our ideas of normal periods to the process of associative re-stimulation—the most fundamental of our nervous capacities. When the duration of a particular experience, or set of experiences, has become fixed by habit or routine, an idea of a change from it—that is to say, of its end—is re-stimulated on the completion of its normal length. So we suddenly come to think that a sermon is longer than usual, or that a call has prolonged itself unduly. It is by this faculty that we are able to apprehend the regularity or irregularity of successive intervals—as in the beating of the heart. It is mysterious that an idea should be re-stimulated by the passage of a period ; but not more mysterious than that it should be re-stimulated by another idea, as in memory. The process is illustrated in physical life by the effect of changes of habit in altering the hours of appetite or fatigue. The intervals at which this periodic re-stimulation occurs may be fixed instinctively, and not by habit. There are certain physical affections that recur periodically. The curious migrations of birds are plainly stimulated by a periodic memorial urging. We are in fact concerned with a law of immense importance—the law which regulates the growth of living things, and reduces the conduct of most animals to a fixed periodic routine. Man has achieved some freedom of behaviour because in him the periods of re-stimulation are established by acquired, instead of inherited, habitudes.

It is, moreover, clear that this process of periodic re-stimulation is affected by the inclination of the moment, whether it be like or dislike. For, if an experience pleases us, no idea of its end presents itself even when its normal length is well past, and its period passes so quickly that we " had no idea of the time "—that is to say we had no normal in mind wherewith to compare it. On the other hand, if a routine experience is disliked, an idea of its termination presents itself prematurely, and throws us into the disagreeable condition of " waiting for " it. Its period, consequently, passes very slowly. We all know how time drags when we are waiting for a train.

We can also roughly estimate the duration of a period by the number of changes that occur in it. For this reason days that are full of incident seem longer than usual, and days that are uneventful pass rapidly.

The measurement of time.—The duration of a period can be measured if it can be compared with another succession. Thus we can measure the duration of a cricket match by the movement of the sun. When a succession is recurrent at equal intervals, it provides a unit of measurement. So the month is defined as a unit by the recurrence of the full moon, and the astronomical year by the alignment of the sun at midday with a particular star. A succession of such units is rhythmic. So again is the dropping of water, which offers a simple, if inaccurate, method of measuring time. Movement can be rendered rhythmic if the distance over which it passes is graduated, and the graduation of distance is, as we have seen, effected by the rhythmic steps of pacing. Movement is also rhythmic if it is vibratory. Hence time is measured at once by the dial hands of a watch and by the oscillations of its balance wheel.

Past, present and future time.—Time must be in past, present or future, since a change must either have occurred, be occurring, or be about to occur. We realize these phases through the process of associative re-stimulation, since this brings before us the antecedent and the consequent of every experience that has impressed itself on the memory. But since both *follow* the experience which re-stimulates them, the past, as well as the future, occurs to us in thought after the present ; they are, so far, similar, and the curious fact is explained that in Hindustani the same word is used to signify yesterday and to-morrow. A past occurrence is a future possibility.

Space.—Places in space are marked by things. But they are not identical with the particular things that mark them, for they persist when these things are changed. The distances between places are known to us through movement, or through inferences from associated experiences of sight and movement. We think that we owe our ideas of distance to sight. But this notion is plainly incorrect since the blind can appreciate distances with great nicety. Sight enables us to " judge distance ". This is because our movements, whether of touch or of progress, are accompanied by visual impressions of different perspectives, and the two become so intimately associated that, if perspective changes, we think that we are moving. So the changing scenes of a panorama produce an illusion of travelling, and the sight of a starting train alongside our own, gives us an impression that we ourselves have started. Our acquaintance with space is based upon movement. If we were fixed in immobility we should have no notion of it.

Accordingly movement is an instrument for discovering space. But space clearly exists irrespective of movement. For we can verify its persistence by touching two places simultaneously ; we can see that places do not disappear as we progress away from them, and we are assured of their endurance by receiving communications from others at a distance. There is, then, no reason to conclude that space is variable, as some modern theories would have us believe. We have no experience of infinitude in space, and the idea of it that is inherent in the abstract concept of " Space " cannot be relied upon. But we cannot conceive of a distance to which a fraction could not be added.

Space is measured by units of distance, which are obtained by movement over distances, as in stepping them. The process of applying these units involves time, and there is accordingly a ratio between measured time and distance (used in the measurement of velocity) through which distances can be measured in time—as involving, for instance, so many minutes or hours. These interconnections have led to an idea that time enters into the dimensions of space. But this notion confuses space with movement in measuring space. The two are, of course, quite distinct. Space is a " frame-work " in which movements and changes occur. To assert that space includes an element of time because there is an element of time in the instrument by which we measure it, is tantamount to maintaining that the area of a table is affected by the foot-rule by which, in successive (or *timed*) applications, we take its dimensions.

We may make a brief digression here to explain that movement must not be confused with *velocity*. For this is a *quality* of movement, and cannot exist without a movement that it qualifies. *As an abstract* it appears to have an independent measurable existence. But abstracts are not realities, and mathematical inferences that are based upon them may lead us astray. When two velocities are concurrent, one appears to affect the rate of the other. An ordinary train, for instance, seems to its passengers to lose pace if passed by an express. But this effect is only apparent, unless the two velocities are contributory, as when a bowler adds by his run to the velocity of his delivery, or a railway passenger increases or diminishes the rapidity of his progress by walking along the train corridor in or against the direction of its movement. Two non-contributory velocities do not affect one another except by complicating measurement. The velocity of a motor-car is not increased or diminished by meeting or passing another ; nor can the velocity of light be affected by the movement of the earth in turning towards or away from its source. If two objects in contrary movement collide, the force of impact is greater than if one of them was at a standstill. But this is an increase, not in velocity, but in the force generated by the discord between movement and resistance to movement.

Direction.—If, with closed eyes, we touch successively a number of things that are outspread before us, our arms align them in directions that are related to a point straight in front, exactly as the hands of a clock connect the dial figures with the line of mid-day. The front, back and sides of the body serve as four cardinal points which can be standardized by substituting the line of the north pole for that of the body-front. Touches that impinge upon the body are similarly aligned in the direction from which they come ; and when blind-folded, we know the direction in which we are moving by the relationship of each turn to the line of the body-front. Vision clarifies these impressions. The head can be swung like a theodolite, the *datum* line being that straight in front of us. The eyes are kept in plane by the semi-circular canals of the ear, which correspond exactly with the spirit-level of a theodolite. By moving the head we can only describe a semi-circle, and it is permissible to suppose that our ideas of direction would be more precise if we could turn it right round, as a bird can.

We have, so far, been considering our knowledge of places outside us. But we are also aware of the positions of the various parts of our own bodies, and of transient feelings, as of pain. It is impossible to conceive how this knowledge could be gained through unrelated consciousness of the body and its conditions, and it seems clear that we owe it to movements of touch. Our bodily feelings are closely associated with movements of touch, inasmuch as if we touch ourselves there is a feeling of *being touched*, and a feeling is commonly attended by a touch, as when one rubs a pain. Recollections of the two become so intimately associated as to be inseparable, as is the case with impressions of movement and perspective. It follows that pains could not be located without experiences of touch. Babies could not locate their pains : and this seems to be the case.

Spatial relationships.—Space includes concepts of surface, volume and shape. The principal surface is that upon which we live. An object which we can handle is bounded by a surface that runs into a continuous whole ; and, through analogies, we extend this conception to masses that are presented to us by vision. Their volume is determined by their height, length and breadth, which, when measured, become their *dimensions*. A vertical line is given by the upright position of the body : by extending the arms straight in front and at the sides we make lines of breadth and length.

Our idea of a *shape*, being derived from a tactile movement with the hands, is actually one of movement in a succession of different directions, each in relation to its predecessor. Shape is, then, a relationship of surface, just as " upon-ness " is a relationship of position. Shapes are reflected upon the retina of the eye, but with such continual changes that, apart from touch, we should have no idea of their permanence.

The abstract shapes of geometry are deduced and generalized from movements of our own. There is nothing in Nature to suggest a square or a triangle. The concept of a plane, apart from a tangible surface, is obviously formed by isolating flatness from a flat surface. But its character, as horizontal or inclined, appears to have been gathered from movements of the arms assisted by sight. For arms are horizontal if outstretched in front, and can be held at any inclination. A forward step followed by one sideways makes a *right angle*, which becomes a triangle if we return to our starting-point, and a square if we repeat the two steps backwards. In walking the hands make *parallel* movements with the feet. By swinging the arms we obtain ideas of *circles*, *curves* and *arches*. Accordingly the elements of the hypothetical space, with which geometry is concerned, are drawn from ourselves. Geometry has arisen from these crude experiences by the discovery of their various *qualities*, and by reasoning deductively from them.

8 The Process of Thinking

Thought appears so inscrutable because it is seemingly bound by no rules. But it is hardly more mysterious than the wireless transmission of electro-magnetic energy ; and since this can, in some measure, be reduced to law, there is no *prima facie* reason why the laws of thought should not be discoverable. But the search for them is exceedingly difficult. Consciousness reveals to us the thoughts of each moment, but cannot pause to analyse the processes by which one idea draws another into the current. As materialized in language, thought, it might seem, could be dissected. But words are not essentially a part of thought. We can think without words, as do beasts and birds, and we not infrequently have ideas in mind for which words are not immediately forthcoming and must be hunted for with an effort. Moreover, the verbal expression of a thought may elaborate it almost out of recognition. A thought which presents itself as " fine again to-morrow " may be expressed as : " We may safely assume that the present fine weather will continue over at least a further period of 24 hours ". It is indisputable that two currents of words may run in mind together—one colloquial, of word-ideas that are spontaneously recalled by the thoughts which present themselves—the other literary, of ideas of words and phrases that commend themselves as polished instruments for the expression of thoughts. The second current is connected with the first by substantial identities of meaning, as is clear when one thinks in one language and expresses himself in another. But this guidance leaves it much liberty of development, since words suggest one another through familiarity of association (as in *clichés*), or may be voluntarily recalled through their suitability in dignity, accent, alliteration or rhyme. So far it is true that we " think in words ". The literary current, being in accord with the artificial tendency of civilized evolution attracts more interest and attention than the " vulgar ". But, being artificial, it affords little indication of the actual current of the thoughts which originate it.

Spoken being less sophisticated than written language, more can be learnt by listening to conversation than by attempting to analyze cold print. But there are confusing complications. The course of thought baffles pursuit by oscillating, like a shuttle, between the past and the future. It is continually swayed by emotions, or feelings, that are stimulated by passing ideas and present themselves as such " thoughts " as *I think, I believe, I prefer*. And many of the links in the chain of ideas are disguised by being *unions*, in which one idea is covered by, or absorbed in, another by reason of its identity with it. The relative " who ", for instance, identifies the subject of an accessory sentence with something in the sentence preceding : the affirmative " yes " identifies the speaker's thought with that of another. It is so difficult to pick thought to pieces that very little progress has been made in analyzing it ; and there is a lack of familiar words to describe its processes.

In two respects the process of thought is extraordinarily anomalous. It is always in the present, although it may be concerned with the past or the future. And, although it may deal with successions in movement and in time, it represents them as a series of coincidences, each follower, so to speak, being simultaneous with its leader. " A long day's work ", " he worked all day ", " at last he went home ", are successions in qualification, in time and in movement. But they present themselves as a series of coincident ideas. These two peculiarities mark the evolution of thought from sensation. For sensation is always in the present ; and if we convert the process into a succession by turning our eyes, the new sensations which we receive are in coincidence with their predecessors. Recollections, it may seem, are in the past, not in the present. But they are indubitably *present* experiences, and represent the past because they refer to things that are placed in a backward direction from us. If we recollect that yesterday we met a friend, the meeting is in the past, because, although *present* in memory, we look *back* at it. We use the word " to have " as an auxiliary for the expression of past time because we seem to " possess " an experience through which we have passed and which can be recalled in recollection. The French use this verb to signify future time (as in j'aimer*ai*) because " having " may also mean the possession of an intention—that is to say, of a *direction*. For thoughts of movements, and of future events, are represented as lying in a forward direction ; and in this form they can be coincident with the present. A journey to London is not a succession, but a coincidence, if its movement is represented as a direction. The future can similarly be coincident with the present if it is figured as something to which we look forward. Hence we use the words " going to " and " will " (intention) to signify future time. It follows that thought deals with time and movement in terms of direction in space. And naturally, for sensation is spatial.

Many of our modes of expression, we have already noticed, are exceedingly ingenious contrivances for converting time into space. Origin and outcome, cause and effect, are successions in time. They are changed into coincidences by treating one of them as a *quality* of the other, using for this purpose the preposition *of*. A conclusion *follows* its reason : we express the reason as simultaneous with it by " because " (by cause) ," since " (looking back), or " for " (in front) ; the conclusion as simultaneous with its reason by " therefore " (thence onward).

Ascription.—In perception not only do we note the apparent or remembered attributes of the objects before us : we attach new attributes to certain of them by referring them to generalizations from experience. We conclude, for instance, that a thing is alive because it moves, and *movement is a sign of life*. This (it may be observed) involves the identification of the particular movement with the general movement which is a sign of life. In rational thought we may follow exactly the same process. Known attributes are used descriptively : new attributes are attached ascriptively by identifying the subject of thought with the subject or attribute of a general rule or law. Thus it is that for every ascription we can always find a " because ". When this law is immediately brought to mind by some quality of the subject, its use is so rapid as to evade detection. But when there is some difficulty in discovering a law, there arises a condition of doubt or hesitation ; we become conscious of the difficulty and can make shift to watch the process by which we endeavour to overcome it. We are successful if we can find a clue which will conduct us to a law. This involves an effort, and our conclusion takes the form of a " judgment ".

Accordingly, both perception and rational thought involve a series of more or less rapid identifications. Indeed, as we have already seen, we only " recognize " an object by identifying it with an idea of kind which we already possess. It is by identification that we connect an object of perception or a subject of thought with a general law that is within our knowledge. We speak of the process as if it was voluntary. In fact, it is the automatic consequence of the re-stimulation of one idea by another through a sameness. This is an intelligent, as opposed to a memorial, process. But it runs of itself unless action is interfered with by a like or dislike.

So far we have been referring to thought, which makes its ascriptions by the use of either experience or intelligence—the kind of thought to which the term " rational " is commonly applied. But thought may make its ascriptions by other means. When we think that we are hungry or tired we ascribe these conditions to ourselves, not as inferences from experience, but *intuitively*, because we feel that they are attached to us. They are " subjectively perceptive ", not reflective, ascriptions. Such thoughts as that " I like him ", " I believe ", " I will go out ", reveal conditions which are, in fact, qualities of ourselves. And, when thought is not of this perceptive or introspective kind, it may still be " irrational ". Its ascriptions may be the consequences of habit, of likes and dislikes, of prejudice, loyalty, or faith, of emotional hopes or fears, or of idealistic aspirations. That is to say, they may be inclinational, or emotional, instead of rational. If we ascribe to a mascot that it " certainly brings luck " it is because we hope that it will do so. Such are most of our thoughts upon politics. Our only *reason*, so called, is that we are attracted or repelled. A man may hold rational and emotional conclusions that are naturally contradictory. He may believe in " the struggle for life ", and at the same time in an All-merciful Providence. They can exist together because they affect different " sides of his nature ", the practical and the emotional.

We have already considered the technique—so to speak—of the process of ascription through the instrumentality of a verb ; but, since it is not easy to comprehend, we may revert to it. The difficulty is in recognizing that in using a simple verb in the past or future, it is the ascription, and not the ascribed condition, that is thrown backwards or forwards. It is obvious that in thinking " he was in town " the condition that is ascribed is timeless. But when we think " he went to town " we seem to ascribe a condition that is itself in the past, whereas actually we ascribe to him in a backwards direction a condition of activity that is itself untimed. " He slept " is precisely the same as " he was asleep ". But the word " asleep " contains no implications of past, present or future time. The Greeks appreciated the timelessness of the condition that is ascribed by a simple past tense and termed it " aoristic ". The simple future, as we have seen, similarily times an ascription by expressing it as a forward intention or purpose, which is itself in the present. Timing is imported into the condition ascribed as well as into the ascription, when a timed verbal participle, or a phrase signifying intention, is combined with an ascribing verb. " He is going ", " he was going ", indicate present and backward ascriptions of a present condition. " He has gone ", " he had gone ", " he will have gone ", connect him with a past condition of going, from a " close-up " point of view, looking backwards, and looking forwards respectively. The verb " to be " is used to impart a sense of continuity. " He has been going " means that he is connected with a continued past condition of going in the present. And since existence implies endurance, this verb can also be used to express a passive signification, as in " he has been beaten ". We have already referred to the implications of potentiality, necessity, obligation and permissibility that are introduced by the auxiliaries *can, must, ought* and *may.*

The process of ascription originates a new condition of relationship —a combination of a peculiar kind. For time as well as space enters into it. It is, of course, the essential element of a " sentence ".

Description.—To permit of the elaboration of a descriptive attribute it may be thrown into the form of an ancillary ascription. This is very commonly linked to the subject or attribute of the main ascription by a coincidence of identity—by a relative pronoun, or

conjunction, or the conjunction " as ". The link is one of combination in succession when the connective used is " that "—a
demonstrative conjunction which signifies " the following ". A
quality of purpose is elaborated by an ascription introduced by
" in order that " or " so that " : a connected cause, or reason, is
ascribed through " because ", " since ", or " for " : a consequence
or conclusion through an " accordingly ", " consequently ", or
" therefore ". When a consequence or conclusion that would
naturally suggest itself would be incorrect, it is contradicted by a
" but " or " nevertheless ", or the attribution from which it follows
is circumscribed by " although ".

An ascription of a thought or speech may be made imitatively (or
dramatically), as in " he said, I will go ". But it is more commonly
expressed descriptively (or according to the jargon of grammar,
" obliquely ") through an ancillary ascription introduced by " that ".
In this case the timing of the thought or speech must accord with
that of the condition which it elaborates : if this is in the past the
thought or speech will be in the past also, and to render this possible
" will " and " shall " are thrown into the past as " would " and
" should ". They are similarly transformed when the ancillary
ascription is of a conclusion that is based upon an impracticable or
unacceptable supposition. " I would go if I could " implies that
I shall not go. The going is excluded from question by being
thrown into the past—behind one, so to speak—and the conclusion
is, therefore, in the past also. A supposition, it may be added, is
commonly expressed in the subjunctive mood, unless its realization
is probable. If the supposition is quite impossible, the subjunctive
must be used, as in " if I were you ".

The course of thought.—The process of ascribing through a generalization, or rule, may, it appears, function automatically, for it will
continue during sleep. But it is normally driven by a motive, and
when this is lacking it declines into aimless reverie. The motive may
be that of inquisitiveness—the spontaneous curiosity of childhood.
We may be urged inclinatively by a like or dislike—the ordinary
motive of " gossipy " thought, which " savours ", so to speak, the
ideas that offer themselves, and in particular those that affect our
self-esteem, or are amusing. Our motive may be an ambition—
the desire of success, which can, of course, be obtained by discovery
of the new, as well as by securing the advantageous. If success be
aimed at through the teaching or influencing of others, thought takes
a demonstrative or persuasive line. It is emotional if it admiringly
appreciates what is excellent in persons, objects and qualities, or

if it takes an imaginative cast. But both appreciative and imaginative thought may come under the influence of the will, losing their
emotional character in the volitional. Whatever our motive be,
it endows thought with a *purpose* by which its course is directed along
a line that we describe as " to the point ". The purpose of a train
of thought acts, in fact, precisely as does an arresting sensation in
confining attention to itself to the exclusion of other impressions
that are assailing the senses. It prevents thought from wandering
off a certain track. But along this track it can progress only by
making use of leads that are spontaneously given to it under the
law of associative re-stimulation in the form of blank ideas, in
relationship to definite ideas, which can be filled up in detail.

By self-observation it is impossible to detect the " technique " of
thought—the process by which one idea brings forward another so
as to form a connected chain. For the current passes too rapidly
to be marked in detail by consciousness, and it involves lightning
identifications which elude us because their two elements become
united. It might appear that the methods of thought are contraries
of those of perception. In the latter we perceive qualities, conditions and activities and attach them to their subjects through
relationships. In thought relationships seem to initiate the linkings
which connect subjects with ideas of their qualities, conditions and
activities. But the relationships themselves are drawn into action
through indefinite, blank, ideas of " something " to which definite
ideas can be attached. It is obvious that all the ideas that are signified
by grammatical parts of speech, other than nouns, pronouns and
interjections, possess " implications "—that is to say, hold in
attachment—indefinite ideas of " something " that are linked to
them by a relationship. The articles, for instance, imply a blank
subject that they describe by number, or particularity. An adjective similarly implies an indefinite possessor of its quality, and, if it
is a comparative, it also implies a second " something " with which
the comparison is made. A verb implies an indefinite subject of its
condition or activity, and, if it is an active verb, also an indefinite
object. Some of these " related " ideas have, therefore, two blank
ideas attached to them. There is a further development. The
definite idea which causes these related implications may be one of
an isolated relationship. In this case it is signified by a preposition
or conjunction. These are generally related to two blank ideas.
" On ", for instance, implies that something is *on* something else :
" as " that something is the same as something else. But they may
be related to one blank only, as is the case with prepositions that

merely complete the meaning of a verb, as in " going out ", where " out " represents a condition of relationship to a vague direction.

Accordingly the idea of a quality, condition or relationship can be attached to a subject if the latter is identified with an indefinite, or blank, idea that is attached in relationship to the qualifying idea. To use a homely illustration, thought progresses through the filling up of blank cheques. If, for example, we are thinking of the weather, the adjective " good " or " bad " is attached by identifying the weather with the " something " that is qualificatively implied by one or other of these attributes. If we think " intuitively " that " I shall go out ", the idea of ourselves connects itself with a future condition of " going " by being identified with a blank something that is linked ascriptively to this condition as its subject, and this again completes itself by the combination of " going " with a blank that is carried by an idea of outside direction. Thought, therefore, proceeds through a series of identifications of definite with indefinite (or blank) ideas ; and since identification involves intelligence, those who are gifted with this faculty naturally think more rapidly than the stupid. Its course is, consequently, similar to that of perception. For this, as we have seen, involves the identification of an impression with a general recollection, which completes it by recalling qualities that are not perceivable by the senses. We appear to think through relationships because the preliminary identifications elude our observation.

Influence of the will.—The will may itself be a motive of thought. This is so when reflections are motived by ambition to achieve success, whether by exploration, by the attainment of expected advantages, or by the influencing of others It is, indeed, by the use of the will that we are able to deceive. In other cases it intrudes itself into spontaneous thought as the instrument for manifesting self-importance, impatience or ill-temper, or for overcoming a difficulty that causes doubt. We can contort the course of thought by filling up blanks self-assertively, instead of accepting the particulars that are offered by common sense—that is to say, by the use of generalizations from experience, or of intelligence. In this fashion we can think as defiantly, and absurdly, as we please. The will acts more sensibly when it assists us in cases of doubt in discovering what should be the particulars to be filled in. It may prompt us to ask a question of another or to make an experiment. It may also prompt us to search for a clue by a reasoning effort. This is a special use of our reasoning faculties. If no doubt " pulls us up ", reasoning thought pursues its course spontaneously. For " reasoning " in itself, is merely the use in thought of general ascriptions that have been established by experience or are dictated by intelligence, and thought naturally uses these ascriptions when it is unswayed by inclination, emotion, or self-assertive effort.

Negatives and contraries The processes of negativing and contrarifying are vital to thought. We negative by reversing the link that connects two ideas : we contrarify by reversing an idea. " He did not go " reverses the connection between him and the condition of going : " dissatisfied " or " disbelieving " are the contraries of " satisfied " and " believing "—and are far stronger than the negatives " unsatisfied " and " unbelieving ", differing from negatives as the owing of five pounds differs from simply not having them. This process of contrarification displays a close analogy with electrical conditions. The two phases of electricity—positive and negative— are contraries. We need not scruple to argue from this analogy, for it has been proved by experiment that a nervous current possesses decided electrical affinities. If, then, we assume that the process of thought involves the passage of an electrical current of some sort, and that the phase of this current can be reversed, the formation of negatives and contraries will be in some measure explained. We know from experience that the primitive cause of a negation is a feeling of repelledness or dislike : a child that is out of temper negatives everything ; and one of maturer years who dislikes an opinion not infrequently negatives it offhand and proceeds to argue " on the contrary ". It seems clear, then, that the " contrariness " of dislike influences the working of the brain by extending itself to the process of thought. Negativing evolves into a higher form when it proceeds, not from emotional dislike, but from the shock that is caused by a discord between an opinion and experience. So one would negative a suggestion that the weather follows the phases of the moon, since this is contradicted by experience. Negatives and contraries once formed are conserved as ideas by the words which express them, and can be used in thought exactly as if they were affirmative.

All conditions of relationship between two things are reversible *in their order*—that is to say, can be contrarified in direction. For a relationship that connects A with B, viewed from another direction, connects B with A. If stars are like eyes, eyes are like stars. If a buttercup possesses a golden colour, a golden colour is possessed by a buttercup. Hence an adjective may precede or follow its noun, and a relationship may be indicated either by a preposition or a case-ending. That A precedes B can be stated as that B follows A. These two phases may be generally described as active and passive.

They are correlatives, and the idea of one suggests the other. The reversability of relationships plays a most important part in the process of reasoning. For the relationship from which we argue can often only be connected with the point in doubt by being reversed. If, for instance, we are in doubt why it froze during the night, the relationship of a clear sky to a frost, as its antecedent or cause, must present itself reversed—as that of a frost to a clear sky, *as its consequence*, before it can link itself to the freezing which excited our doubt.

Reasoning.—This is the process of thinking through a relationship —or " ratio "—the relationship being the analogy which connects a point in mind with a generalized ascription—that is to say, a rule, law or axiom, as, for instance, when we think that bread will rise in price because wheat has risen in price and the *cost of one is dependent upon that of the other*. No such reasoning is required when an ascription is forced upon the mind by actual perception : such a thought as " I feel ill ", or " I think " is not *rational*. Nor is thought rational when its conclusions are based upon a like or dislike—that is to say, are opinions or beliefs.

The generalized ascriptions upon which reasoning depends are, in fact, " laws ", of the same kind as the " law of gravity ", although, it may be, of humbler reputation. They may have been established by past experience, which links itself to the experience that is before us ; or they may arise from samenesses or analogies that are evident to the intelligence. In the first case we argue *through* them, in the second *from* them. Experience is the basis of such proverbs as " birds of a feather flock together ", " a red sky at night is a shepherd's delight ", " a handful is a sample of an asses load " ; whereas the truth of " what is sauce for the goose is sauce for the gander ", " things that are equal to the same thing are equal to one another ", " twice two is four " rests upon samenesses that are recognized by the intelligence. We use a law of experience if we conclude that a man who is on his way to the station is going on a railway journey, since we know by experience that people generally go to the railway in order to take a train and past consequences are future contingencies : we argue from an intelligent law when we decide that we shall have breakfast earlier than usual in order to catch an early train, since the earlier we start the earlier we shall arrive. In both cases, it will be observed, we arrive at our decision by identifying an idea that is in mind with one or both of the ideas that are coupled together ascriptively by a law.

When the laws that dictate the ascriptions of thought are spontaneously recalled by the sensations or ideas of the moment, thought runs so rapidly and smoothly that we are unaware of their assistance. When they are recalled through the intermediate agency of a *clue* that has suggested itself, the clue enters into thought as a " because " —as when we think that the door must be open because we feel chilly. The *law* upon which this ascription is based is that a draught follows from an open door. But this hardly presents itself in consciousness. When, however, a law fails to present itself because a clue to it is lacking, the course of thought is checked by a doubt, and its character is changed. It becomes voluntary, or " effort-ful ", instead of spontaneous. For, as we have seen, an effort is stimulated by a discord, and doubt is discordant.

Every doubt that arises is as to the completion of a blank in an ascription. And, since every ascription consists of three terms— the subject, the attribute and the relationship that connects them— the doubt may be as to the particular idea which should complete a *blank* subject or attribute, or as to the existence of a relationship (that is to say, a coincidence, a succession or a sameness) between a *known* subject and attribute. It may be (A) as to the identity of an unknown thing which is in known relationship with another known thing or (B) as to the existence of a relationship between two known things—as, for instance (A) Why was it so cold last night ? or (B) Has he gone out ? In the first case we are in doubt as to the identity of a cause : in the second, as to the existence of a relationship between a certain person and a condition of going out. The indefinite can be particularized only by the assistance of two definites. Failing them, our resource must be guess-work. The idea of whose identity we are in doubt may be of many various kinds : it may be an individuality, a class, a condition, action, purpose or method, a quality or quantity, a point or interval in time or space, a cause (or origin) or a consequence (or outcome). The relationship of whose existence we are in doubt is an ascription of some sort the propriety of which is uncertain.

These two cases of doubt are recognized and distinguished by our methods of expressing them. Doubts as to the identity of a thing are expressed by sentences commencing with interrogative particles —" who " or " what " ? (of what individuality or class) ; why ? (from what cause or reason) ; how ? (in what manner or by what instrument) ; where ? (in what place) ; when ? ; how long ? ; how much ? Doubts as to the existence of a relationship are expressed by the use of the particle " whether ", or by reversing the order of the subject and the verb. (I doubt whether he knows ? **Does he** know ?).

A doubt of either kind is solved if we can discover a clue leading to a law with two terms of which the two known terms can be identified or assimilated—that is to say, in *case A*, the known subject, *or* attribute, and its relationship, and in *case B*, the known subject *and* attribute. The third term of the law will be that of which we are in search. A morning frost (*Case A*) is explained by experience if we have noticed that the preceding night was clear ; for *a frost follows a clear sky*. So if a bird, of whose kind we are in doubt, has a curved beak, it is recognized as being probably of the hawk kind, since, in experience, *birds with curved beaks are generally hawks*. If, again, we would know the cost of 3½ tons of coal, and the clue is a rate of 42/·, the amount is given by the " intelligent " law, 3½ x 42—£7 7s. Our doubt (case B) as to whether a friend has gone out or not, is solved if we notice, as our clue, that his hat is missing, since it is a law of experience that one who goes out takes his hat with him.

The effort that is involved in settling a doubt is, then, in the discovery of a clue. Its service in guiding us to a law is immensely facilitated by the fact that all laws are reversible, and, therefore, present two points of junction. Every activity can be reversed into a passivity. " A movement follows an effort " can take the form of " an effort is followed by a movement." The clue is discovered amongst things that are connected with the doubtful point, either in coincidence, or as its antecedents or consequences : or it may be suggested to the intelligence by a sameness. We identify a doubtful flower by discovering a quality which leads to a law. If someone has taken our umbrella, our clue to his identity is the fact that he who took it must have passed through the hall since it was last seen there. If we are in doubt whether we should go out in the rain, the *consequence* of rain in wetting us recalls the law that a wetting may be followed by a cold. If we would know whether a friend called during the morning or the afternoon, we have a clue if his card is below a letter that came by the mid-day post, since this calls to mind the law that the undermost is the earliest. In all these cases our law is one of experience. We use a law of intelligence when we settle the hour of starting for a train by using the distance of the station as a clue to the time which it will take to walk to it ; or when we identify electricity with an " energy " because it leads to movement, and, in regard to our own movement, there is a law which ascribes it to energy.

The fundamental reason for our conclusion is the law with which the point in doubt has been connected. The clue is also however, a " reason ", and it is generally the only reason that is expressed in language, since the law is so well known, or appreciated, that it is needless to quote it. We may express the clue-reason either before or after the conclusion : in the first case the conclusion that follows is introduced by a " therefore ", in the second case the clue-reason is introduced by a " because " or " since ". The latter order is the commonest, since the conclusion is the main point, the reason being only explanatory. In the terminology of formal Logic the law is the major and the clue the minor premiss.

The validity of laws.—If the law from which we are arguing is one of experience, its value depends upon its comprehensiveness or regularity. This is graduated by the experiences that establish it. If a quality is *invariably* possessed by a kind, the law gives it as possessed by " all " or " always " : if its possession is less general, it is graduated as being " sometimes ", " often ", " rarely ", etc. : if it is peculiar it is distinguished as " only ". When a law relates to an occurrence which precedes or follows another, the regularity of the succession is similarly graduated. The character of our conclusion, as certain, probable or possible, depends upon the graduation of the law that leads to it. The measure of one is that of the other. Our capacity for reasoning correctly from relationships of experience must, then, depend upon the breadth of our experience—that is to say, of our knowledge.

If we are reasoning from a sameness that is apprehended by intelligence, similar graduations affect the extent of its application. It may vary from complete identity to a distant analogy that affords but a slender foundation for extending the qualities, antecedents or consequences of one thing to another. Identities are the instruments of mathematics in defining and cancelling one term by another, in substituting one term for another and in contrarifying ; and, if the identities are real, and not merely assumed, inferences arrived at by these processes must be correct. Euclid's axioms *must* be true because their ascriptions repeat and are identical with, the meanings of their subjects.

Effort in forming conclusions.—A conclusion, or decision, follows inevitably from a law. Yet we are conscious of some effort in forming it, for it is the final phase of the struggle into which we are thrown by a doubt, and may be compared with the grip with which we take hold of an object for which we have been feeling in the dark. And a still stronger effort is felt if our conclusion involves a break with a past belief, opinion or habit of mind, or if it rejects the lead of reason in favour of such an established predisposition. We can discern signs of this conflict in the facial expression of one who has to sacrifice his prejudice to his reason, or his reason to his prejudice.

Inductive and deductive reasoning.—The use of a clue to discover a law renders our reasoning "inductive" : we are *led* to the law. We may proceed to argue from the law "deductively". If, for instance, we have decided that a friend whom we saw on the railway station road is probably going to Wembley (" because most excursionists are going there "), we may deduce as an antecedent that he had been given a day's holiday, and, as a consequence, that he would have lunch there—deductions which follow generalized ascriptions that have been established by experience. We are deductively extending a process which commenced inductively. But the reasoning which is ordinarily referred to as " deductive " starts with a law and draws conclusions from it. If the law is based upon general experience, or rests upon an identity which grips the intelligence, its conclusions are as reliable as those that may be formed inductively. Thus we may argue deductively, fairly enough, that, since things which are alike in essentials are alike in origin, willing and movement have evolved from the same source, because they both involve effort. But the laws used in deductive reasoning are commonly drawn from " the nature of things ", which is, in fact, hardly discoverable, and may lead in this case to very fallacious conclusions. We form " abstract " ideas, for instance, under the impulse of an idea that everything must be formed by a pre-existing material—an idea which is quite erroneous if " things " are, in fact, peculiar conditions that are produced by certain causes. By a similar process it is deduced that the world must have a Creator ; and one may proceed to argue that since there is evil in the world, and " evil is that evil does ", its Creator must be malignant. Again, if we start with the assumption that the immaterial is indestructible, we arrive deductively at the conclusion that the souls of all animals must be immortal.

Mathematical reasoning is deductive. But its laws are, as a rule, self-evidently true—that is to say, they rest upon samenesses that are not disputable or variable. The first four rules of arithmetic rest upon identities between two numbers and their added total, and between a number and its multiplied product, differing from it only in repetition. Subtraction and division are the contraries of addition and multiplication. Mathematical *reasoning* begins with the rule of three—that an unknown quantity can be discovered from a known quantity if the two are related to one another in the same relationship of proportion (or *ratio*) as that which connects two other given quantities, since the correlation of *ratio* is independent of magnitude. It follows, then, precisely the same course as the reasoning of everyday life.

Supposition.—We reason from supposition or hypothesis when we make use of a possibility (introduced by " if " or " unless ") in order to lead to an antecedent, or consequence, that will be a reason for a conclusion, or for conduct. A possibility may be of two very different kinds. It may be a *chance*—something which may occur by luck : or it may be an *effort*—an exercise of *power* which gives to the word " possibility " its original meaning. Such a thought as that " if it rains I shall not go " supposes a chance : the suppositions of Rudyard Kipling's *If* are all efforts of will. Possibility is a relationship of immense importance which constantly suggests itself, especially in conditions of doubt—as, for instance, " if I run I shall get hot ". But it is commonly employed in hunting for a clue to a law—as, for example, " if it has six legs, it is an insect ", and in this case leads to further observation, or to an experiment. It is also used in deducing an antecedent or consequence from a conclusion, as in " if democracy gives expression to a salutary ambition, it must promise better than the monarchies of the past, and the wider is the suffrage the better ".

Contrast and contradiction.—Our most useful safeguard against error in reasoning is the apprehension of illustrations, or parallel cases, which, introduced by a " but ", contradict the universality of our law—that is to say, are exceptions to it. They present themselves through samenesses, and their recall is a mark of instructed and unbiassed intelligence. Socrates would not have concluded that man is specially distinguished from the lower animals by his capacity for breeding all the year round if the thought of rabbits had occurred to him. Naturalists would not find a " protective law " in the colouring of some butterflies if they reflected that some of the commonest kinds are startlingly conspicuous. Politics must be a compromise inasmuch as the laws or " principles " which are its battle-cries can generally be invalidated by experience. Trades unions, for instance, have undoubtedly done much good ; but they are also harmful in deadening the individual energy which is the life-spring of industry. So disconcerting are contradictory illustrations to those who pin their faith to general laws as to have prompted the monstrous fallacy that " the exception proves the rule "—a saying the only sense of which is that if an " exception " occurs to us we must have had some rule in mind.

When two descriptions or ascriptions follow one another in succession, and the second is out of accord with the natural inference from the first, it is sharply contrasted with the natural inference, either by marking it as exceptional by *but* or *nevertheless*, or using *although* to circumscribe the bearings of its predecessor, as in " she was black but comely " or " although black she was comely ".

Grammar.—If our conclusions as to the technique of thought are true, they should explain the complexities of grammatical syntax. That this is so has been repeatedly illustrated in the foregoing pages, and a very brief review will now suffice.

All the grammatical " parts of speech ", except the nouns and the personal pronouns in their nominative cases, represent ideas that are furnished with " connecting-catches ". They are ideas related to a blank—or to two blanks—possessing either one or two blank attachments or implications, through which they can be linked into connection. This connection may be ascriptive or descriptive. The instrument of *ascription* is the verb—generally a highly complex " idea-combine " that is related in blank to an indefinite subject. Intransitive, neuter and reflexive verbs are " subjective " : active verbs are " objective ", and are related in blank to an object. In the passive form they are reversed. The so-called " impersonal " verbs may merely be devices for inverting a sentence so as to emphasize or amplify their subject. But in such a phrase as " it rains " there is real impersonality. For " it " signifies a cause of whose nature we are ignorant.

The remaining parts of speech are *descriptive*. Adjectives and verbal participles are ideas of qualities or conditions related to blanks. Adverbs are qualifications related to a blank that can be applied to conditions or qualities : they include attributes of place and time because these have the effect of qualifying a condition. The articles, demonstrative and possessive pronouns, describe a thing, respectively, as one of a class, as a " particular ", by its position or by its possessor. In the relative pronouns a blank relationship of identity is attached to a subject that is described by its gender or case. The interrogatives express doubts on various points that are similarly related in blank identity to something in particular. The distributives express degrees of comprehension in the distribution of an ascription throughout a group—concurrently (all, some) or successively (each, every). Akin to them are the adverbial distributives (always, often, sometimes) which define the comparative regularities of successions.

The prepositions and conjunctions carry two blank attachments, or implications. The former have already been discussed in some detail. Conjunctions are of two kinds according as they connect in combination or through identity. " And " conjoins in coincidence two subjects in description or ascription, or two qualities in attribution ; " that " links demonstratively in succession as " the following ". " Or " and " as " illustrate connection through identity—the former links two things together as mutually replaceable, the latter expresses *manner* related in blank identity to what precedes, so that it can be vulgarily employed as a relative pronoun. The relative conjunctions (*when*) are also of this kind. The hypothetical conjunctions *if* and *unless* put a suppositious condition either by " giving " it (*gif*), or by defining an intention as contingent upon not being " lessened " by something. The contrastive conjunctions *but* (" by-out ") and *nevertheless* (" at no time diminished ") specialize the second of two successive descriptions or ascriptions by signifying that it is exceptional : *although* and *albeit* produce a similar effect by invalidating the causality of its predecessor (" whatever be its strength "). These conjunctive expedients illustrate the vulgar but artful ingenuity which has taught us to express ourselves. The *particles* of a language are far more characteristic than the nouns and verbs which it borrows so freely from others. They are chips of mosaic that have come down to us from the long past.

Logic.—The mental processes which we have been describing may be difficult to understand for the reason that they conflict with preconceptions. But, in themselves, they are direct enough ; and their simplicity is in violent contrast with the fine-drawn complexities of the science of Logic. It is characteristic of evolution that it converts instruments into objects. Their usefulness enables them to attract admiration to themselves. We see this tendency illustrated in a hundred fashions. Language is an instrument : it becomes an object of literary cult. Government is an instrument : it is incessantly becoming complicated by formalities because its processes are so interesting that they stimulate a taste for " red tape ". In like fashion the various possibilities of deductive reasoning have been elaborated, with immense ingenuity, into an art. But to no practical purpose. Logic has hardly ventured to claim that its study has improved man's reasoning capacity.

The judging of evidence.—Doubts as to the value of particular evidence are solved, like other doubts, by using clues to connect the evidence with general laws. One of these laws is that statements should be suspected when they are in accord with a witness's interests, prejudices or beliefs, and that, on the other hand, they may generally be trusted when they run against these influences. Another law is that sensation is fallacious—and indeed this is not surprising when we reflect how little is supplied by sensation, and how much by thought in the process of perception. In ancient days the testimony of two witnesses was commonly accepted as proof positive. With broadening experience, testimony from perception and recollection carries less weight than good circumstantial evidence.

The effect of inclination and emotion upon reasoning.—Throughout this discussion we have been assuming that thought is free to follow its own lines. But this only seldom happens. The brain is the instrument of the body, and its processes are strongly affected by the likes and dislikes that are the fundamental impulses of our physical nature and gives a *practical* bent to our emotions. A sameness is not apprehended if it would lead to a conclusion that is disliked or would violate a like. We cannot, for instance, put ourselves in the place of an enemy and regard a situation with his eyes, or accept as a parallel case one which conflicts with our dignity. Such blindness to similarities completely distorts the course of reasoning, since every step involves the identification of the particular with the general. And even when the brain apprehends a sameness, and we cannot shut our eyes to the conclusion to which it leads, we may still feel that there is another point of view from which we should not be convinced. We may hold that reasoning is a less reliable guide than the predilections that we mistake for " intuitions ". Or we may think " in compartments ", accepting, in a rational mood, reasoned conclusions, and, when touched by inclination or emotions, the views that are forced upon us by our feelings.

Amongst the strongest of our likes are those which accompany the trustfulness of faith. We owe to them the emotional conclusions which we call " beliefs " and " opinions ". Our faith in another impels us to imitate him in a mental obedience which reasoning can hardly unsettle. Without faith the young would learn but little from their elders. It is the instrument by which knowledge is transmitted from one generation to another. It is the guardian of civilization ; but resembles a nurse that spoils her children. For it instils the false along with the true. And habit renders the one as ineradicable as the other. For habit is liked because it is familiar and, therefore, harmonious. Hence anything that conflicts with it has but a struggling chance of acceptance. It is through habit that mankind has been obsessed by the superstitions of magic and witchcraft, which would have been disproved immediately had the fancies that led to them been dispassionately compared with experience.

Particular likes and dislikes are dignified by the name of " pre-

judices ". They engender beliefs that can altogether incapacitate
us from reasoning. We are as blind to shortcomings that affect our
pride, whether individual, class or national, as we are to the merits
of those whom we dislike. We reject conclusions that are derogatory
to our self-esteem. The discovery of Copernicus that the earth
moves round the sun, appeared humiliating to mankind, and Sir
Thomas Browne, the accomplished and versatile author of the
Religio Medici, writing a century later, refers to it only " as Copernicus will have it ".[1] In our own days the idea that evolution applies
to man is still bitterly resented. Can God's noblest work be related
to the apes ? And, indeed, having regard to the sordidness and
indecency of life as it really is (amidst, be it said, very much that is
generous and refined), it is not surprising that we should close our
eyes to the truth. We must render it lip-service, for there is
humiliation in being contentedly deceived. But our practical
attitude is that of Clough's *Human Spirits* :

> We know not—what avails to know ?
> We know not—wherefore need we know ?
> *Dost thou not know that these things only seem ?*
> I know not, let me dream my dream.
> *Are dust and ashes fit to make a treasure ?*
> I know not, let me take my pleasure.

Truth is indeed so disconcerting that we not unnaturally prefer to
" make believe "—to *play*—until there comes at last the inevitable
hour of bed-time. Human progress would otherwise have been far
more rapid and continuous. For improvement is the fruit of
repentance, and this involves self-abasement.

9 Applications of Thought

In tracing out the processes of thought we have found the laby-
rinth of the subjective at its obscurest. There is still an angle to be
explored before we emerge into the daylight, and pass to the discussion of our objective activities. We have to consider the uses
to which thought is applied by our various motives.

As a spontaneous process, thought, as we have seen, progresses
rationally, making its ascriptions through generalizations that are
derived from experience, or are dictated by intelligence. In this
dispassionate form it may even function during sleep. If there is a

---

[1] *Religio Medici*, II., 14.

difficulty in finding a generalization, the will comes to its assistance. But its ascriptions may be distorted by inclination, volition, or emotion, if an idea arouses a prejudice, an ambition or an enthusiasm. The influence of these motives may, moreover, extend further. They may affect thought, not incidentally, but essentially. They may, so to speak, capture it and use it as an instrument for their purposes. That is to say, a course of thought may be dictated by an inclination, ambition or emotion. In this case thought becomes an " applied " activity. It is put into harness to serve a motive. But, as we well know, our motives may be " mixed ". We must not think of inclination, volition and emotion as separate streams with well-defined banks. They are currents in the river of life, that may send rills across into one another's paths. Emotional enthusiasm may find its way into thought which is primarily inclinational or volitional. And imaginative thought can become deliberately " clever ".

Thought is inclinational when it is of the kind commonly called " gossipy "—dignified in literary criticism as " human ". It " savours " ideas that stimulate like and dislike, as we savour our food ; and, in default of a better established term, we may call it " gustative ". It is distinguished from " appreciative " thought by its lack of emotional admiration. Thought becomes volitional when it is motived by ideas of success which re-stimulate effort' " ex-revulsively " in the form of persistent ambition. Success may be won in hundreds of different ways, which it is difficult to classify under heads that are mutually exclusive. But we may distinguish success that is achieved by discovering the truth, from that which is represented by the gain of an advantage, and this again from the success that is involved in dominating others. Volitional courses of thought may, then, be distinguished as *explorative, acquisitive* and *dominative*. Volitional thought, being purposeful, is always concerned with the future, whereas gustative thought is most characteristically occupied with the past. Thought is *appreciative* when it is inspired by admiration of persons, things or qualities : *imaginative* when admiration for qualities has the effect of creatively endowing them with a subjective personality or an objective appearance.

Gustative (or " gossipy ") thought.—As might be expected from their origin, thoughts of this description constitute the main-stream of our reflective life. We " savour " our own qualities when we think of ourselves. A man's whole heart may be in his work ; yet his thoughts will wander to the credit which it may be expected to bring him. Even our misfortunes afford us the pleasures of a dog that licks its wounds. We draw a like satisfaction from thinking over the circumstances of others. For our ideas of their conditions are derived from ourselves : they are " objective " only in that they are recalled by outward manifestations of behaviour or speech : in themselves they are " subjective ". Consequently, the fortunes and conduct of others always represent themselves as possibilities of our own. But gossip has many other attractions. It may afford us the " Lucretian " pleasure of feeling superior to those whose conditions are inferior to our own, and the revulsive self-satisfaction of resisting the shock that is given by suggestions of another's superiority. It is, consequently, inclined to be scandalous, since injurious impu- tations not merely give vent to dislike, but exalt, correlatively, our own respectability. It ministers to our insatiable curiosity as to the causes of things---our impulse to complete in detail ideas of ante- cedents that present themselves in blank—which (if the pun be excused) gives to gossip the character of a " causerie ". Disguise it as we may, there is an attraction in the indecent. And horrors of any kind make an extraordinary appeal to the interests of mankind. For they are all possibilities of self. There is, moreover, the amuse- ment which comes from passing shocks to habitual feelings and thoughts. Many and various are the sensibilities which anecdotes and scandal tickle.

So it comes that fiction is so popular, and that biographies are so much more interesting than essays and poetry. The chronicles of Pepys and Boswell have a perennial charm. We attribute it to the " human feeling " which they display. But this merely means that they stimulate a " gossipy " interest. For the same reason we are not content to accept an artist's work in itself, and to admire it. Literary criticism occupies itself with the discovery of every little detail of his private life, forgetting that genius has no connection with what is called " character ". For this implies self-repression in some form or other, whereas the artistic temperament must " let itself go ".

Explorative thought.—Curiosity arises as a spontaneous reaction against the shock of a doubt. In this elementary form its strength decreases with advancing years. A child is inquisitive about every- thing, the cause of which is not apparent. " Why ? " is always upon its lips ; and so disconcerting are its questions that it is customary to reprove them. This insatiable curiosity generally loses its per- vasiveness : it confines itself to certain interesting subjects, or may vanish altogether. Several causes probably contribute to this remarkable change of mentality. In the first place, nervous sensibility is at its acutest during childhood, and loses delicacy with age : a child's imagination, for instance, is so vivid as to keep it almost continuously in the world of " make believe ". Consequently, strange experiences give a shock which is immediately antagonized by an involuntary effort of " wonder ". Secondly, the explanations that are given us during childhood, however incorrect, serve at least to concatenate our ideas : a thunderstorm is explained if ascribed to the Almighty. And, thirdly, as we become more and more impressed with the future, we turn our eyes towards consequences and away from causes. It is consequences that are useful to us ; and we are content to ignore that which offers no hope of profit, unless it is in striking disaccord with past experience. It is then " mysteriously " stimulating, and impels us to assign it a cause in the mysterious.

Generally, however, the curiosity which may persist in later years is volitional, not spontaneous. It is a deliberate effort to win success by discovery, which, when habitual, is called the " spirit of enquiry ", Being deliberate—that is to say, actuated by an inclination which directs an effort of will—it is practical : it relies upon experience. and uses reasoning as its instrument. Of this kind is all scientific thought which can keep itself divorced from the influence of emotion. There is emotion if we pursue truth as an ideal. For an ideal is an aim which excites admiration. We may admire truth either for its harmony, or for its power in dissipating error. But a spirit of enquiry that is influenced by admiring emotion is apt to discard reason for " intuition "—to argue from abstract conceptions that have no basis in experience and lead to conclusions that are impressive but unsubstantial. Science is constantly tempted into metaphysical speculations of this sort. There is scientific as well as religious mysticism.

The spirit of deliberate enquiry may be prompted by a desire to obtain useful, or profitable, consequences, as well as by the simple ambition of discovering truth. In this case, however, it is not explorative, but acquisitive. Its object is not knowledge, but advantage.

Acquisitive thought.—Exploration conquers the unknown by discovering it ; acquisition the known by annexing it. The object of our desire need not be material : it may be distinction, popularity, or respect : we may even " acquire merit ". But the tendency of modern civilization is to rank material above " moral " success ; and hence the propensities called " acquisitive " are generally understood as urging us to amass material possessions, and as reaching their climax in " profiteering ".

They commence as a spontaneous, or " naïve ", desire to appropriate things that give pleasure in themselves, and are thrown away, like discarded toys, when they cease to be enjoyable or amusing. Desire passes into volition when possession is regarded as a means of adding to one's successful qualities—as, in fact, a symbolic guarantee of some form of success.   This is, of course, the main attraction of wealth, and its trappings in fine clothes, large houses, imposing equipages and costly furniture.   In very many cases these give their possessors no other pleasure than this—may indeed bore them—to be gladly thrown aside for the simple life, if this can be adopted without loss of dignity, as in travelling and sport. But they are prized because they are comforting, and enduring, assurances of achieved superiority.

Civilization, by proscribing violence but encouraging competition, has made the acquisition of wealth infinitely more complicated than in primitive times.   It generally involves exploitations or exchanges which depend for success upon a vast number of factors—possibilities that are constantly stimulating the deliberative faculties. The use of advertisement, for example, has become an instrument of success which must be seriously studied in the pursuit of wealth and distinction.   The practice of deliberation is prudence, and it is a truism that man becomes more prudent as he becomes more civilized. Prudence need not be material.   It may avoid the subjective penalty of shame as well as the objective penalty of a loss of money.   But, with the increasing materiality of our interests, prudence tends to become more objective.   It rejoices in the motto, " business is business ".   It is rational, for it follows the lessons of experience. It has conferred immense practical benefits upon society.   But it is dangerous, since it lessens the hold of ideal motives upon us. This is, however, a development which may be considered more conveniently when we are concerned with conduct.

We may, however, refer to two points.   Prudence is constantly occupied with the balancing of rival considerations, and as their clash involves a discord, it is of a serious, not joyful, complexion. Man owes to it his social and material progress.   But he pays for these advantages in a distinct loss of happiness.   And it is prudence which counsels man to deceive his fellows.   Spontaneous, or " heartfelt ", conduct is truthful, unless it is influenced by fear.   But deception may very often be a useful instrument of success : and prudence, if unchecked by idealism or by habit, may quite reasonably choose to employ it.

Our motives, as has been mentioned, are very frequently "mixed ", and acquisitive thought may take an emotional complexion. This is so when it is stimulated, not by reasoned expectations, but by hopes or fears. These are the incentives to speculation and gambling. And, *salvâ reverentiâ*, they enter very largely into the consolations that are offered by most religions.

Dominative thought.—To have power over others is obviously one of the most impressive phases of self-assertion. It may be desired for humanitarian reasons—to improve the material condition of our fellows, to impart knowledge to them or to teach them right beliefs and convictions. But it is also valued in itself—with no idea of benevolence—and the desire for it is one of the strongest of human impulses. To have power becomes a voluntary ambition when this presents itself as a gage of success.

Power may be obtained by violence. But this method is out of accord with the orderliness of peaceful civilization, and there has been substituted for it a more subtle, but not less effective, instrument—the influencing of the mind through ideas that are communicated by words. This process gives effect to an impulse which is primarily spontaneous. Man is ordinarily surrounded by companions. We may doubt whether, apart from his thoughts, he is a " social animal ", since he changes his companions very easily—sometimes, indeed, preferring dogs or horses to his own kind—and can live contentedly in solitude. He seems to have no *instinctive* preferences, and to owe it to the memorial and intelligent re-stimulation of ideas that he is disposed towards those who have become familiar, and those with whom he has any sameness of interest. But his mental life undoubtedly inclines him very strongly towards the society of his fellows, and he is very greatly concerned in influencing those who are about him He wishes to comfort and be comforted, to assist and be assisted : in influencing others, he has a means of satisfying self-assertion or of making money : if he is inspired by an ideal, he longs to convert others to it : antagonism may prompt him to argument, contradiction or insult. These are all means of success and become voluntary motives. Hence it comes that a very large proportion of our thoughts are concerned with speaking to, or writing for, others.

Our words may affect others by instructing, commanding, convincing, persuading, inspiring or amusing them. In instruction and command we use authority, and trust to faith for acceptance. In convincing, we use argument, reasoning about the known as if it was unknown : in persuading, we rely upon likes or dislikes that are pre-existing prejudices or are stimulated by our words. We depend upon enthusiasm to inspire others artistically or idealistically, that is to say, to communicate our own admiration to them. To amuse we give a slight shock that will stimulate a rebound of pleasure.

When we are concerned with instructing, commanding or convincing others, our thoughts are concentrated upon the knowledge that we mean to instil, the conduct upon which we insist, or the truth of our own convictions. We are not disturbed by any great desire to render our words palatable, although it must be admitted that scientific writers not infrequently endeavour to arouse admiration by appealing to the *grandeur* of their subject. When our object is to persuade, our reflections are much more complicated. For we have to take into account, not merely the merits of our case, but the inclinations, dislikes and prejudices of those whom we wish to influence. In teaching, ordering or demonstrating, we are concerned with things in themselves. In persuading we must rely upon their consequences in stimulating like or dislike, approval or disapproval. Accordingly persuasion involves the balancing of considerations— euphemistically termed " political " or " psychological "—which involve the use of the art vulgarly known as " humbug ". The art of advertisement is persuasive ; so are the inducements which are used in " propaganda ". It follows that in meditating over a speech, or an article, which is to persuade, the question is not so much of the truth of our position, as of the means of inducing others to accept it. A politician or journalist must, therefore, astutely realize the limitations of human nature, and understand the prejudices, hopes and fears upon which he must play to be successful.

He may, however, take another tone—may endeavour to persuade by inspiration—that is to say, by exciting admiration for an ideal. Provided that this is *strong*, it may be malevolent as well as benevolent, self-assertive or self-impressive, revengeful or merciful. An idealistic orator is generally more inspiring when he trusts to the enthusiasm of the moment rather than to the rhetorical force of prepared eloquence. And persuasiveness is, of course, immensely assisted by wit or humour. For those who are amused by another become disposed towards him and his opinions.

Appreciative thought.—Emotion, as we have seen, may enter incidentally into gustative, explorative and acquisitive thought. It is the essential element of appreciative thought ; and we are now concerned with emotion as contrasted with inclination and volition. The emotion is that aroused by any phase or quality of success or failure, harmony or disharmony, and may take the form of admiration, pity or disdain. The origin, stimuli, and effects of these feelings have already been discussed in Part II. But, in view of their revolutionary influence upon the disposition, some repetition and elaboration may be permitted. They determine what are called the " values " of life—that is to say, the objects and qualities which we hold in esteem. Some of these are variable : others constant. But in either case it is man's emotional attitude towards things which are not immediately concerned with the practical objects of life that raises him most distinctly above the lower animals. In strength many of them are his superiors : in skill the insects are more wonderful. But in his emotional aspirations man stands supreme.

As to the nature of these emotions, it suffices to repeat that they are generally re-stimulated " spiritual " *replicas* of the conditions of exhilaration and depression that are the instinctive and invariable accompaniments of success and failure in ourselves—to which a practical like or dislike is superadded by the physical element of our nature. Their effect upon us is very much greater than consciousness leads us to suppose. We may judge of its strength from the shouts of applause, the cries of execration that are evoked by objects of popular adoration and contempt—by the courage and loyalty that are inspired by admiration and pity. We so far recognize the *power* of admiration in that, under the name of " love ", we enthrone it above all other emotions.

Admiration produces two very remarkable effects upon us, one mental, the other emotional. It impels us mentally to decorate or " glorify " what we admire ; emotionally it causes us—quite involuntarily—to imitate the object of our admiration. It acts, in fact, upon our feelings like the flux that is employed in metal founding : it melts us into sympathy with its cause. Pity has a similar sympathetic effect. It is uncertain why admiration and pity should affect us in these fashions. But it is certain that they do so, and that their action is so regular that it can be generalized as a *law*.

The stimuli of these emotions may be qualities in themselves, or persons and objects (including ourselves) with whom these qualities are associated or combined. Actually a quality is inseparable from that to which it belongs. But, through the mental process of comparison, we isolate it from its possessor, and form an idea of it as a thing apart. And, since thoughts are *stimuli*, these ideas powerfully influence both feelings and behaviour. The sources of these ideas of qualities may be objective, subjective, or conditions of relationship. They are all phases or qualities of success, or of harmony. The former are exciting because success is at once a vital necessity and an instinctive stimulant : the latter because harmony appeals to one of our deepest natural sensibilities. Success is, indeed, itself a harmony between aim and achievement. Amongst its qualities are those of power and excellence. Beauty is a blend of the excellent, the harmonious and the pleasing.

We have already given some attention to these stimuli in treating of their emotional effects in Part II. We may amplify our description a little. First of *objective* qualities. There is power in muscular development, in agility, adroitness and skill, in elegance (for this is strength with economy of material) and in velocity—the charm of the horse and the motor-car. Eloquence is doubly powerful, for it is persuasive as well as skilful. It is successful to be popular, and to be esteemed by others. Age affords an implication of power, since, during the early years of life, power is associated with largeness of size and length of experience. Rank and authority are obviously powerful : we associate with them ideas of grandeur and majesty, and stand in awe of them if our admiration includes an element of fear. A thing has power if it possesses value, since this enables it to " overcome " other things in exchange. Wealth is power. There is an idea of success associated with the peculiar, eccentric or exclusive, since, by " standing out " from other persons or things, they are superior to them.

Harmony exists " objectively " in perception and in movement. There is harmony between colours and shapes that meet our eyes : also between sounds—whether in succession, as in melody, or in chorded coincidence—the artistic development of which is the technique of music. Harmony in movement is rhythm—the succession of intervals that are equal and regular, however much they may be subdivided—a charm which music has annexed, but is illustrated most fundamentally by the movements of dancing. But there is also " subjective " harmony that is not less admirable— that which may exist between two ideas in consecutive relationship, and gives their " inspiring " character to our concepts of justice, gratitude, and righteousness.

Beauty is so difficult to define because it is a complex of three elements : there must be an appeal to the senses, an element of excellence, and an element of harmony. Excellence depends upon the standard by which we measure, and since this is very largely artificial, ideas of what is excellent may vary greatly from one time and one people, to another. Indeed, we may come to regard as excellent what is merely grotesque, unless our standards of excellence are controlled by the limitation that they must fundamentally be based upon nature.

Secondly of *subjective* qualities. When ideas of these are admired they become "ideals". Our emotional dispositions clearly exhibit power and weakness, harmony and discord. There is power in self-assertive willing, and accordingly we admire such ideals as those of Self-determination, Liberty, Nationalism, Patriotism, and can hardly refuse admiration to Revenge. But there is also power in self-repression, whether carried to an extreme as Asceticism or as the motives of the virtues of Purity, Sobriety, Sincerity, Patience, Honesty and Humility. The Loving-kindness of broad-minded sympathy is admirable because it is harmonious : it is also powerful, for it is the cause of union, and union is strength. In Magnanimity self-control and sympathy join their forces, as illustrated by Forgiveness, Mercy, Tolerance, Loyalty and Generosity. Justice, and the Gratitude that manifests a sense of justice, are, as we have seen, admirable because they are harmonious. It is very remarkable that self-repressive and harmonious virtues, so defined by philosophic analysis, should be identical with those that were insisted upon by Christ.

Thirdly of *qualities of relationship*. By these are meant such qualities as those of the Good, the Just, the Right and the True. They are *accordances* between two things. A thing may be good from the personal, moral, or ideal point of view, according as it harmonizes with a like, with custom or convention,'or with a subjective quality that we admire. The just is a harmony between what precedes and follows ; the right a harmony between conduct and intention or obligation. A thing may be true or false according to a *reasoned* or a *visioned* standard. Reasoning, as we have seen, goes by experience and intelligence, and, judged by it, truth is that which accords with experience, or is endorsed by intelligence. By " vision " is meant an imaginative conviction that presents itself with a force transcending that of reason because it is admirable. These two forms of truth are poles apart. Religious beliefs, for example, are not endorsed by simple experience : we cannot infer from the course of worldly affairs that they are directed by an Authority who possesses the human attributes of justice and mercy. But the idea of such a directing power incites enthusiasm because it involves protective strength. Those to whom it seems to be transcendentally true will judge as false any allegation that conflicts with it. The inspiration that it affords counts for more than experience or intelligence.

The effects of fashion and of education.—There is a vast difference between the objective (or æsthetic) values of art, and the subjective values of idealism. The former are artificially acquired and may, therefore, change their objects : the latter are innate, and are consequently enduring. Æsthetic values must be *evolved :* idealistic values need only to be *intensified.* Our ideas of the beautiful are almost as changeable as fashions in dress. The present day is convinced of the beauty of mountain scenery : two centuries ago it was quite unappreciated. The advanced painting and music of the present day would have been scouted fifty years ago, and appears childish to those whose tastes were formed so far back. But the values of our emotions are unchangeable. Art which concerns itself with them, as the poems of Homer, can never lose its hold. Man has it in him to be ascetic and magnanimous as he has to be sensual and self-seeking ; and art which is purely " naturalistic " (as the pourtrayal of our lower impulses is called) is therefore imperfect. The perfect artist sees the idealistic side also. This is the difference between Anatole France and Thomas Hardy. It is to be added, however, that the influence of ethical ideals depends very greatly upon their intensification by education. But this adds nothing new to human character : it merely brings certain elements out into relief, as particular notes of an orchestra may be emphaized by resonators.

The effects of the admirable upon thought.—Such are the stimuli of appreciative thought. Whether we are thinking of these qualities in themselves, or of ourselves, other persons or objects, as possessing them, our reflections follow a " decorative " line : we magnify or glorify them by emphasising or exaggerating their qualities. On the other hand we vilify what we despise. Admiration for an ideal presses us not only to extol it, but also to think of spreading its cult to others. In regard to ourselves this tendency is naïvely illustrated by the boastfulness of self-conceit. If it is another person whom we admire, we think of enhancing his merits and of extending his influence : if it is a thing, we insist upon its excellencies. Our thoughts in all these cases are emotional, and, if they make use of reasoning, it is only for incidental purposes. Criticism of art and literature, when it extends beyond mere qualities of technique, is simply praise or blame, more or less appealingly expressed.

Appreciative thoughts, moreover, possess the quality that is called " sentimental ". This is given them by the involuntary—automatic —imitation of the admired object, be it a subjective feeling or a person. We are impelled to copy those whom we admire, in conduct, speech and even in dress. We also copy them in feeling. If we admire a virtue we shall experience it : it becomes a " heart-felt " as opposed to a voluntary motive. If we admire the courageous or victorious, we shall feel courageous or victorious : if we pity the unfortunate, we realize in ourselves the effects of misfortune. This admiring sympathy reaches its climax in love. When our interest in another is less real, our sympathies are less vivacious. But they are the very life of the charm which is exercised upon us by the drama and fiction.

Imaginative thought.—The imagination, by individualizing qualities, creates a world of its own. It is the most wonderful of human faculties. For it is so *unpractical,* and its existence is so discordant with the accepted law of evolution. It is of no assistance in the struggle for life : so far from adapting us to our environment, it creates an environment of its own—a fairy-land which transcends experience and does not conform to it—a world in which facts are supplemented by fancies. It is the ultimate source of Art. But this is a " grace ", not a necessity of life. The imagination seems to stand mysteriously outside the course of evolution—to be an inspiration, not a development.

But, in fact, imaginative sensibility can be traced to a very primitive phase in which it is plainly a very curious product of emotional excitement. Ghosts are imaginative creations : they are the products of fear. The visionary phantoms of ecstasy, the hallucinations of delirium, similarily spring from emotional exaltation or irritation, and it seems probable that dreams arise from " escapes " of emotion into the brain. Alcohol and drugs certainly beget illusions. In all these cases the mind runs a similar course. It generates " living " existences out of qualities—it constructs individuals out of attributes. It is, therefore, creative.

This creativeness shows itself in the artless play of children, understanding by " play " games that are imaginative and are not merely instruments (as is Blind Man's Buff for example) for the procuring of shocks of amusement. Play becomes Art when it is skilled : we recognize this evolution when we speak of an artist as " playing with his subject ", or of the theatre as the " playhouse ". The imagination, like our other conscious faculties, gradually changes its character as it comes more and more under the domination of the will—a tendency which is clear beyond doubt if we compare the impulsiveness of children with the deliberateness into which they grow. Imaginative ideas, whether playful or artistic, must be " executed ", and their execution requires the use of the will as an instrument. But, from this foothold, the will makes an annexing invasion. It becomes the motive energy of art instead of being merely its instrument.   Art, in fact, is born as an inspiration and grows into an ingenuity.

To begin with, we will consider it in the first of these phases. Imaginings are " playful " in childhood, and " inspired " in maturer years, when they are excited by the emotions of admiration or pity. The themes with which children play are those which they admire. The enthusiasm of the inspired artist is generally admiring :

> Tell me where is Fancy bred.
> It is engendered in the eyes
> With gazing fed.

Admiration, as we have seen, is also the stimulus of appreciative thought, and it is not always easy to distinguish between the appreciative and imaginative attitudes of mind : much poetry, for instance, voices praise unassisted by phantasy.   The two attitudes differ from one another in that appreciation shows its effect upon subjective feeling, whereas imagination stamps itself upon thought in the forms of objective sensation.   Consequently, while appreciation need not declare itself—for one may remain silent in the most ecstatic devotion—imagination must manifest itself in sensory form. The artist must express himself and cannot rest until he commences to do so.   His admiration moves him to imitate his mental creations, and since these have sensory forms, he must imitate them sensorily, or describe them in terms of sensation.   He wins success by using art—or skill—in his imitative expressions.   Hence execution is so vital to artistic spirit that we think of art rather as a dexterous activity than as a condition of mind.   Artistic execution is a phase of behaviour and will be touched upon in the next section.   But it, of course, implies that there is a current of imaginative thought in the background.

Artistic imagination, then, assimilates thought to sensation by individualizing qualities that excite admiration or pity.   This process will lose something of its mystery if we realize that in our ordinary life we only " perceive " the individuals and objects around us by mentally investing them with individuality.   Imagination extends to thought a process which is an ordinary accompaniment of sensation.   When the admired qualities are subjective—conditions, that is to say, of feeling as opposed to sensation—the effect of individualizing them is to " objectify " or " sensorify " them : a feeling becomes an individual which *illustrates* it.   When the qualities are objective, their individualization involves their being " subjectified " or *animated*.   Accordingly imaginings may be described as personifying either the subjective, through illustration, or the objective through animation.   A subjective quality, such as courage, becomes illustrated as Mars : an objective quality, such as the starriness of the sky, becomes animated as the myriad eyes of the night.   It is obviously easier to apprehend the objective than the subjective ; and children's play, therefore, generally animates the objective—either by representing objects or actions in lifelike fashion, or by investing with life things that are inanimate symbols. In " playing at horses ", lively expression is given to a number of objective qualities : a doll is a symbol of objective qualities to which life is given.   The artist draws his themes—that is to say, the qualities that inspire him—from both subjective and objective worlds.   In his *Blessed Damozel* Rossetti illustrates affection that can outlive death ; Hood's *Song of the Shirt* illustrates the pitifulness of sweated industry ; Gray's *Elegy* the peacefulness of evening and of death, and the feelings that arise from thoughts of them ; Browning's *Prospice* the strength of courage.   On the other hand, Keat's *Ode on a Grecian Urn* animates the decorations of a vase ; Shelley's *Cloud* and *Spirit of Night* animate beautiful natural features.   But the two modes can readily be combined, since illustrative figments of the imagination may be treated as objects and be animated with feelings and thoughts.   By such a combination the drama has evolved.   Painting and Sculpture may illustrate feeling, as when they deal with religious subjects ; when they pourtray actualities they are animative.   For a portrait or a landscape is inspired only if it is infused with human feeling.   So it shines " with a light that never was on sea or land ".

   In illustrating or animating a quality the imagining mind may be led by the intimate connection between cause and consequence. Thus Shelley fancied a wave as " panting " under the West Wind because panting is the cause of rising and falling.   Linkings of this kind are drawn from experience.   But the principal instruments of the imagination are analogies, or samenesses, that strike the intelligence.   Their use can be exemplified from almost every verse of poetry.   The resemblance between a flat plain and the sky suggested to Francis Thompson his " long savannahs of the blue " ; Swinburne writes of " the feet of the day and the feet of the night " because one advances and the other retires ; Rossetti could imagine the cadence of church bells to be an " echoing stair " between heaven and earth.   So children (may the comparison be excused !) when they " play at bears " go on all-fours.

   Imaginings, however inspired, or enthusiastic, are not artistic

unless they are skilfully expressed, and the element of skill introduces
a new complication.   For we may admire skill in execution quite
apart from the ideas that it executes.   An artist's skill is admirable
as well as the subject which inspires him, for his skill is a triumph.
It is won by voluntary effort, and since we can voluntarily make use
of any mental process of which we are conscious, we can subordinate
imagination to volition ; we can deliberately summon to mind
subjects that will inspire us, or even imagine in cold blood without
any inspiring motive.   If these imaginings are ingenious, and
are skilfully expressed, they will rank as art.   Much modern poetry
is of this ingenious type.   It may be clever, but it is not " convincing ", because it has no emotional foundation.   Painting
similarly tends to become a " tour de force " : its subject is an
opportunity rather than an inspiration.   The Saga, with its themes
of heroism, gives place to the story, with a purpose, not of elevating,
but of interesting.   So has developed the art of fiction.   It is so
popular because it amuses as well as excites, introducing an element
which would be as out of place in a heroic or romantic atmosphere
as laughter in church.   Accordingly modern fiction characteristically
appeals to those interests which we have termed " gustative "
rather than to admiring appreciation.   It may be violently
emotional.   But its object is to excite rather than to inspire.   There
are, of course, exceptions.   The " romantic " school centres its
fancies round an ideal of nobility.   But the interest of most popular
fiction is purely " gossipy ".

There is, of course, the strongest possible contrast between art
of this kind and that which is stimulated by enthusiastic admiration
or pity.   The one is practical, the other emotional.   How far was
imaginative *ingenuity* from Shelley's mind when he appealed to the
Skylark !

> Teach me half the gladness
> That thy brain must know ;
> Such harmonious madness
> From my lips would flow
> The world would listen then as I am listening now.

Emotional imagination resembles appreciation in producing
imitative sympathy with its subject.   This may occur even when
the subject is drawn from features of the material world, if the artist
animates them with human sentiments.   He sympathises with the
feeling that he imagines to exist, and attains the sentimental experience of being " one with Nature ".   So Francis Thompson could feel

> Heavy with the evening
> When she lit her glimmering tapers
> Round the day's dead sanctities.

And so Shelley experienced in himself the " fierceness " with which he imaginatively endowed the West Wind.

We have not referred here to dancing and music because these arts stand in a class apart. They are developments of expression, not of thought : they are not evolved through the action of emotion or volition upon ideas of qualities, but are elaborated from the movements and utterances by which emotion is manifested. They arouse admiration by their excellencies. And they also stimulate other emotions through auto-suggestive effects. But they are the products, not of feeling, but of its manifestative *consequences*.

10 The Influence of the Mind Upon Motives

Life without thought is spontaneous, or "instinctive", in its motives, and automatic (or "reflex") in its actions. This is illustrated, not only by the natural history of the humbler animals, but by the functioning of our own internal organs. Motives follow one another as they are stimulated, and each produces action that is appropriate to the occasion—and is fitted to it by inherited concatenations of nervous processes. Spontaneous, or instinctive, life has, however, two instruments at its command by means of which it can improve upon hereditary routine. It can respond to a difficulty, or discord, by an effort which, if successful, will automatically repeat itself upon a like occasion. So a mindless animal may *struggle* into success and acquire new reactions. And by unconscious imitation it can learn from others, although it cannot be consciously *taught* by them.

Thought introduces a new force into life by converting outcomes into origins. A thought or idea is the outcome of an experience. By presenting itself as a future possibility, it becomes the origin, or stimulus, of a similar, or analogous, experience. We order a fried sole, or purchase a theatre ticket, because we have pleasurable ideas of the consequences of these actions, which are either memorially derived from past experiences, or are linked to past experiences by analogies, or by the words of others. Being associated with certain actions, they re-stimulate them. Ideas may have this causal, re-stimulating effect when they differ very considerably from the recollections of any *particular* experiences that have been undergone. It suffices that they should represent an essential *quality* of an actual stimulus. An idea of power, or of superiority, for example, is as moving as one of success, since power and superiority are qualities of success. Hence desire and aversion can be stimulated by ideas of things which differ in many respects from things that have been actually experienced : fear by a thought of indefinite danger : anger by the imagination of a slight.

Our attitudes towards our fellows which seem to be " instinctive " are really the products of *mental* processes. Ideas of qualities are mentally associable with ideas of individuals : hence ideas of kindliness attach us to our relatives and friends ; ideas of identities stimulate class affections and fellowships ; and ideas of antagonism arouse rivalries and hatreds.

Thought entirely changes the character of the discord that stimulates effort. It is no longer an automatic conflict between an inclination and resistant emotion, as in spontaneous courage or anger. It is a clash between an inclination and *an idea*, as, for instance, between an impulse and the thought of its non-attainment, or of its ulterior consequences. It is this *mental* discord that gives rise to conscious efforts of will. Reflective, or willed, courage, for instance, arises from a discord between fear and ideas of pride or self-respect ; and it is a remarkable fact that it will enable a man to stand fast when spontaneous courage fails him. Mental discords of less poignancy—disharmonies between inclinations and their non-attainment—are continually stimulating us in this fashion. Consequently, as our inclinations expand, the will extends its influence.

In the same fashion curiosity comes into being as a *willed* reaction against doubt—not a mere clash between sensation and memory, but a deliberate endeavour to fit a new experience into a generalization from the past.

Through the re-stimulating effect of ideas, revulsive effort and emotion undergo a remarkable evolutionary change : they may be resuscitated without a preceding discord, as when ambition is optimistically kindled by an idea of success, or amusement is created by the repetition of a time-worn pleasantry.

And thought revolutionizes the basis of muscular activity. Actions are stimulated by ideas of them, instead of proceeding from instinctive concatenations of internal and external impulses.

Nevertheless, the motives and activities which are thus initiated by reflection revert into a phase which is almost as mechanical as that of instinctive life. Motives become habits : activities become automatic. So, having been introduced by thought to higher spheres of motive and activity, we adapt ourselves to these new conditions in a fashion that was stereotyped before reflection commenced.

It is a matter of common knowledge that deliberation—that is to say, prudence—gains upon spontaneity as one advances from childhood towards maturity, since thought restrains impulse by suggesting ideas of consequences. We see the same change in the development of a nation. As it advances in civilization a prudent materialism replaces the impulsiveness and romance of earlier days. It is, then, easy to draw an analogy between the mental development of a nation and that of an individual. But the causes are different. The growth of reflectiveness, which is natural in the individual, in the nation is artificial, and results from the education of the young. Prudence is instilled as the most reliable of virtues : and each rising generation is, therefore, exposed in increasing degree to an influence from which its less sophisticated predecessors were free.

But deliberation cannot annihilate the primitive spontaneous impulses of human nature. It can check them, and nothing more. We remain subject to a number of instincts which shepherd us towards the essential requirements of life. Courage and anger can " thoughtlessly " invigorate the most reflective of men. There are " unreasonable " likes and dislikes. And, below the surface of our refinements, unreflective instinct urges us imperiously to reproduce our species, and to provide ourselves, in some way or another, with food, drink and shelter.

PART IV

BEHAVIOUR

1 The Evolution of Conduct and Speech

We include under the term "behaviour" all man's external activities—the manners and methods of his speech as well as of his actions. Utterance, like action, involves muscular movement; and hence we can define "behaviour" scientifically as the various kinds of movement that are the consequences of motives. We are conscious of our own motives as we are of our movements. But the motives of others must be inferred from their movements. In respect to them we are under the same limitations as those which straiten our knowledge of ethereal forces—as of gravity and electricity. These disclose themselves only through the movements that they produce. We perceive the waves of radio-activity merely through the mechanical effects that they occasion in our receivers. There is, however, this great difference : Motives can be observed directly, and apart from their consequences, in ourselves. Else this book could not have been written.

Nervous energy must, it seems, find a material outlet. Its channel of escape may be that of secretion. But it generally vents itself in movement. That produced by feminine energy is *inclinational*—towards a stimulus or away from it. Masculine energy liberates itself *expressively*. The one is practical or purposeful : the other is emotional. But just as emotion intensifies inclination, so inclination directs emotion, leading into practical channels activities that are primarily manifestations of excitement.

The purposeful and the expressive.—It is, then. a law of evolution that the emotional tends to change into the practical—the romantic into the prudent. The fundamental difference between the two becomes obscured. The most striking exemplification of purposeful activity is the functioning of our internal organs. But purpose is also illustrated by the spontaneous, "tropistic", movements

of babyhood towards the favourable and away from the unfavourable. Expressive activity is illustrated as primitively by our
spontaneous manifestations of emotion—smiles and frowns, gestures
and ejaculations. In themselves they are objectless except as
an escape, although, when brought into harness by feminine
" practicality ", ejaculations have developed into language, and
changes of feature make the fortune of cinema stars. Behaviour
is purposeful, or practical, when it avoids the disagreeable, and
seeks the agreeable ; when it is actuated by fear, fellow-feeling,
courage or anger ; when it voluntarily seeks success through self-
assertion, or self-repression, or the many forms that ambition
can assume. It is expressive when it signifies pleasure or displeasure ; when it manifests our own dignity or self-abasement,
or gives expression to the feelings of admiration, reverence, faith,
contempt or pity that are aroused by other persons or things,
or by qualities. Art, in its various phases, expresses the imagined
by materializing it imitatively or descriptively. Idealism similarly
expresses the admirable in feeling by materializing it in conduct.
The social usages called " manners " are in great part expressive :
politeness expresses the disavowal of either a disdainful feeling of
superiority or a resentful feeling of inferiority. Similarly expressive
are the ceremonies which figure so largely in religious and political
life.

The expressive evolves into the purposeful when compliments are
used as instruments of persuasion. Self-control and idealism take a
practical form in the conventional morality which affects respectability or avoids punishment. Art becomes an instrument of
ambition, or a means of livelihood. Worship becomes purposeful
in prayer. Speech which begins in ejaculations and expletives
grows into a purposeful instrument for communicating with others.

The artificiality of behaviour.—In the simplest movements of the
arms and legs, as in feeling, grasping, rejecting, shrinking and pacing,
as well as in the various expressions of emotion, behaviour has an
instinctive, spontaneous or involuntary origin. But the methods
which are grafted upon these simple impulses are artificial. This
is a momentous difference between man and all the animals that are
inferior to him. They are born with tendencies, actual or potential,
which fetter their activities by confining them to certain definite
lines. A thrush must strengthen its nest with mud : a blackbird
cannot do so. Subject to certain seasonal variations (and in some
cases to imitative aptitudes) each kind of bird possesses a hereditary
" language " of its own. The language of man is simply that which

he has been taught.   Amongst the insects these innate concatenated
habits are extraordinarily rigid and precise.   There are possibilities
of change in successful efforts of venture, and in automatic imitation.
But these liberating capacities seem to be limited, or even atrophied,
by instinct, so that an insect is little more than a puppet controlled
by cords that are interwoven with its nature.   For if successful
actions are effortlessly linked to their stimuli, the avenues to
development are closed.   There is no discovery by efforts of
venture, and no winning of the exhilaration of success, with
its consequences in volition, ambition and the appreciative
emotions.   As the animal kingdom developed, the chains of
hereditary habit were gradually loosened, so that animals could
profit more and more by tentative experience and by example.
In man the chains were almost entirely cut away.   It is owing to
this that he, alone of all animals, exhibits such extraordinary
differences of manners, and that the human species can put forward,
at the same moment, the man of fashion and the cannibal.

It may be urged that we exaggerate the cramping influence of
heredity upon the habits of the lower animals.   For many of them
can be taught elaborate tricks—or to perform useful services—which
are quite out of accord with their natural behaviour.   Instincts,
as we have seen, can be varied by efforts of trial, and these may be
stimulated by the association of pain with failure or of pleasure with
achievement.   So a dog is taught to " sit up ".   But these accomplishments, being out of accord[1] with natural promptings, do not
afford the pleasure of pride : they may be compared in man with
artificial hair and teeth, which, however convenient, are not things
to boast about.   Hence a dog has no inducement to practise its
tricks or teach them to its young.   A child, on the other hand, does
not feel that its acquirements in manners, speaking and reading are
unnatural : it is proud of them, and has, therefore, an incentive
to practise them and display them to others.

We are, very naturally, proud of our civilization and are disposed
to think that it must have made some hereditary mark upon our
methods and manners.   This would, however, reverse the course
of evolution : it would limit man's freedom.   And, as a matter of
fact, there is nothing to show that a baby is born more sophisticated
in London than in Patagonia.   The children whom Darwin brought
home from Tierra del Fuego acquired under education the usual
habits of Europeans.   We cannot, of course, argue that a baby has
no instinctive potentialities because it does not exhibit them, for

[1] See on this point Köhler's *Mentality of Apes* (p. 70), Kegan Paul.

faculties that are undoubtedly hereditary may be delayed in development so as not to show themselves until long after birth. A newly-hatched cuckoo, for example, does not resemble the full-grown bird in its voice or its movements, although it ultimately develops the peculiarities of its kind in spite of being nurtured by hedge-sparrows. But a baby has no such clear-cut destiny before it. The language which it will speak is determined by its surroundings, and if these are dumb it will speak no language. It is clear, then, that the multitudinous languages of mankind are not hereditary dispositions, but accomplishments which are learnt after birth. The manners of different peoples are, of course, less discrepant than their languages. This may be taken to show that they are less artificial, and owe something to hereditary tendencies. The use of the hands for feeling, gripping, tearing and striking, and of the legs for the rhythmic movements of crawling and walking, seem to be instinctive—that is to say, determined by innate promptings which develop after birth. But in methods of detail there are striking differences between one people and another. Orientals, for instance, turn a screw counter-clock-wise, and show respect by uncovering the feet instead of the head. These are, however, simply the results of differences in education : it has been established by experience that an Indian foundling brought up in a European asylum perfectly acquires European manners. There may be innate differences of *character*. But˙ we are not at present concerned with them. The question is as to language and customs. If these were innate, man could not relapse into barbarism so rapidly as occurred on the break-up of the Roman Empire. There is, moreover, conclusive evidence that man's civilized habits—and even his upright carriage—are not inborn, but acquired—evidence that can be ignored only by refusing all belief to the many well-authenticated cases of children that have been carried off by she-wolves in infancy, and subsequently recovered. In India[1] three of such cases have occurred within the last thirty years and are testified to by reliable European observers. All agree that these unfortunates exhibited no trace of human manners : they ran on all-fours, and actually preferred the society of dogs to that of men. They were, moreover, unteachable, and never learnt to speak—not even one who was under the care of a Medical Mission at Agra from 1897 to 1903.

It seems, then, that man is able to civilize himself because there is so little in his hereditary disposition to reject any novelties that

---

[1] More detailed information regarding these " fairy tale " experiences will be found in the *Science of Ourselves* (p. 279).

suggest themselves tentatively or imitatively. His strength, in fact, lies in his nakedness.

Learning for oneself.—Every acquirement in action or utterance is the result of a nervous association which will bring the accomplishment into play when occasion for its exercise arises. These new associations may be established by involuntary experience, by accidentally successful efforts of venture, by the appreciation of analogies, and by imitation. *Involuntary experience* comes into play from the moment one is born. A baby's earliest movements are actuated by inherited habit. But every movement creates a series of associations that include an idea of it, and this idea can re-stimulate the movement. Of the involuntary re-stimulation of movements by ideas there can be no doubt : it is demonstrated conclusively by one who " talks to himself ". An idea of a *feeling* in itself cannot re-stimulate the feeling : we are not made angry by an idea of anger : our thought must include the idea of a *stimulus*. But, unless checked by the will, an idea of a movement re-stimulates the movement because, we may surmise, thought is intimately connected, through its origin, with movement. Again, by frequent simultaneous occurrence, certain impressions of sight become so closely associated with certain movements that the sight can guide the limbs automatically. When running upstairs we unconsciously and without effort adapt our steps to the winding of the staircase. And, by the same process, visioned things are invested with solidity and distance. A baby is constantly occupied in forming these visual and tactile associations by touching what it sees. So again, simultaneous impressions of sight and hearing are of immense importance, since they enable sounds to recall ideas of their causes and so pave the way to the use of spoken words as symbols. Thus barking, or its imitation, recalls the idea of a dog, and a scolding suggests the idea of another's crossness, or, it may be, of one's own naughtiness. A child's first words are imitations of sounds which have accompanied the objects, conditions or movements that it wishes to indicate.

Efforts of venture, as we have seen, are the result of conditions of discord, and are primitively expressive rather than purposeful. This is, indeed, the reason why they are capable of developing into the multiform phases of willing. But they may succeed. The material progress of mankind owes far more to accident than is generally realized : the greatest of all discoveries—the use of fire—must have been accidental. And was not gunpowder invented by mixing charcoal, nitre and sulphur " to see what would happen " ? An effort which wins success has a good chance of being remembered.

For success excites emotion, and this has a very striking effect in fixing events in the memory. A schoolboy who has been caned for a false quantity does not easily forget his error ; and, if we think of any such strong emotional experience as a declaration of love, or an anguished parting, it comes back to us, not alone, but set in an elaborate scene of unforgettable detail.

By the *appreciation of analogies*—that is to say, by inteligence— an effort which has proved successful on one occasion is repeated on a similar occasion. The greater the intelligence, the less close need be the resemblance between the two. Intelligence is not confined to man. A kitten obviously appreciates the resemblance between a drifting leaf and a mouse. But its appreciation of analogies is limited. A dog which has learnt by accident to push up a gate-latch can rarely apply its knowledge to the opening of other gates. A child has no such difficulty. Moreover, by intelligence, degrees of comparison are apprehended : a jump which has fallen short can be lengthened by the expenditure of greater energy. And by the use of analogies efforts of venture grow into considered experiments : in endeavouring to reach a fruit, one does not thoughtlessly jump at it, but tries to gain height by means which have been found effective in quite different connections.

The success of an effort stimulates one to practise it, and by practice the nerves which connect movements into actions become so intimately associated that each will re-stimulate its successor automatically. So actions that it needed effort to initiate, run of themselves in effortless continuity.

We commonly think of *imitation* as a voluntary process. But in its primitive phases it is involuntary—the re-stimulation of an activity by an idea of it that is recalled by seeing or hearing others. It is not voluntarily that we yawn when others are yawning, pick up tricks of manner from others, or are led by them into applauding indifferent performances. This spontaneous kind of imitation plays a part of immense importance in the self-education of a child. It is its first introduction to the manners of civilized life. Voluntary imitation is, as we shall see, the process by which we assimilate instruction. This leads us to a separate question—the transmission of knowledge by education. But, education apart, man has, by voluntary imitation, been able to profit by the example of the lower animals. He has, in savage or childish play, been delighted to mimic them. It seems probable that he learnt from them to climb and to swim, and he may be indebted to them for his first notions of moulding, weaving, house-building and even of singing. This possibility will not seem far-fetched if we recollect that in our own times aviation has admittedly been copied from the birds.

Learning from others.—Thus far of the artificialities that can be acquired by an individual unaided by instruction—the progress that could have been made by man in a state of uninstructed savagery. By instruction, the acquirements of each generation are transmitted to its successors ; the course of evolution is profoundly modified, since progress is rendered cumulative. We are instructed either by the teaching of another or by his example. In both cases we imitate. When we assimilate lessons we imitate memorial associations that are in the teacher's mind ; when we obey precepts we imitate in action the ideas of actions that are conveyed to us. And we obviously imitate another when we follow his example. So the speech, morality, feelings, knowledge and dexterities of one generation are handed on to another. Words are associated with things by persistent repetition under a mother's lead. Decency and " goodness " are learnt by associating, under pressure, certain acts or resistances with particular occasions. Feelings (or " prejudices ") are acquired by the attachment of ideas of certain stimulating qualities to ideas of particular personalities. An idea of power stimulates reverence ; of excellence, admiration ; of danger, fear ; of usefulness, like ; of harmfulness, dislike. So one learns to fear God, honour the King, to be afraid of snakes, to be kind to some animals and cruel to others. Knowledge associates certain individuas with particular ascriptions, as that the Roman occupation of England lasted three and a half centuries, and that the nettle is akin to the fig. The words of a teacher or writer extend these associations from his own mind to those who learn from him. Dexterities are similarly acquired by imitating the actions of another, as one studies a stroke at golf by watching a professional.

The ingraining of acquirements.—When these new associations are strengthened by practice, they become part and parcel of one's nervous equipment. It is difficult to realize that one does not " see " solidity, that such words as " jump " and " shriek " are imitative, and that one's beliefs and prejudices are not innate, and may be wrong. The instinctive " feel " of these artificial associations may be due in some measure to the fact that we remember nothing of the first three or four years of life, during which the process of acquiring them was established. No one, for instance, can remember learning to speak. The associated ideas and actions which constitute our habits run their course so smoothly that we are almost unconscious of them ; and we become quite unconscious of the complicated, rapid and accurate movements that form our dexterities. When a pianist plays from score, his fingers are, so to speak, electrified by his eyes. Yet he can achieve admirable *technique* whilst his thoughts are far away from the music.

Conduct and language.—To analyze behaviour in further detail we must divide our subject under two separate heads—the development of conduct, and the evolution of language. Conduct differs essentially from language in that, being derived in most part from movements that are instinctively, or innately, *purposeful*, it develops along more or less similar lines throughout all peoples of the world. There are minor differences. But these are of no moment compared with the astonishing heterogeneity of human language, which artificially divides mankind into groups that are for practical purposes almost as distinct as species. It is really amazing that creatures of the same kind should use such different utterances. This diversity arises from the fact that language is derived from manifestations of emotion which, being purposeless, are plastic.

2 The Development of Conduct

Phases of conduct.—We have already emphasized the distinction between the spontaneous, the deliberate and the habitual in conduct, showing that these three phases are stages of evolutionary progression, each of which is not entirely superseded by its successor, but continues to compete with it. And we have insisted upon the fundamental difference between purposeful and expressive conduct, which subsists in spite of the endeavour of purpose to convert all expression to practical ends. Evolution cannot obliterate a difference which springs from the fundamental duality of our nature. Purpose is the effect of the feminine ; emotion—and consequently emotional expression—the effect of the masculine element within us.

Methods of conduct.—Passive conditions such as those of feeling, perceiving and thinking are sometimes included in "conduct". But we are now dealing with *activities*—that is to say with movements. Amongst them are the rapid changes in the muscles of the throat, tongue, lips and face involved in speaking, singing and emotional expression. These will be noticed when we come to treat of language. Our present concern is with the muscular functions

of the arms and hands, legs and body.   The primitive uses of the
arms and hands are for feeling (or fingering), grasping, rejecting
(or throwing), shifting things, and placing them.   The actions of
eating, dressing, sewing and golfing merely involve dexterous
combinations of these movements.   We use our legs naturally for
walking, running, jumping, and dancing—adding the artificial
accomplishments of climbing, swimming and riding.   The body
muscles are generally involved in the actions of shrinking, pushing,
pulling and carrying.   The purposeful elaboration of these simple
movements into the complicated " businesses " of civilized life
commenced very generally in purposeless or expressive activities
that primarily only manifested emotion.   Take, for instance, the
manners that play so large a part in social life.   The pride of success
is accompanied by an involuntary bracing of the muscles—by a
strut—and accordingly we associate rigidity with a feeling of dignity ;
this evolves into stateliness of carriage, and the crook of the little
finger that is commonly held to dignify the lifting of a teacup.
The reaction from dignity occasions a muscular relaxation which
is at its maximum in the prostration of respect.   The passage of
this into forms of salutation strikingly illustrates the course of
evolution.   It is less irksome to lift earth to one's head than to level
oneself to its surface, and the Oriental salaam obviously expressed
this idea by a gesture which, modified in the interests of military
precision, became the soldier's salute.   Since dress manifests the
dignity of decoration, respect may be manifested by removing something of it, as the hat or the shoes.

A further cause of complication was the discovery of instruments
and processes which required special kinds of conduct for their use.
And conduct is, of course, also differentiated by the motives which
underlie it.   With this factor, however, we are not at present
concerned.

Judging from the anthropoid apes—the nearest of man's humble
relatives—there is nothing in human nature which prompts one to
make things.   But man is extraordinarily imitative in that he
can isolate the qualities of objects from the objects themselves,
and can, therefore, through a quality, make an imitation which,
to a lower intelligence, would not seem to be imitation at all.   There
is no real resemblance between a child's sand castle and the castle
of actuality.   It is very probable that man's first essays in " making " were playful imitations of natural objects.   Play, which
seems a mere pastime, is, then, an important step on the ladder of
evolution.   If the imitation possessed any utility, the practical side

of man's nature would at once take hold of it, and convert an expressive into a purposeful activity. *Working* would evolve in the same fashion. We can hardly assume that to work is instinctive with man. Children and savages are naturally indolent unless their imitative or imaginative capacities are aroused. It may seem that voluntary labour distinguishes man from all mammals except the beaver by a gulf which could never be bridged by reflective evolution. But, commencing in play, it would evolve into business by a prudent appreciation of its consequences. Man, however much civilized, works for the most part because he is pressed by self-interest, or led by habit. Idealism may urge him to work for the service of his fellows. But this is a motive of *expression*, and experience shows that it cannot maintain its ardour against the chilling effect of practical considerations. This is the argument against Socialism.

Another distinctive propensity of mankind is to *possess* things. We can trace its evolution if we realize that a thing which is possessed by a person becomes an artificial *quality* of his, and is appreciated by himself and others as natural qualities are appreciated. A necklace, for example, is a peculiar and admirable quality, just as a graceful neck, and enhances in the same way the attractiveness —and the dignity—of its possessor. Amongst the most notable impulses of savages is that of self decoration : they eagerly seize hold of anything peculiar—such as a top-hat, for instance—in complete unconsciousness of its absurdity. It gives an air (or quality) of distinction, and this suffices. In tattooing, a decorative quality is actually grafted on to the body. Possession becomes particularly attractive when it involves power over another. This was, no doubt, an inducement to the taming of animals and the capture of slaves. Possessions which were useful as well as decorative or distinctive would appeal to the purposeful side of human nature. They would be turned to useful purpose—and, their utility demonstrated, there would be a prudential motive to accumulate them. There was, then, an inducement to *hoard*, and the distinction declared itself between rich and poor. Hoarding involves transporting, and a new practical question presented itself for solution.

Building may very well have been initiated by analogies drawn from casual experiences of shelter from sun or rain. A hut provides imitatively the protection that is naturally offered by a cave or a tree. It may appear that the rudiments of *fighting* by blows, kicks or bites are innate in mankind. But it seems likely enough that these efforts are not originally purposeful, in the sense of revengeful, and merely externalize irritation against its causes. Their retaliatory success would, however, lead to their voluntary adoption ; and, since the most primitive times, man has endeavoured to improve upon them by experimenting with more effective means of causing injury or death.

Instruments.—Man has been defined as a " tool-using animal ". But there is no good reason for assuming that this capacity is innate. He may have discovered the use of some things—a sharp stone, for instance—by an effort of venture. But, having regard to the general course of evolution in other respects, it is probable that his first tools were playthings, which were perceived to offer practical advantages. The use of a stick would be discovered in play ; by an accidental improvement it would become a club. The idea of cutting would similarly arise from the manipulation of a sharp flint ; it gradually improved its material as man passed through the Stone, the Bronze and the Iron Ages. The bow uses the elasticity of the branches that one bends back in passing through a forest. The original pick-axe was a forked branch, or a deer's horn ; the primitive plough is a pick-axe drawn by animal instead of by human effort. It is not difficult to suppose that the drum and pipe were accidentally discovered in the course of playful manipulation.

If man (as appears to be certain) commenced his artificial evolution under tropical conditions, the potter's art could have been suggested by the usefulness of gourds. These could be imitated in plaited fibre smeared with clay. It is noticeable that the bases of primitive vessels are often rounded, not flattened, as would obviously be most convenient for standing them upright. So the flat surface of a leaf would suggest a fabric made by beating out glutinous fibres into a sheet—an expedient still practised in Polynesia. Weaving could have been learnt from the birds. A nest of crossed sticks remains compact ; and once it is realised that it is the quality of being crossed that keeps the sticks together, the quality could be applied to fibre. The instinctive industries of birds and insects surround man with an exhibition of skilful designs that have been perfected in the course of spontaneous evolution, and literally represent the wisdom of the ages.

Means of locomotion probably evolved from the slave-litter. It is more dignified to be carried than to walk. When animals had been domesticated, the use of their drawing and carrying powers would be suggested by obvious identities of quality. Riding is a comparatively recent accomplishment ; it was evidently unknown in Homer's time. The use of boats arose from the experience that wood floats in water. That man should have taken to the water is one of the most surprising of his artificial developments. It may have commenced in imitative play. Or we may discover in it evidence to show that his original habitat was a region which volcanic subsidence gradually changed to an inland archipelago. Such a change has actually occurred in the South Seas.

Dress.—There are tribes who still go naked and unashamed. But, generally, a sense of decency has prescribed the use of some covering for the body. From a means of concealment it has passed into an instrument of display. Its use is not essentially dependent upon climate. For men and women are as particular, and as fantastic, in " dressing themselves up " in Polynesia as in Paris. In hot, as in cold climates, the most primitive of ambitions is to mark one's superiority and distinction by decorating the body. As man migrated northwards, he felt the need of warm covering, and, by an easy analogy, he clothed himself in the coverings of the beasts that he killed. If dress only served this necessity it would have remained an easy *negligé*. But, in fact, there is hardly any discomfort too great, or unfitness too glaring, to be suffered, if it will confer a sense of dignity or distinction. The body itself is pressed to assist. It is trimmed—and even tortured—like an ornamental box-tree—by shaving and hair-dressing, painting, tattooing, circumcising, boring the ears, nostrils and lips, filing the teeth, flattening the skull, and cramping the feet. Civilization has freed us from the worst of these artificialities. It grasps the opportunities for winning distinction that is offered by variety, and delights in constantly changing the fashions of clothes.

Processes.—We live in a torrent of tremendous forces which our senses—very fortunately—are unable to perceive. We know of them only through their material consequences, and these are obviously quite different to the forces themselves. In some cases we can summon these energies to our assistance by material means ; we can, for instance, kindle fire and set up electrical conditions. But over the force of gravity and the course of the weather we have no control whatever. The material consequences of these forces conform to definite laws. That is to say they are " processes " of which we can take advantage. For instance, we utilize gravity in pouring out tea, although we are profoundly ignorant of what gravity is.

In agriculture and stock-raising we turn to account the living forces of reproduction and growth. The art of cultivating plants could have been discovered through the accidental germination of grain that had been collected for food. The raising of live stock is a prudential application of experience that may have been gained in the domestication of pet animals. The use of fire stands as the greatest of man's inventions ; it enabled him to extend his dietary enormously, and to migrate to localities where, without artificial warmth and cooking, human existence was impossible. Previously to its use he could only have subsisted in places with a warm, equable climate where edible fruits, roots or nuts were in season all the year round. And since accidental and useful experiences could only have occurred upon a lava field, man's original habitat must have lain in a region of volcanoes. It is remarkable that, having learnt to generate heat, mankind halted so many ages before applying this discovery to the production of steam, chemical and electrical power, and this, too, although in other respects nations attained very high degrees of civilization. It is only within recent years that the value of considered experiments has been appreciated. Earlier civilizations were content to argue deductively (or mathematically) about the forces of Nature ; and this, however fruitful in metaphysical or religious conceptions, does not extend the range of practical knowledge. For we can learn of these forces only through their material consequences, and these must be elucidated inductively by patient experiment. If we take the history of the inventions that have revolutionized modern life—those which have enabled man to enslave the powers of steam, of oil gas, of electricity, and to rival the birds in aerial flight—we find that they have been gradually perfected by the experimental aptitude of practical men —often of artizans whose ingenuity has passed unnoticed because its fruits, in money and in credit, have been grasped by others, and whose earliest efforts were actually ridiculed at the time. Less than half a century has passed since the experiments of the brothers Wright, which were the beginning of aviation, were referred to by the *Scientific American* in terms of indulgent contempt.

Amongst the natural forces that are utilizable are those of human nature. Authoritative government rests upon the feelings of respect that are aroused by superior authority, or upon the fear of a ruler's power. The dread of punishment is utilized, through the criminal law, for the promotion of orderliness, and the instilling of a morality, which at first demands a reflective self-control for observance, but soon becomes habitual. Inclinations—likes and dislikes—are also energies that are used in the process of persuasion. One is *persuaded*, when, under the influence of an awakened—or instilled—like or dislike, he acts in a fashion which he would otherwise not have adopted.

Persuasion is the motive force of commerce, and of popular government. These two very different modes of activity are alike in the force which drives them ; and it is generally true, as shown by experience, that a nation is incapable of prudently governing itself until it has developed the commercial spirit, that is to say, until it has emerged from the emotional into the practical, or prudent, stage of development. The exchanges in which commerce consists are actuated by a preference for something that is offered over something that is possessed. The former " over-comes " the latter ; this is its " value " (or valour)—appraised in terms of that which it overcomes. Both parties to an exchange profit by it, but only through the defeat of their liking for the things that they give in exchange ; and it is this " correlative contrariety " which renders economic questions so difficult to understand. If one has nothing else exchangeable, he offers his labour. Thus man comes voluntarily to work for hire. The value of a thing is more conveniently computed in money than in the terms of that for which it is exchanged, since money valuation reduces all values to a common standard. Judging from history, and from war-time experiences of our own days, coins were at first tokens, issued by private merchants, as giving definite credits upon them for the supply of certain quantities of goods. They possessed, therefore, a guaranteed exchange value. The process of exchange was immensely facilitated by this expedient. Ambitions were attracted into commercial channels with effects that have revolutionized society. This change took place within historical times, for money was evidently unknown in the days of Homer. As an enterprise of the State, the issue of money could be exceedingly profitable, since the State could use its authority, in place of goods, as a guarantee of validity. Minting consequently became a State monopoly, and governments have very generally been unable to withstand the temptation of debasing the currency by using the privilege of coining to pay their debts.

The power of money is immense. It gives a security to future expectations of any material kind. In fact it materializes or " objectifies " expectations. And it gives birth to a new order of expectations—those of receiving money—which have developed into our complicated systems of credit. Moreover, money has a high sentimental value as a symbol of power ; and it consequently stimulates exertion, quite apart from the comfort and luxury which it affords.

It is the boast of democracy that it substitutes persuasion for force as the fundamental instrument for the control of society ; and it is certainly true that prudential persuasion represents a development which corresponds with the evolution of motives from the spontaneous to the reflective stage. Persuasion may be, however, rhetorical as well as prudential. In the first case it appeals to *absolute* values that excite unreflective enthusiasm ; in the second, the values upon which it insists are *relative*, and can be temperately balanced one against the other. The efficacy of these two kinds of appeal depends upon the mentality of those to whom they are addressed. Rhetoric touches the *heart* of the emotional ; prudent arguments influence the *choice* of the reflective. Accordingly, democracy takes one or other of two forms according to the stage of mental development upon which it plays. Amongst emotional peoples, who are moved spontaneously by such feelings as respect, faith, loyalty, class prejudice or revenge, it degenerates into despotism pure and simple—despotism that is in continual danger of revolutionary attack. It is obvious that people of this mentality will listen to no persuader against whom they are antagonized ; attempts to introduce popular government in India under British tutelage have been very disappointing. Democracy is less unreal when popular judgment is amenable to prudential arguments. But here again there is a lion in the path. The prudential interests of rich and poor alike are—and must be—opposed, and these two classes are, therefore, moved by contrary arguments. As soon as the poor realize their power, they are tempted to make demands upon the rich which render it impossible to accumulate capital or to compete in foreign markets. In a country whose life depends upon imported food, this tendency, if it passes beyond control, must end in widespread starvation.

3 Lines of Conduct

Conduct is classified in lines when it is distinguished by the motives which it materializes in movement. Motives have already been discussed with some fulness in Part II of this book. We are now concerned with their manifestations. But these cannot be separated from the motives which underlie them, and it is unfortunately impossible to avoid a good deal of repetition. We may clear the ground by rehearsing some fundamental points that have already been made.

Our motives are blends of the practical and emotional, in which one or other takes the lead. The former has been identified with the feminine, the latter with the masculine element in our nature. The practical is that which inclines us towards or away from persons, things or experiences. As a leading element it endows us with *inclinations*—likes and dislikes—which give conduct a *purposeful* drift. Emotion is associated with them as the pleasure and displeasure that are the consequences of their satisfaction. Experiences of pleasure and displeasure serve to develop new inclinations, and recollections of pleasure and displeasure re-stimulate inclinations. Emotion, on the other hand, is the leading element in such *appreciative* feelings as admiration, pity and contempt. The emotion may be of the kind—commonly styled " spiritual "—that is re-stimulated by ideas of *qualities* of success and failure, such as power and weakness, excellence or inferiority. The practical element which enters into these appreciations inclines us towards or away from the persons, things and qualities which arouse them. The conduct which is motived by them is, nevertheless, not purposeful, but *expressive*. We have no purpose in view when we are proud of ourselves, or honour the King. Briefly, in our inclinations, the practical is the chief and the emotional is the subordinate : in our appreciative emotions the contrary is the case.

Purposeful and expressive motives each undergo two very important developments or metamorphoses. Purpose becomes *antagonistic* when it is distracted by discord, *ambitious* when stimulated by ideas of success. Expression becomes *idealistic* when it translates into conduct a subjective quality that arouses admiring appreciation, *artistic* when it gives objective expression to imagined individualizations of qualities. Purposeful (or practical) conduct may then be distinguished as inclinational, antagonistic and ambitious : expressive (or emotional) conduct as appreciatory, idealistic and artistic.

There is, however, a further complication. Conduct of whatever kind may take one of three evolutionary phases : it may be spontaneous (sometimes called " naïve "), deliberate, or habitual. There is a law of development under which action tends to pass from one of these phases into its successor. Spontaneous steadies itself into deliberate conduct, and this becomes automatic under the force of habit.

Inclinational conduct is that of ordinary everyday life. The experiences towards which we gravitate may be the sensorily gratifying, the interesting, the amusing or the flattering. It would be a mistake to regard all inclinational conduct as " sensual ". The pleasure that we receive may be of the revulsive, or the " spiritual " kind, as well as sensory. Our amusements and many of our interests please us revulsively—through the pleasurable intensifications that are caused by passing shocks. Flattery and compliments, on the other hand, afford pleasure of the ex-revulsive kind that is stimulated by qualities of success. Our attachments and affections are inclinations, motived by ideas of kindly feeling towards us, or of identities in interest. But they generally include something of the spiritual element of admiration. This is pre-eminently the case with sexual love.

We instinctively avoid pain and illness. Pain is a condition of acute nervous discord that automatically stimulates a movement of recoil from its cause, when this is external and is immediately associated with it in sensation. When the cause is within us, or is not directly apparent, we are urged to discover it. The medical profession is maintained by the anxieties of its patients. Pain takes an immaterial form in shame. We avoid this when we are influenced by " conscience ", and also when we are swayed by thoughts of " what the world will say ", since an ashamed sense of failure is aroused auto-suggestively by experiences of others' disapproval. This is the strongest of the buttresses that support conventional morality—stronger than " self-retributional " shame, because it is the consequence of " objective " experiences. Legal punishment uses material pain or discomfort as a means of influencing choice, so that those who are tempted to infringe the order upon which society depends, may have a strong inducement to refrain from doing so. After a time their restraint becomes habitual. But it is doubtful whether, without punishment, civilized life would have evolved. Idealistic teaching can work wonders. But ideals are apt to fade in disillusionment.

The tendency of inclinations to become habitual " passions " is illustrated by such vices as drunkenness, and not less strikingly by the obsessing influence of games. To a golf enthusiast there is no other interest in life. So again with the passion for society. Man is not instinctively " gregarious " in the sense of living in a crowd. He can live contentedly in a very small circle of associates. But, when habituated to society, a day spent in the quiet of home seems to be a day wasted. Anxiety about one's health may in like manner become the only motive of existence.

Antagonistic conduct.—One can, as we have seen, antagonize oneself as well as other persons. Courage, whether spontaneous or deliberate, opposes a timorous dislike : it may grow into a habitual disregard of danger. There is self-antagonism in both self-assertion and self-repression, the effect of which is writ large in history by such very different cults as those of liberty and of asceticism. Both of these movements have, however, owed their energy rather to an idealistic admiration of their strength than to a mere spirit of antagonism—in other words, they have been emotional rather than practical. In everyday life self-repression is self-control. We antagonize others in emulation of all kinds, and industry contains an element of combativeness. Both may be deliberate as well as impulsive. Antagonism becomes irritated in anger. This is ordinarily a passing fit of contrariety. But it becomes chronic in war, although, here again, idealism—the admiration of the power of one's own country, and the strength of its defiant attitude—is the main source of energy. Anger cannot be deliberate, since it is the response to an *injury*. But the retaliation which is its consequence may be divorced from it, and be deliberately employed, in the form of punishment. Discipline, whether in the family or the State, is the product of the dispassionate use of the retaliatory promptings of passion.

Ambitious conduct.—Success is a necessary instrument for the procuring of satisfaction. But, being so pleasurable an experience, it becomes an object in itself as the motive of ambition. This may be accompanied by idealistic aspirations for the good of others, as, for instance, the ambition of an earnest political reformer. But success is always the fundamental, and often the sole object in view. What is there but success, pure and simple, in climbing Mount Everest, or in winning a race or a decoration?

Curiously enough, a satisfying assurance of success may be won by conduct that is not in itself " successful ". For it may be gained from the esteem or respect of others, although this may be quite undeserved. To seek popularity is, then, a common line of conduct. It may also be gained as a " reflected " lustre—from association with the great or wealthy. For their *liaison* with us becomes, so to speak, an admirable quality of our own by which our dignity is enhanced, as by the wearing of fine clothes. For the actual winning of success hundreds of routes are open—in education, industry, art, politics, games and sport. The goal upon which most eyes are fixed at the present day is the phase of power that is involved in *possessing* things, and for this reason modern ambitions are often stigmatized as " material ". But, in fact, possessions have always been in esteem since private property first came into being. What gives modern ambitions their peculiar bent is the overweening desire to *make money* by exchange. This is impossible on a large scale until material civilization is well advanced—until the means of exchange are extensively developed and there is, above all things, a reasonable confidence as to the security of future prospects. These assurances not merely render money-making possible : they act as stimuli to money-making by presenting clear visions of future profits.

Money-making involves *prudence*, that is to say, careful deliberation over possible losses as well as possible gains. "Business" is accordingly infected with anxiety : there is a lack of the happiness that is given by optimistic impulse. Consequently it is not inspiring. Impulsive ambition may be effectively dramatized. But no playwright can make use of the prudent "man of affairs" except in satire. The development of commercial life has entailed a distinct loss of general happiness. We endeavour to make the loss good by multiplying amusements.

Success may be won by research. But it is only within the last century and a half that the value of observation and experiment has become apparent. Philosophy had previously been content to argue deductively from laws that were dictated by self-respect, not by experience. Consequently, since its premises were fanciful, it arrived at very varied and discrepant conclusions as to the character of natural forces. At various epochs the value of experience has struck advanced intelligences—those of Aristotle, Galileo, Francis Bacon and Voltaire, for example. But it is more inspiring to argue than to experiment, and practical science was long in gaining favour. Now, however observation and experiment have become the fashion of the day. We are inclined to ascribe this revolution to a tendency of human faculties towards "progress". In reality it has resulted from a far more definite cause—the discovery that exact science could be profitable as well as interesting. Science is valued because it can be *applied*. We rarely find a scientific book, addressed to the general reader, that does not insist upon the practical use of the discoveries which it describes. There are, of course, men of science whose ambition is to discover truth for truth's sake. But, speaking generally, it is because the truth may be *profitable* that their efforts are respected and assisted.

Emotional conduct.—It is a remarkable fact that (apart from some instinctive mannerisms) emotional conduct is always *imitative* when it is urged by admiration or pity. For we imitate another when we sympathize with him, and also when we obey him, assist him or make a likeness of him. Obedience clearly imitates the ideas with which it complies. If we assist another, propitiate him, or please him, we are imitating what we suppose to be his wishes or aspirations. So again, if we "decorate" or glorify him. We like to enhance our own qualities by adornment, and, in embellishing another, we imitate actively what it must be his desire to experience passively. Sympathy can be only spontaneous. But in its other phases imitation may be either spontaneous or deliberate, just as applause may be heart-felt or " forced ".

Appreciatory conduct.—This is moved by the emotions of admiration, pity, contempt, respect and faith. We can be actuated by these emotions towards ourselves. Man has some excuse for his self-admiration (or pride) since it is by a continuous series of successes that he maintains his level above the lower animals. Pride automatically braces the muscles : a sense of superiority shows itself in a stiff aloofness of demeanour. In the passion for self-adornment, and the boastful exaggerations of self-conceit, we can trace the tendency to decorate what is admired. Shame, or a sense of inferiority, on the other hand, is attended by muscular relaxation : it is deferential and strives to escape from itself by excuses and apologies. Deferential manners can be deliberately used to conciliate others, since an admission of inferiority is an acknowledgment of superiority. They are a useful instrument for the purpose of commercial persuasion ; and for this reason trade seemed to our forefathers to be humiliating. This prejudice has now passed away. And, indeed, self-depreciation that is correlatively flattering to others is simply a form of politeness, and is as useful in ordinary society as it is in commerce.

Admiration for another shows itself spontaneously in applause. It becomes reverence or respect when it is tinged by a sense of inferiority ; and faith, when there is also a sense of the other's protective benevolence. Faith manifests itself in spontaneous obedience. Upon this emotional response rests the structure of society, whether in the family or the State, until its place is taken by prudence. Obedience then becomes *calculated*. But it lacks the energy of spontaneity. " Intelligent " loyalty and the loyalty of mere habitude are but fragile bucklers for an authority that is seriously menaced. And they do not give the happiness of the whole-hearted impulse—the cheerfulness of a regiment to which its colonel is a " creed ". Reverence also manifests itself in propitiatory manners, presents and ceremonies, and in an impulse to glorify its object by praise and propaganda.

These external manifestations of admiration are, however, much less striking than the sympathy which it spontaneously begets, for this is the *cause* of obedience, propitiation and glorification. The emotion of pity has precisely the same effect. For this feeling, as we have seen, resembles admiration in that it is correlatively

P

aroused by a feeling of superiority—the superiority being our own
instead of another's. It is through its sympathy that pity is
benevolent and charitable. And through its " expansiveness " it
is strong. There is no more inspiring incentive to courage. Man
attains the climax of his strength when he pitifully risks his own life
to save that of another.

Idealistic conduct in its typical enthusiastic phase, impulsively
expresses a subjective quality that is admired. The idealist is
inspired by his ideal, and is energized by one of humanity's strongest
motives. A physical inclination may be irresistible : but we are
its slaves. Will-power is impressive ; but it cannot still the tremblings of fear or anger : it can control action and speech, but is
powerless over feeling. Idealism, on the contrary, fills a man with
the feeling which is its stimulus in idea—to the exclusion of all others.
He is urged by an uncalculating enthusiasm which we call " fanatic "
when its ideal is other than our own. So he becomes capable of
things that materialistic philosophy cannot explain. As an ascetic
he can renounce all that seems to make life worth living : as cham-
pion of a cause he can mock at death : as a martyr he can welcome
it. On the other hand, zeal for a self-assertive, national or religious
ideal can stifle all feelings of pity and endow him with the unreflecting cruelty of an insect. Ambition and prudence can do none of
these things. But they endure, whereas idealism fades, as hot iron
cools. Emotion is liable to fatigue. Prudent inclination is tireless.

Ideals are " regenerative ", and man is free from all " practical "
trammels when he is inspired by them. They must be " strong "
to arouse admiring enthusiasm. But they may be innocent or
benevolent, as are those enjoined by Christ. On the other hand,
they may be diabolically demoralizing and pernicious. Revenge
may be idealized as well as mercy. For both are strong.

An ideal is followed deliberately when it becomes a canon of
morality. Many of our moral rules are idealistic in their origin.
So conduct which is accordant with idealism may become habitual,
and Christian ideals, if taught in all sincerity, might really change
the behaviour of mankind.

Artistic conduct.—The artist executes his ideas by imitating or
describing them. Imitation is simplest, and most direct, when it is
mimetic—that is to say, when it dramatizes feelings and thoughts.
But the delineation of sculpture and painting are also imitative.

Artistic talent may present to us the fruits of either inspiration
or ingenuity. In the former case it has an emotional quality which
" touches the heart ". The admiration which dictates it is infec-

tious. Ingenious art is motived for the most part by ideas of success. It may be admirable for its technique, or its originality : it may be interesting through its subject, or amusing in its incidents or methods of treatment. But it does not " carry one away ".

Acting, as in children's play, seems to be the most primitive form of artistic expression. There is, as we have seen, an intimate connection between thought and movement, and ideas of action and utterances automatically materialize themselves as they occur. The imitation involved in delineating things, either in the round or on the flat, is more sophisticated. It involves the appreciation of analogies between form and movement, and the skill that is required to imitate one through the other. Delineation is decorative when it is used for the purpose of enhancing the qualities of an object. Its design may be borrowed from nature, as in the acanthus leaf border, or be suggested by the shapes of geometry, as in the " key " pattern.

Descriptive expression has the advantage over dramatic acting that it can represent feelings and thoughts more naturally than is possible in the dramatic soliloquy or " aside ". These may be of the artist himself as well as of his fancied characters. In poetry descriptive expression is embellished by being thrown into the harmony of rhythm : rhyme and alliteration are additional ornaments.

Dancing is rhythm pure and simple : music is harmonious sound that is controlled by rhythm. Both stand apart from dramatic, descriptive and delineative art. For they elaborate and materialize, not ideas, but *expressions of feeling*. Emotion naturally vents itself in rhythmic steps and in vocal utterances. These are the materials which the arts of dancing and music elaborate. Their basis is not reflective but manifestative ; and they make so strong an appeal to the feelings of mankind because they are evolved from the ventings of feeling, that are natural and instinctive.

Religious conduct.—A passing reference must be made to the religious observances and activities which figure so prominently in the manners of all races of mankind. In religious feeling, reverence for mysterious power, and an idealistic admiration for what seems excellent, are imaginatively combined. Divine personalities represent the majesty of ultimate *causes*, the existence of which is deduced from experience, but the nature of which is unknown. They may affect the passing dispositions of man (as Venus was supposed to inspire love) or the changing courses of Nature. Reverence for them manifests itself in such services of propitiation as would be offered to human potentates, by the self-abasement of worship, by ceremonial adoration and the establishment of a hierarchy of priestly intermediaries between the human and the divine. The impulse to decorate, or magnify, expresses itself by the use of all the ornamental possibil.ties of jewelry and dress, painting, sculpture, architecture and music : it also prompts the glorification of its divinities by spreading their influence through warlike or persecuting forces, missionary propaganda, or pious fiction.

All religions but the most primitive contain an element of admiration—of idealistic enthusiasm for transcendental qualities, that may express itself in ecstatic meditation, or in metaphysical enquiry. This has not infrequently led speculation into doctrines that are frankly nihilistic, yet are, nevertheless, inspired by an imaginative glow.

The will makes its contribution. Prudence—the outcome of deliberative reflection—suggests the enlistment of supernatural forces to one's own advantage by means of services which would propitiate the divine, or identify man with the divine—by sacrifice, prayers and sacraments. Finally, as occurs in all phases of living activity, the spontaneous and the willed pass into the habitual, and religious beliefs and observances become the lifeless products of convention.

Religion has claimed to be an indispensable mainstay of morality. But this is not born out by experience. Sceptics may be amongst the most virtuous of men. And, were it true, morality would have been lost by the mass of the English working-classes, for whom religion exists but in name.

4 The Growth of Culture

The origin of our culture has been the establishment of new combinations, or associations, of ideas and movements, by the means of *successful* experiences. These may have presented themselves either accidentally, or as the results of efforts of trial, or of the intelligent recognition of identities between two different things. By education these combinations are instilled into others, so that they do not perish with their discoverer but are spread far and wide. Example is an *accelerating* force since it is infinitely easier to learn than to invent. It also has the effect of spreading a discovery *accumulatively* in as much as each convert becomes an example to numbers of others. It can, then, extend very rapidly to a people the acquirements which particular individuals have gained from successful or fortunate experiences and the use of intelligence.

Before passing to the consideration of language, it will be interesting to review very briefly the development of morality, politics, art and modern civilization in the light of the facts that have been set forth in this section. Our comprehension of these wonderful achievements will be assisted if we bear in mind seven laws, or " tendencies ", the existence of which has already been demonstrated. *Firstly*, that the energy of effort is generated by discord, which may be that of failure or adversity. *Secondly*, that deliberation—that is to say, the will—gradually ousts spontaneity, and itself gives place to habit ; and it is to be noticed that the will, by enabling man to control his expressions, endows him with the faculty of deceiving others. *Thirdly*, that conduct and utterances which are primitively expressive, tend to evolve into the practical or purposeful. *Fourthly*, that the objective—the material—tends to become more attractive than the subjective, or spiritual, partly because of the influence of the will (for this is an objective force and cannot affect feeling), and partly because objective sensation is capable of almost indefinite refinement, whereas subjective feeling cannot be so elaborated. *Fifthly*, that the power of another, when reflectively apprehended, suggests a galling idea of one's own correlative inferiority, the discord of which excites an effort to achieve "liberty": another's weakness similarly suggests a pleasing idea of one's own superiority which fosters the sentiment of pity. *Sixthly*, that instruments tend to become objects in themselves, since they attach to themselves the interests of the objects which they serve : language, dress and manners are all primarily instruments, but they become cults in themselves. *Seventhly*, that one instrument or process that resembles another in an essential point can be substituted for it through identification : so musical instruments can replace the voice.

5 Morality

Behaviour is " moral "—in the literal sense of the word—when it conforms to custom—that is to say, is in accordance with an accepted rule of conduct. One may conform to a rule because one wills to do so, because one is habituated to do so, or because one admires the ideal upon which the rule is based. It follows that moral conduct may be volitional, conventional, or ideal. Conduct that is purely heart-felt, " natural ", or spontaneous, may be good or bad. But it is not *moral*.

Accordingly morality involves the inter-action of two correlatives —a set of authoritative rules and a disposition to obey them. Each of these implies the other : there is no authority without obedience, and no obedience is possible unless there is an authority to be obeyed. It will be convenient to refer in the first place to the genesis of the disposition to obey. In children we call this " goodness ". It may commence as " goodness of heart " : a child obeys its mother because it admires, or loves, her, and consequently sympathizes with her wishes. But this disposition is not proof against fits of ill-temper, and some further security is required. This is given by the fear of punishment, taking the word in a broad sense so as to include any kind of unpleasant consequence, as, for instance, the shame that follows a mother's displeasure. When this presents itself in thought as the consequence of an action, there is hesitation, and the child *chooses* in place of acting impulsively. Its conduct becomes deliberate instead of spontaneous. It shows a sense of " moral responsibility " or " obligation ". *But this sense is generated by an apprehension.* " The fear of the Lord is the beginning of wisdom ".

Choice involves the energy that is stimulated by discord. But the conduct to which it leads soon crystallizes into habit, since it is associatively re-stimulated when it has become familiar. Hence moral conduct that is primarily willed passes into the conventional. The child becomes " well-behaved " through discipline, and from the social point of view " goodness of heart " appears to be superfluous.

We feel, nevertheless, that goodness of habit, however convenient to society, is not admirable. For one thing, it may be hypocritical or deceitful. Morality is on a far higher plane when it is the outcome of an ideal which is obeyed, or followed, not by an effort of choice but in admiration of its excellence. In this case the ultimate motive of conduct is not apprehension, but appreciation ; and, since admiration breeds sympathy, one is moral, not merely in action or speech, but in feeling. " Natural " goodness of disposition is the product of admiration or pity for a person—feelings to which we commonly give the name of " love " : goodness becomes " ideal " when it proceeds from admiration, not of a person, but of a quality. Ideal morality is, however, more difficult to establish than volitional, insamuch as it generally involves the development of admiring appreciation, and it is harder to educate a capability than to instil an apprehension. It is easier to alarm than to inspire : the threat of a slap stops a child from teasing the cat more effectually than a lesson upon loving-kindness. And experience seems to show that admiration is not as powerful as apprehension in withstanding sudden onsets of cupidity or anger. We may, incidentally, draw an important conclusion—that the League of Nations, so long as it has no punitive powers, will hardly be able to hold its own against outbreaks of national feeling, or to render peace as habitual between nations as the fear of the law has made it between individuals.

Rules of willed and conventional morality.—Passing now from moral compliance to the moral authority that is complied with, let us very briefly review the precepts which grow into a system of conventional morality through the influence upon the will of the consequences of disobeying them. *In the first place*, they insist upon respect for constituted authority, and reverence for the dead—observances that are dictated by natural feelings ; for authority that is powerful always commands respect, while the majesty of the dead is probably the earliest, the most general, and the most enduring of religious convictions :

> Be near us when we climb or fall;
> Ye watch, like God, the rolling hours
> With larger, other eyes than ours,
> To make allowance for us all.

A cemetery is probably the most ancient of *temples*—places " cut off " from the world—and is still one of the most popular.

Secondly, moral rules seek to enforce lessons that have been taught by experience—acts and forbearances which have proved essential or useful to society, and are consequently dictated by prudence, such as, for instance, the eschewing of violence, theft and adultery, the practice of honesty, and the use of consideration and politeness in our manners towards others. And, since man is prone to argue from fanciful, or " magic ", analogies, actions may seem to be imprudent for reasons that, judged by experience, are ridiculous. It is probable, for instance, that Jewish morality prohibited the eating of hares and pigs because it was thought that their flesh would carry with it something of their character, making man cowardly in disposition and filthy in habits—an idea which lingers in India, where a morsel of tiger's flesh is held to be a sovereign stimulant of courage. *Thirdly*, morality prohibits behaviour that is inconsistent with decency and modesty. These are motives which are peculiar to mankind : there is little trace of them amongst the lower animals. They have their ultimate origin in mental deductions which man draws from the internal antagonism of which he is conscious—the conflict between his physical and his spiritual impulses. This endows him with anti-physical tendencies—spiritual protests against humiliating physical impurities. The sordid necessities of the body are out of accord with man's high ideas of himself : they are degrading to his dignity and seem to pollute it. Hence have arisen ideas of purity and impurity which, judged from a purely naturalistic standpoint, are absurd. They have been fantastically elaborated and carried to the extreme of imaginative exaggeration. To the zealous ascetic all purely physical actions, including those of reproduction, are impure. The Hindu sees dangers of pollution in the act of eating, and his " caste " rules—or rules of " chasteness "—fence it about with meticulous precautions. The blood which seems to be the life of the body, carries a taint, and there is one Iudian caste which eschews lentils because their pink colour suggests it. But this distinction between the pure and the impure, however fanciful have been its developments, is the origin of man's notions of modesty and decency.

There is a *fourth* element that enters into conventional morality—the prescription of certain peculiarities of behaviour that originate in the desire to assert the distinctiveness of one's class—to claim for it the excellence of not being " ordinary ". It is, for instance, wrong for men of a certain station to appear in public without a collar and necktie, or attend a funeral in a " bowler " hat. The officers of certain regiments " don't dance ". We euphemistically ascribe these peculiarities to " class consciousness " : they are actually manifestations of class-conceit. For lack of a better term we may call them " class-distinctional ". They are extraordinarily elaborate amongst schoolboys : they dominate the lives of savages, and are never absent from the mind of an Indian caste. In the air of democracy they naturally tend to fade away.

Ideal morality.—A gulf lies between conventional—or practical—morality and the moral aspirations of the idealist, for he is swayed by the spirit, not by the law. The character of his behaviour depends upon the ideal that he admires ; and, since there are as many possible ideals as there are strong qualities in human nature, idealistic aspirations may be so varied as to be contradictory, and may be either harmful or beneficial to mankind. St. Francis, Savonarola, Robespierre and Lenin were all idealists. The idealism of Christ is super-excellent in that the qualities which it sets before us are innocent—in the sense of innocuous—if not actively beneficent. They are strong, but harmless. Sympathy, or loving-kindness is admirable because it is the cause of harmony and unity. If one admires it, he will acquire a " goodness of heart " which will reinforce—or even supply the lack of—natural good-feeling. Purity, Sobriety, Sincerity, Patience and Humility all involve the strength of self-control, but of a self-control that does not set itself blindly against all man's natural tendencies, and is content to create virtues that are beneficial to the individual and to society. Self-control is combined with sympathy in the magnanimous virtues of Forgiveness, Mercy, Tolerance, Loyalty and Generosity. Justice and Gratitude are strong because they are harmonious : they render what follows accordant with what precedes. They are of immense value in smoothing the relationships of social intercourse. Had these ideals been systematically impressed upon Christians as the vital elements of their Master's teaching, Christianity would beyond doubt have been a far greater force for human improvement. For habits may spring from idealism as well as from prudence. But they have lain almost obscured behind a veil of dogma and ceremonies.

It may certainly be urged that idealism is unpractical—that it is out of accord with the material objects of life. The ideals of Christ, whole-heartedly adopted, would reduce his followers to submissive poverty. But they were never intended to over-ride all of man's other propensities. They were expressly compared to leaven, which lightens bread but does not take its place—a comparison the meaning of which is not invalidated by the fact that, to enforce their importance, they were paradoxically illustrated. Prudence is necessary for the affairs of everyday life. Idealism plays its part as an inspiring admixture.

Moral responsibility.—The distinction between spontaneous (or unreflecting) impulse, reflective will and crystallized habit is the pivot upon which turns the much-debated question of " moral responsibility ". If impulse bars the very commencement of reflection, there is no responsibility : accordingly children and lunatics are not held amenable to the criminal law. There is similarly no responsibility if one is completely dominated by habit : a slave to the drug habit cannot help but dope himself. There is, in fact, no responsibility unless there is a capacity for deliberately choosing—that is to say, unless the consequences of an act are realized with sufficient clearness to balance themselves against the idea of it with some chance of success. This chance is naturally improved by the decline which occurs in impulsive excitement as one grows from childhood to maturity. It is also improved by an increase in the severity, or the certainty, of the counter-balancing consequences. It has been proved over and over again by experience that the spread of a particular crime can be checked by increasing the degree of its punishment—as, for instance, by the prescription of whipping.

It is obvious that the orderliness of society depends upon the checking of impulse by the will, or its mechanization by habit. The possibility of checking it is innate in man, for the duality of his constitution leads to self-antagonism, and this being *strong* seems to be admirable, whereas weakness in self-control is penalized by a feeling of shame, the apprehension of which is conscience. But this is idealistic morality : ideals generally tend to fade, and something more durable is needed to check the impulses of the ordinary man. The first suggestions of impulse must be so closely associated with ideas of deterrent consequences that one cannot present itself without the other. It is the function of laws and moral conventions to effect this association, the one attaching punishment, the other reprobation to impulsive conduct. With the development of national civilization, and the desire for possessions, another penalty gains force—the fear of material loss to which we give the name of " prudence ". These deterrents, acting together, produce automatic habits of orderliness and respectability, which end by altogether excluding any ideas that are not consistent with law and morality. So man may become, not merely capable of acting respectably, but incapable of acting otherwise than respectably.

6 Politics

History, as commonly written, is imaginative, not scientific : it is a study, often very incorrect, of outstanding personalities who are represented as " laws unto themselves ". We endeavour, nevertheless, to discover general tendencies that regulate the political development of mankind. But we search for them only in geographical or economic—that is to say in *objective*—circumstances, closing our eyes to the infinitely more important laws that determine the course of our " subjective " feelings.

There must be government of some kind if man is to profit by the experience of his forebears. For this involves teaching, and teaching is authoritative. And the lessons of the past would be fruitless if violence were uncontrolled, and no limits were set to the selfish intensity of the struggle for success.

Government is the product of two correlatives—authority and obedience—one of which cannot exist without the other. The simplest, and most natural, of all authorities is that of the father of the family. Its acceptance is spontaneous and unreflecting—an act of faith. To unite families into a tribe, the obvious instrument is a council of fathers, or " senate ". But this, to be efficient, must have an executive chief or head. His election by his fellows was man's first experience of *voting*—that is to say, of measuring another's worth by computing arithmetically the amount of his popularity. There are tribes on the Assam frontier who have not made this evolutionary step. Their tribal council has no president. They are consequently at the mercy of neighbouring tribes, greatly inferior in numbers, who are commanded by *rajas*. This leads to the reflection that the authority of a king is far more often derived from conquest—that is to say, from a manifestation of power in its crudest and most impressive form—than from any voluntary process of election.

Power, however obtained, maintains its involuntary influence over mankind only if it is supported by strength of character, since this is the subjective form of power that we idealize. But strength of character is more often ascribed to rulers than possessed by them, and they have generally felt the need of something beyond their personal qualities to secure them in their authority. The maintenance of an armed force was an obvious expedient. But the influence of religion could be as effective. The king became high priest—or allied himself closely with a priesthood. The doctrine of " divine right " followed. Such a mysterious privilege would naturally pass from father to son, and kingship became hereditary, with a prestige which completely overshadowed the privileges of any senate that existed.

But, unless supported by pre-eminent ability, the absolute authority of a king is questionable by the intelligence, especially if it fails to win success for the nation. The intelligent are few and may be silenced for a time. But should anything occur which produces a national sense of failure, their opinions spread rapidly. There comes general disillusionment. When man's respect fails for a ruler, his authority becomes discordant with their ideas. Discord (as we have seen) leads to an exercise of the will. This takes form in revolt. And another element contributes to the spirit of unrest. When a king's superiority ceases to inspire admiration, we become aware that it implies a displeasing idea of our own inferiority.

Revolt need not be rebellion. It may be a deliberate attempt to lessen the royal prerogatives by withdrawing from them the right to make laws and to levy taxes, and reserving these powers to a senate. Or, if religious beliefs had been organized, a priesthood could effectively interpose itself between a king and his subjects, cloaking its human imperfections in the mysterious privilege of knowing, and being favoured by, the Divine. The king could make a counter-move by summoning into council representatives of the rank and file of the population. These might win election through the emotional effect of their prestige or popularity. But they might also secure election by promising certain benefits to their constituents. This introduced a new element into politics—the deliberate influence of prospective advantages. The judgment of votes would be swayed, not by impulsive feelings of loyalty or admiration, but by prudence, and a practical regard for self-interest.

Since all men love power, the people's representatives could not be expected to rest content with the part of a make-weight. By an intelligent use of State difficulties, they could gradually obtain an influence which completely eclipsed that of the king, the senate and the priesthood. They might retain the king as a symbol of national unity, or replace him by an elected president. But the practical result was the same. The policy of the State became subject to popular likes and dislikes. This is democracy.

The process of election offered a new opening to ambition. The instrument of success was the obtaining of votes. They have not uncommonly been frankly purchased, either in hard cash or in State appointments. Less cynical inducements were rhetorical appeals to sentiment and prejudice, and the " practical " persuasiveness which addresses itself to " reason "—that is to say, to an intelligent appreciation of future advantages. The first stimulates spontaneous emotion : the second deliberate choice. Both are combined in the electoral appeals of the present day. But the latter is tending to preponderate. Reflective choice is gaining upon impulse.

Acting alone, popular representatives are capable of very little indeed. They have, generally, little personal influence. Indeed, the expedients to which they must resort in canvassing for votes involves a loss of personal dignity that is fatal to the authority that is given by power. They must consequently regiment themselves into groups or parties, and this has the incidental advantage of arousing a spirit of emulation which immensely increases the enthusiasm of the voting public. Men who cannot define the difference between Conservative and Liberal will be stirred by the distinction between Blue and Buff, as they are by the rival colours of the University Boat Race. The simplest line of party division is suggested by the comparative attractedness of the old and the new—

of vested interests and reform. But a profounder distinction is that between rich and poor—between capital and labour—and there are signs to show that this will obliterate the emulative, or " sporting " interest of party feeling. For it arouses reasoning will as opposed to spontaneous impulse. Experience has shown that the immediate interests of capital and labour are diametrically opposed. The one desires hard work and low pay, the other light work on high pay. It can be shown beyond a doubt that capital is as necessary to produce wages as labour is to produce profit. But this leaves the fact untouched that they act upon one another through discordance.

This change will assuredly impart a graver note to politics. So long as they are based upon emulative feelings they have the nature of a " game ". And, as in a game failures are not taken seriously, so politicians can survive mistakes which would ruin the prospects of a " business man ". But in a struggle between rich and poor there is little room for the play of the " sporting spirit ".

In the democratic system of government two correlatives— authority and obedience—are assimilated. The ruler is identical with the ruled ; and it follows that the only discipline that can be imposed is that which is accepted by those who are to suffer it. Judging from experience this will not be very severe ; and, unless the wisdom of the past is utterly misleading, one cannot regard the future of popular rule with much confidence. In Italy and Spain it has broken down entirely. But one must not argue from Mediterranean nations to those of the North. Owing, it may be, to climatic influences, northerners have a larger share of that prudent will-power that is called " common sense ". In the South this can make no head against impulsive feelings. There, politics have always been purely emotional, and democracy has never developed the people's *will* as opposed to their prejudices. It may be that in the North this element may suffice to protect popular government from its natural consequences, by inducing men to sacrifice their immediate interests for those that bear fruit " in the long run ".

There are signs that even in this country confidence in democratic government is gradually lessening. But its most cynical critics cannot deny that, as voting power has been extended, the needs of the poor have received increasing attention. The outstanding social change of the last century is the extraordinary amelioration of the conditions of the working classes. They may have lost in contentment, but life offers them such amusement as it never did before.

Nationality.—At the present day national patriotism has become so habitual a sentiment as to appear to be instinctive. But the idea that men are bound together in unity because they inhabit the same tract of country is quite artificial, and is obviously of much later origin than tribal or caste sentiment. As a matter of fact, mere proximity may be no more of a tie between men than between beasts and birds. In London one concerns himself not at all about his next-door neighbours. In India neighbourliness leaves the barriers of caste quite unshaken ; and the Turks are developing their nationality by expelling their neighbours instead of by assimilating them. History shows that tribes have gradually coalesced to form nations under the influence either of enthusiastic resistance to conquest, or of the suffering of conquest. Nationality is, in fact, the product of war. The bond of territorial union is strengthened by sameness of religion and language. But it requires to be also reinforced by fanciful theories of racial brotherhood ; and it tends to disintegrate under the stress of discrepant class interests. A very large number of the workmen of this country are Trade Unionists first and Englishmen afterwards.

Tides in evolution.—The history of civilization, so far as it is known to us, is a record of " tidal " changes. Society crystallizes into orderliness and comfort to dissolve again into turbulent simplicity. Out of anarchy emerges a controlling power, and the " moralization ', of discipline : disillusionment and demoralization follow ; and there is a reversion to anarchy. A contributory cause of this decadence is, no doubt, the loss of spiritual (or masculine) energy that is entailed by material comfort. This places a sophisticated community at the mercy of a hardy invader. But decadence occurs without the catastrophe of conquest. A natural impatience with superiority that is unreal provokes a continuous attack upon any governing authority which has lost respect, and demoralization sets in as control is weakened. The influence of religion may delay disillusionment ; and respect for controlling authority may be revived by a commanding personality. But this process of integration and disintegration appears to have been so regular as to be a law. The tide may go out more slowly in some cases than others. But its final retreat may be with a rush. The Roman Empire of the West became barbarized within the space of two generations. In these days the danger of barbarian invasion seems very remote. But there are some signs of a process of internal disruption.

7 Art

" Art " primarily means *skill*. But in the sense with which we are now concerned, it signifies the skilful expression of harmonious or inspiring feelings or ideas—that is to say, the achievements of artistic talent. These achievements serve to give pleasure to others. So employed, art is " impressive ", as opposed to expressive.

Art as an expression.—Artistic expression must have an energizing motive, which may be either self-suggested, or deliberately adopted. In the former case the artist is " inspired " by it : in the latter he *chooses* it. His instruments of expression are gestures, utterances and imitations. All these have their ultimate sources in spontaneous life : a smile spontaneously expresses pleasure as a bird's song the joy of life. Imitation itself, as we have seen, commences as a spontaneous auto-suggestive process. These " objective " activities are all phases of movement, and can, therefore, be taken hold of and elaborated by the will, under the impulse of a desire for success, and be gradually developed into automatic dexterities. They assume, however, a spontaneous complexion when they are used by an artist to " liberate his soul ". In this case we may term them " emotional " : the force that urges them is involuntary. When they simply give effect to an ambition for success, they lose their emotional character, and become " practical " or ingenious.

Apart from increasing efficiency in *technique*, these instruments of expression have gradually been moulded into artistic methods through the operation of three laws. In the first place, they have been elaborated by the refinement, or education, of sensibility that comes from the attentive exercise of the senses. The history of music illustrates this process very strikingly : with the refinement of musical taste combinations of notes are appreciated which would afford no pleasure to an uncultured ear. Secondly, by efforts of trial, the results of which are conserved by memory, distinct processes may be combined, as rhythm is blended with music, or, in the case of poetry, with speech. And thirdly, through the intelligent appreciation of identities, one process can be substituted for another if they have elements in common. So musical instruments have been substituted for the voice, and verbal description for dramatic imitation.

Art as an impression.—The typical effect of the artist's work upon

others is to produce a feeling of admiration or pity.   But this is only
one of its products.   It may excite emotion by associative recall,
and the recall may be through natural (instinctive) or artificial
associations.   Thus quick time in music recalls cheerful feelings, and
slow time sad or solemn feelings, because we naturally move quickly
in joy, and slowly when affected by sadness or reverence.   Certain
musical sequences and chords naturally move us excitingly or
sedatively because they have identities with the vocal inflections
of joy and sorrow.   On the other hand, it is through artificial
associations that certain feelings are recalled by hymn tunes, for
instance, or by the national anthem.   Art may also interest us by
ministering to the pleasure that has been styled " gustative ".   And
it may be amusing.   But its characteristic effect is to arouse
admiration.   This admiration, however, may be compelled, either
by the artist's theme, or by his technique.   It is only in the first case
that it is emotionally " inspiring ", in the sense of moving us to
sentimental sympathy.   Admiration for *technique* contains a practical, as well as an emotional, element.   The difference between
the practical and the emotional can, then, be traced, not only in
artistic expression, but in the impression which the artist's work
makes upon others.

Dancing and music.—These stand apart from the drama, poetry,
fiction and painting, because they are developed through the
elaboration, not of emotional or interesting themes, but of methods
of expression.   They spring, not from emotion, but from the
consequences of emotion.   The ideas from which they spring are ideas
of expression, not of motives.   They are, primarily, elaborations, not
of objects, but of instruments.   But a composer is undoubtedly
assisted in elaborating them by an emotional frame of mind :
indeed, it is only when they are evoked by sentiment that his com-
positions are " inspired ".   Being intimately associated with
emotion, the rhythm of movement, and sequences of sound act
auto-suggestively as emotional stimuli.

Rhythm.—This is the basis of dancing—the most primitive of our
artificial manners of ecstatic expression.   But it gives music its
" time " and poetry its " metre ", and is employed by decorative
art to regularize patterns.   It is, then, one of the artist's most
attractive materials.   It is first appreciated as harmony in movement—the harmony of equality between progressive intervals that
maintains itself irrespective of their sub-division.   Our primitive
ideas of it are gained from ourselves, for we are naturally rhythmic
in our movements of walking and running.   Feelings of rhythmic

movement appeal to a fundamental liking for that which is continuous, and is, therefore, accordant with expectation.

This is *sensory* harmony. There is also an *emotional* harmony in rhythm—that between emphasis or rapidity (and their contraries) and particular states of feeling. In certain moods our actions and utterances are instinctively more lively than in others : from earliest infancy there is a natural correspondence between feeling and energy of expression. The movements of grief and regret are slow and languid : those of joy and triumph quick and well-marked. A funeral march and a dance are harmoniously appropriate to the moods which they represent. But, through their auto-suggestive effect, they may make themselves harmonious by stimulating the feelings that go with them.

Since the harmony of rhythm is æsthetically pleasing, man has found pleasure in elaborating ideas of it. In dancing one actively expresses them, and at the same time is auto-suggestively—that is to say passively—impressed by them. This passive enjoyment can be obtained by watching others dance. By the combination of two or more persons, dancing gradually evolves into the modes of the ballet and the ball-room. And, since rhythmic steps occasion, and are accompanied by, rhythmic sounds, rhythm can use sound as its vehicle. The attraction of the drum is world-wide. In like manner rhythm extends itself to speech ; if, in the course of a processional march, one recites as he paces, his words adapt themselves to his pacing and become metrical. So the Sagas were cast in metre, and metre became, so to speak, the vehicle of emotional speech. By a similar process rhythm was imported into music as its " time ". And, finally, a rhythmic effect is produced to the eyes by the repetition of a decorative pattern at regular intervals. It is not improbable that these repetitions were originally intended to symbolize movement—that they were man's first attempt to obtain the effect of the cinema.

When rhythm accords with feelings, it possesses a " subjective " harmony which is one of its greatest charms. The slow beat of Handel's *Comfort ye*, the wavering time of Chopin's Nocturnes, are, for instance, in inspiring accord with feelings of distressed endurance, and with the vague sentiments that follow one another with varying intensity during lonely *reverie*.

Music.—This can be very simply defined as the harmonious in sound. But it is not so easy to define the precise nature of musical harmony. It is a fact that musical notes are rarely pure—that they are generally accompanied by a number of over-tones, or harmonics, which can be distinguished by one of good musical ear. The constitution of a note is, therefore, complex : it includes a number of elements which could prompt a composer by suggesting one another. It is also a fact that in the simplest harmonious intervals (the fifth, the fourth and the third) the vibratory rapidities of the two notes are in simple ratios to one another, so that one leads to the other more or less easily. But these acoustic realities are far from explaining all the intervals that are used in musical composition, and, in particular, the introduction of discords. Moreover, the " tempered " scale of European music is out of precise accord with them. It is, then, obvious that the harmonious relation of one note to another must depend a great deal upon " subjective " feeling ; and harmony in music can, it seems, be most adequately explained as the connection between two notes that leads one to suggest another, arising in part from the acoustic relationship of the two, and in part from a familiarity between them that is brought about by an acquired habit of ear—that is to say, by a refinement of musical discrimination. The effect of familiarity in " generating " harmony is shown by the fact that most people welcome music which they *know*—that is to say, the successions and chords of which are *expected*. And since habits crystallize the results of efforts of trial, they may vary greatly from one people, or period, to another, and we can understand why Europeans and Asiatics are each incapable of appreciating the other's music.

The tendency of one note to suggest another that is in acoustic or conventional accord with it would account for our insistent demand that a discord should be resolved harmoniously. Its resolution is pleasurable ; and it, accordingly, appears that music owes much of its charm to the process of intensification by shock. A vast number of its progressions and chords are in themselves unsatisfying : standing alone, or ending a phrase, they produce an uncomfortable sense of incompleteness which is dispelled by the notes which follow them. This is particularly the case with discords. They are deliberately introduced in order to be resolved.

Music must have commenced with singing—very possibly with attempts to imitate the cries of animals or the songs of birds. The " chanty " and the " folk-song " were the earliest artistic developments of melodic possibilities. The pleasing effect of chorded notes, and of certain chords in succession, was discovered through a combination of voices, some of which were at variance with the others in phrase or in time. Instruments could be substituted for the voice when it was discovered that they could render the same notes as the voice. Time introduced itself either through marching as one sung or played, or through a drum accompaniment. From these humble beginnings modern music has evolved in stages that are definitely traceable. Musical composition is, of course, mainly a deliberate process. But it must have emotion behind it if it is to be doubly harmonious—if it is to develop the harmony between music and feeling as well as that between one note, or phrase, and another. This emotion may be a feeling that has arisen independently of the composition and is expressed by it, as, for instance, in the case of a love song. Or it may be a sentiment that is auto-suggestively stimulated by the composition—a consequence which has the effect of rendering it emotionally expressive, instead of being merely an ingenious arrangement of pleasing sounds. It is through this process of auto-suggestion—arising from either instinctive or conventional association—that music becomes " emotional " to those who listen to it.

The drama, fiction and poetry.—Dancing and music express and stimulate emotion by the elaboration of expressions of emotion. The drama, fiction and poetry express and stimulate it by imaginative elaboration—by the creation, or invention, of personalities and attendant circumstances. Both personalities and circumstances may be founded on fact, as well as wholly imaginary. In poetry the poet's own feelings are often the chief subject of his meditations.

Apart from subjective feeling, a personality is only a marionette, and the artist, to be " convincing ", must be sympathetically inspired by the feelings of his characters. Feeling can, however, only be presented objectively—through the movements of speech, facial changes, gestures or conduct. These may be presented by the artist from one or other of two standpoints—that of the actor or the spectator. In the first case, its presentation is *imitative*, for he imitates in speech or action ideas of speech or action that are in his mind. In the second case it is descriptive. And, as a spectator, he may comment upon his characters and circumstances, and criticise them.

The actor can present by imitation facial changes, gestures and conduct as well as speech. Attendant circumstances are presented theatrically, in semblance. Acting begins with children as a spontaneous, almost thoughtless—mimicry of what has been seen or heard, inspired by admiration for it. Children play with the " grand ", not the ordinary. But their ideas of grandeur may not be those of adults. To them the engine-driver may appear to be more powerful than a king. Play becomes more elaborate as it passes from the spontaneous into the effortful. The dramatist can imitatively present his characters only through their speech, using written instead of spoken words. So far he impersonates, or " acts ", in turn, each of his characters. For the presentation of facial changes, gestures and conduct—and of attendant circumstances—he uses description, passing from the stage to the seat of a spectator. The novel or romance carries the use of description still further. All pretence of dramatic " play " is abandoned, and the author reverts to the descriptive art of the " story-teller ". This in its primitive stage as old as " play ". It began in such spontaneous—almost thoughtless—fancyings, as are illustrated by the fairy-tales and legends of ancient days, and has always demanded a gift of imaginative sensibility, which, under the guidance of the will, evolves into the artistic creativeness of the novelist. This may be used to interest, amuse or inspire. In the latter case the author must be moved by emotional sympathy with his characters : he must admire or pity the behaviour and thoughts which he personifies.

The drama and the story assume a poetical form when their descriptions are thrown into metrical language, or embellished by the harmony of rhyme. Poetry is commonly distinguished as epic, and lyric—terms which indicate differences of origin. Epic poetry began in the bardic rhapsody, declaimed to such pacing as is illustrated by Highland pipers : lyric poetry in song chanted to an instrumental accompaniment. But a more practical difference between the two is that epic poetry deals with several personalities, lyric poetry with one. The former is an *ensemble :* the latter may be likened to a *pas seul.* The character that is personified in lyric poetry may be the poet's self : his work thus assumes a " meditative " cast. But, indeed, whether he writes dramatically, epically or lyrically, it is his own feelings and thoughts that he describes. He is *acting* in all cases ; and it is as unreasonable to judge his real character by his imaginative sentiments as to assume that a comedian is happy at home because he keeps an audience in roars of laughter.

Painting and sculpture.—These also express by imitation, but by imitation that records itself in material. For when a painter represents a subject, whether perceived by his senses or figured in his mind, he imitates its outlines by movements of his hand and fingers. There is an identity between form and movement, for it is only through tactile movements that we realize form. Imitation of this kind is more difficult than the dramatic or descriptive, and has evolved by slower steps.   In all time the excellence of the Homeric poems will hardly be surpassed ; but when they were composed, Greek painting and modelling were in their infancy.

Architecture.—This is an artistic expression when it serves no material purpose.   The uses for which a temple, a church, and a cathedral is designed are immaterial, and these buildings are amongst the flowers of Art—indeed, a Gothic cathedral is perhaps its finest flower.   Their construction was inspired by religious admiration—one of the strongest of sentiments : exalted by this feeling—at a period when dwelling-houses were generally mean and inconspicuous—man reared religious edifices which surpass the most magnificent structures of the present day.

Applied Art.—When architecture sets itself to dignify the useful, it is applied, not pure Art, and we rank its effects on a lower plane, since the practical is less inspiring than imaginative enthusiasm. But our debt to applied art is immense.   We owe to it all that is beautiful in our dwellings, our furniture and our dress.   The application of art to embellish the useful is the natural consequence of the evolutionary process which has led to the development of modern civilization.   Under the pressure of this tendency romance learns to subordinate itself to utility, that is to say, to become ancillary to prudence.

Canons of Art.—The appreciation and criticism of Art is influenced so greatly by the fashion of the day that one may doubt whether there are any enduring standards by which to judge it.   In these days, poems, pictures and music are commended which, fifty years ago, would have been ridiculed.   It seems, however, that there are three canons which the artist must observe if his work is to be judged as " High Art ".   In the first place, his principal theme must either be *admirable* through its strength or harmony, or must arouse pity or pathos ; it must be an idea that excites emotion, apart from the *technique* of its expression, and it must not merely astonish, amuse, or entertain us.   In the second place, its expression must be skilful. And thirdly, its expression must conform to Nature *in its relationships*, however artificial it may be in its personalities, its materials, or its colouring.   Shapes and positions must be as they are in experience.   Movements must be correctly indicated.   If life is depicted, the sequences of emotion and thought must be natural. The theme which music develops must not violently conflict with acoustic relationships, and should have some subtle connection with a spontaneous expression of emotion.   If Art scoffs at Nature in these essential qualities it rapidly degenerates into the grotesque.

8 Modern Civilization

Modern civilization differs sharply in a number of characteristics, not merely from those of antiquity, but from that of two centuries ago. New ambitions have opened out as experience has discovered new avenues to success—through titles, possessions, art, literature, science, politics and sport ; and these new interests diversify men's aspirations as new tastes do their dinner tables. But these complexities of pursuit are of small account compared with the change of mentality which comes about through the systematic subordination of impulse to reflection. Amongst the consequences of this change are two of outstanding importance. By the reflective comparison of himself with others a man becomes conscious of his own inferiority, if they are his superiors. He resents this discordant feeling by asserting his independence or " liberty ". His disposition towards the power or authority of others is very different to that of the days when men accepted the state of life in which it had pleased God to call them. And, in the second place, reflection breeds prudence, which grows as prospects become assured and the future is discernible with greater probability. At the same time there is a tendency to materialism which shows itself in the preference of objective to subjective values—that is to say, of sensory pleasure to that of feeling—and is particularly evident in a desire to make profit by the industrial or commercial exchanges that are offered by the development of money and credit. Another distinctive feature of the present day is the attention paid to science. This is fostered by the utility of science in increasing comfort, pleasure and amusement, and in yielding a commercial profit. The wonderful scientific discoveries of our time are, in great measure, the products of these incentives.

We may, then, distinguish the most notable peculiarities of modern civilization as the growth of independence, of prudence, of materialism, of commercial exchange, and of science.

It is difficult to make a dispassionate comparison between present conditions and those of which we read—or which we may remember —in the past. For, in the first place, our reverence for the old inclines us to depreciate the new—a feeling that has led to the romantic conception of a Golden Age that has passed away. And, secondly, the bent of the present days is practical rather than ideal, and the latter is by far the more inspiring, and, therefore, the more admirable, of the two. Prudence lacks the fire of enthusiasm: it is useful, not joyful. And, if our conclusions are correct, it represents the domination of the masculine by the feminine element.

Independence.—This feeling evinces itself in a desire for " self-realization " or " self-determination ", and in the growing power of what are called " class consciousness " and " national consciousness ". These vague words euphemistically signify a jealous anxiety not to feel inferior to others—an attitude which illustrates very strikingly the effect of a growing " objectivity " of outlook. For one whose thoughts are not engrossed by his environment obtains superiority or dignity " subjectively " through himself. But those whose thoughts are mainly of their surroundings feed these feelings " objectively " by comparing themselves with others : indeed, they appear to lose their powers of " subjective " self-observation. Self-appraisement by comparison breeds jealousy. For the impression of another's superiority calls up the correlative idea of one's own inferiority. This is distasteful and is resented. Hence in these days the poor disclaim inferiority to the rich by imitating their dress and manners—pretensions that would be scouted in the East, and were, until recent years, unknown in Europe. They would rather be herded in the slums than see houses built for them with accommodation that falls short of the " respectable ". They resent charity that implies patronage, whereas in India no dignity is lost by the acceptance of famine relief. Progressive government is therefore far more difficult in England than in India, since practical good sense must be balanced against sentimental prejudices, that are, after all, but the outcome of self-conceit.

Liberty represents freedom, not so much from authority, as from the galling sense of being inferior to others. Accordingly a Trades Unionist can pride himself upon its possession although he is actually in servitude. The desire for it yields to feelings of respect, whether heart-felt or merely habitual : discipline is not resented in the regiment if the colonel attracts respect by his character, or the habit of respect has not been undermined. In the East the idea of liberty evokes no more enthusiasm than it did in the Middle Ages. Its cult is a sign of advanced " objective " civilization. It can be reconciled with the acceptance of another's authority if this is derived from ourselves. We are not inferior to one who has been elected by our votes. Nor are we humiliated by the defeat of our side at the polling station, since we are defeated, not by an individual, but by numbers. For a similar reason we prefer the authority of a committee to that of a person.

It does not seem, then, that anything particularly " noble " has evolved from the modern tendency to appraise ourselves, not subjectively in ourselves, but objectively through comparison with others. But it has borne very excellent fruit in widening our feelings of pity. For, since another's inferiority implies our superiority, we turn to his assistance with pleasure. We are, consequently, disposed to feel compassionate towards all whose conditions are inferior to our own—including " dumb " animals. The East is a stranger to this broad sympathy for the poor, afflicted or weak ; there, if one gives, it is for a " subjective " reason—to " acquire merit ". And the Middle Ages seem to have been untouched by this feeling. It may degenerate into a " flabby " indiscriminate sentimentality. But it is an honour to human nature, nevertheless.

A less estimable consequence of the appraisement of dignity by comparison is the development of strong class and national consciousness. The dignity of our class and our country is our own, since we are identified with them. But when this dignity is not an absolute existence in itself, but is relatively established by a comparison with others, it is jealous, and urges class against class and nation against nation in an antagonism which is an ever-present danger to hopes of peace. And this attitude of aggressive self-assertion bears other unwholesome fruit. It is fatal to the " knowledge of oneself " which philosophy has set before us as the highest of ideals. For we cannot bear information or arguments that lessen our self-esteem. *La bêtise humaine* is due more to self-conceit than to stupidity, and is by no means dispelled by modern civilization.

Prudence.—To be prudent is to be influenced by the future. That there is a future is impressed upon us by the process of associative re-stimulation. The more regular are our memories of the past the more definite will be our expectations of the future. For the future is a " forward " reflection of the past. There is action and reaction between prudence and the future. For the clearer is the future the greater is the incentive to be prudent ; and prudence declines if the future becomes obscured, as was shown very clearly by the effect of the war upon manners of life. On the other hand, prudence conduces to the regularity of our experiences, and is, therefore, constantly stimulating its own growth by rendering the future more and more definite. As a people becomes more civilized, it becomes more prudent, and, as it becomes more prudent, it becomes more civilized.

Prudence is in the strongest possible contrast to both impulse and idealism. Such mottoes as " Safety First " and " Business is Business " are the contrary of idealistic ; and, whereas idealism admires, prudence is disposed " nil admirari ". It is prudent in war to lessen an adversary's chances by overwhelming numbers ; and one is astonished in these days to read of generals, at the time of the Renaissance, who, on discovering that their forces outnumbered those of an opponent, reduced them, so as to fight on equal terms. During the Maori war our savage antagonists, seeing that our ammunition was exhausted, ceased firing until a fresh supply was brought up. A victory won by numbers is effective. But it is not romantic, and we can understand why the peoples of India and Egypt were not greatly impressed by our conquest of the Germans. And prudence is less happy, and therefore less inspiring, than idealism or romance. We acknowledge this in calling it a "bourgeois virtue". If we scan the faces of our fellow travellers in a city-borne train, how little do we see of the gaiety of life I Can the people of " Merrie England " have looked so glum ?

And it seems clear that prudential habits of mind have a depressing effect upon human energy. The prudent no doubt possess the feminine attribute of pertinacity. But they lack the masculine spirit which can rise to meet great emergencies. Their chosen instrument being persuasion, they over-value the effect of diplomatic speeches, and are taken aback when confronted with obstinate hostility. The civilizations of antiquity fell, it seems, before barbarian conquests because they temporized in order to save immediate interests, putting their faith in conciliatory expedients, and failing to recognize that active opposition must be met in an active spirit. Modern civilization is threatened by dangers of another kind—those of communistic revolution ; and one may doubt whether it will be able to maintain itself against the attacks of the multitudes who consider themselves to be victimized by vested interests—attacks which spring from jealousy, but are strengthened by idealism.

Contracts, or agreements, are instruments for assuring prudence, and prudence consequently regards them with immense respect. The " sanctity of contract " is ever upon our lips. But, in itself, an agreement—even when it is based upon mutual persuasion without pressure on either side—has no greater sanctity than generosity, gratitude or loyalty. These cannot, however, be enforced by law. As securities they are, therefore, imperfect, and prudence regards them somewhat cynically.

But, if the will can devise instruments for securing honesty, it is none the less true that it is the origin of deceit. For we deceive others by the voluntary repression or reversal of spontaneous manifestations. Very small children not uncommonly tell falsehoods. But these are the spontaneous outcomes of apprehension which reverses positive ascriptions into negative. " I did eat it " becomes " I did not eat it ", as " I will jump it " becomes " I will not jump it ". Deliberate deceit is the fruit of the will—and generally of prudent calculation.

We must, however, be fair to prudence. It gives us inestimable blessings in the peace, orderliness and comfort of civilized life. The wider is our acquaintance with the history of the past, the less likely shall we be to under-rate these advantages. Prudence has given us modern law, and has marked itself upon morality. It is more dependable than idealism. For this grows cold, whereas prudence increases with its exercise.

The mind and the body are so closely connected that a change in mentality may not improbably affect bodily functions. One of the most striking features of modern civilization is the decline in the birth-rate. This occurs only amongst the prudent classes of the population. With our prejudice in favour of the objective, we attribute it to voluntary material causes. But one can hardly be satisfied that these are adequate explanations of so vital a change, which may well be the effect upon the reproductive organs of a habit of mind that is out of accord with man's natural promptings.

Materialism.--The commonest reproach urged against modern civilization is that it is " materialistic ". By this is meant that the things which are known to us by the senses are valued more highly than those which impress us through feeling—that the objective comes to rank above the subjective. There can be no doubt that a change actually takes place in this direction—that, as man becomes sophisticated, there is a growth in his appreciation of sensory pleasure and a decline in his appreciation of the " spiritual ". This remarkable evolutionary trend may be attributed, in part, to the influence of the development of the will upon our sensibilities. For the will is emphatically an *objective* force : it sways our behaviour independently of feeling—operates so to speak, the transmitter and receiver without the intervening current. There is a contributing cause in the fact that sensory sensibility is continually developing new tastes, whereas that of feeling is stereotyped. A good conscience may be worth more than a glass of beer, but not so much as a chance of champagne to one who has acquired a taste for it. Sensation tends, therefore, to eclipse feeling by multiplying its pleasure. Food, dress and amusements offer us a hundredfold more attractions than those which tempted the ancients of Homer's time or our ancestors of the Middle Ages.

Of all these changes the most important is the recognition of *possession* as the material, " sensible ", symbol of power. Individual proprietorship—save, perhaps, for things in actual current use— is not based upon any instinctive promptings. Man has no such irrational impulse to hoard as may be observed, for instance, in jackdaws. His first conception of property was that of something which belonged to the tribe, the village, or the family. Even cultivated fields were only occupied for use, and were liable to be periodically redistributed. Under the joint family system that still survives in India, a man of however exalted station remits his income to the head of his family—to his elder brother it may be— and receives from him an allowance for his private expenses. Property has tended to become individualized because all men desire power and the " possession " of things expresses power in a visible form. Viewed in this light a man's possessions are estimable *qualities* of a material kind : they are attached to him as are his features, his agility or his courage, and augment the esteem in which he is held by himself and others. This evolution has not yet completed itself in India. There the millionaire still ranks far below the ascetic : material power is outclassed by spiritual. This was also the opinion of the Middle Ages : the friar was honoured, the money-lender abhorred. It has faded into an unpractical sentiment. The sanctity that is now honoured is that of property.

This fundamental change of mentality is imperfectly realized by us because it is so difficult to put ourselves in our ancestors' place and feel as they felt. For ideas such as theirs are smothered by the educational influences to which we have been subjected from childhood. They still find some sympathy amongst the poorer classes : men who have no expectation of riches look for power elsewhere. But amongst the better classes wealth is almost synonymous with power. It is not merely an instrument of pleasure, but an object of ambition.

We can find many other striking illustrations of this evolutionary tendency to prefer the objective to the subjective. Conventional morality earns more credit than Christian feelings because it is more " practical " and impresses the senses. Decency is thought more of than virtue. Skill is more attractive than inspiration, for one can *see* it. Merit is less valued than popularity, for popularity is the visible recognition of merit. Shame is less feared than reprobation, since failure does not become " objective " until it is " found out ".

Indeed, one can avoid objective discomfiture by " putting a good face " on his actions—that is to say, by palliating them. To be popular, journalism must find excuses for national errors of the past, and must not attempt to draw lessons from them.

Industrial and commercial exchange.—The process of exchange lies at the very root of industrial life. A cultivator obtains his crops in industrial exchange for his labour and skill, precisely as a factory hand earns his wages. There is also an exchange of energy or skill for something material when services of any kind are rendered for pay. But in this case the exchange is termed " unproductive " because nothing new is created. In a commercial exchange both of the things exchanged are material—goods of some kind, money, or a claim to receive money with its correlative obligation to pay it. They are exchanged because each of them " overcomes " the other— that is to say, overcomes the owner's reluctance to part with it. This capacity to overcome is expressed as its worth or " value "—a word which is, of course, akin to " valour ". Accordingly, an exchange is a correlative relationship between two things, each of which is superior to the other ; the value of each thing is primarily measured by that which it overcomes. If a pair of boots can *command* 20 loaves of bread, they are " worth " 20 loaves.

An exchange is, therefore, profitable to both parties : otherwise it would not take place. But in addition to this two-fold " motiving " profit, there is generally a *surplus*, interceptible, profit of very considerable amount. The bootmaker may be willing to give a pair of boots for 18 loaves : the baker to offer 22 loaves for them. The minimum value of each product is its cost to its owner : its maximum value is determined by the other's desire to obtain it. The existence of this surplus profit stimulates other persons to intervene for its capture. It is the incentive of commerce—the origin of capital—as surplus energy is the cause of evolution in life. It is increased by the rise in " desire-values " which follows the growth of wealth. Consequently, since it is the pro-ducer of wealth, it is continuously increased by the action of its own product. It is the source from which the professional, as well as the mercantile classes, ultimately derive their income—and from which taxes are met. Its distribution between the various classes that live upon it may be adjusted by competition, or commanded by " combines ". Unfairness in its distribution is the perennial cause of economic unrest.

Until the invention of money—some 3,000 years ago—exchanges could hardly be of much commercial importance. There was not much inducement to intercept surplus profit when it took the form of goods of some kind. The discovery of money ranks with that of fire in its revolutionary effect upon human manners. By giving objective existence to the *quality* of value (and thereby *materializing* surplus profit) it immensely stimulated and facilitated the process of exchange. It has undergone many evolutionary transformations. To begin with, it was metallic " cash ", which, by reason of its universal attractiveness, could be substituted, in the process of exchange, for goods of any kind. For, being universally desired, it represented and materialized value in the abstract. And, since pieces of metal can be subdivided without any loss of value they could be employed to make up a graduated measure of value. Tokens, which guaranteed a claim to receive definite things or services, could be substituted for the precious metals, since they possessed the value of what they represented. When the State assumed the business of coining, it could use its authority to issue official tokens. These might be guaranteed by their convertibility into precious metal. Or they might be unguaranteed except by the influence of the State in rendering them conventionally acceptable.

Cash in the precious metal is valuable in itself. Guaranteed tokens are also intrinsically valuable because they represent cash or valuable goods and can be changed into them. But the value of conventional unguaranteed tokens simply depends upon the proportion between the number current and the number required, and is violently disturbed if they are issued too liberally. Governments have been continually debasing money by the issue of tokens as an inexpensive means of meeting their obligations—to the prejudice of the country's trade. For a measure of value that fluctuates defeats all commercial calculations. The shilling, which was once 1-20th of a pound of silver, is now less than 1-80th of a pound. The debasement of money has, however, had an incidental effect that has been productive of public good, although of great private hardship. It has alleviated the load of debt which, whether through extravagance, foolish speculation, or unavoidable misfortune, tends to outgrow the endurance of a community. It has, in fact, acted like proceedings in bankruptcy or the Mosaic jubilee.

Just as the quality of value can be abstracted from a commodity and be materialized in money, so can the value of money be abstracted from it, as an expectation of receiving money, and be employed in exchange. This is " credit ". One who purchases on credit gives an " obligation " as his payment, and the tradesman receives a correlative " claim " against him. The expectation may be that of receiving interest in place of repayment. So has grown up the enormous structure of modern " investment ". Invested expectations become the objects of exchange in themselves (as in buying and selling stocks and shares), and their fluctuating value has stimulated a gigantic system of gambling which differs in no essential particular from betting on races or football matches.

" Wealth " is not, of course, welfare or happiness. It consists in material things which are objective assurances of certain potentialities. These may be of enjoyment, such as of comfort, dignity or amusement. Or they may be potentialities of production, that render it possible to create more wealth. They are realized by the " investment " of wealth—that is to say, by its conversion into *capital*. So employed it reproduces itself like a living organism, whether it is devoted to making things or exchanging them. For each exchange produces a surplus profit, which would not exist without it, and is materialized in money.

We ordinarily think of capital as consisting of things, such as buildings, machinery, raw materials and money, the latter being very generally borrowed on the strength of an obligation to pay interest. But it may be wholly immaterial, as when it takes the " subjective " form of the influence over a number of customers that is called " good-will ". And it is similarly immaterial when it is a " money-value " that is unsupported by money. This is so if it is raised by an over-draft upon a bank. When trade is flourishing and capital is in demand, a bank can create it by permitting a client to overdraw, since his demands can be met very simply by making contrary entries in his account and in the accounts of the clients who present his cheques. Transactions between the various clients of a bank can be settled without any money payments. A bank can, therefore, lend " money-value " in excess of its assets, and draw profit from the loan of money which does not actually exist.

Capital is productive by employing men or machines to make or procure things which are valuable because they are desired. Without a desire there can be no value. The difference between the " cost-value " and the " desire-value " of the product—that is to say, the surplus profit—may be shared between labour, the capitalist who employs the labour, or distributes its products, and the consumer. The latter may, in favourable circumstances, enjoy a considerable portion of it, by being able to purchase at a lower price than he is willing to pay. There are then three competitors for the profits—

labour, capital (producing and distributing) and the consumer. Unless the working classes can protect themselves from the effects of an overcrowding of the market, they receive little more than bare subsistence, for they respond to offers of employment by increasing their numbers, so that there are more who want work than can obtain it. They have been ruthlessly exploited by capital in the past, and the slums of modern cities still abound with such misery and degradation as one can hardly find in savage life. Trades Unions have raised wages by limiting competition, and by the use of strikes as a means of extorting concessions. They have a third instrument at their disposal—the limitation of output. But this obviously stunts the growth of capital, and must in the long run be injurious to the employed by restricting the openings for employment. Capital, again, combines against the workers by " lock-outs", and against the consumer by the formation of rings or trusts which raise prices much above competition limits. Modern methods of manufacture afford the workers no opportunity for ambition, except under piece-work rules ; and these are discredited because rates are reduced if industry is too successful in earning money. Work becomes intolerably dull. Hence, under the name of Socialism, labour demands the abolition of capital. Commercial civilization gives us peace in the streets. But it shakes the foundations of communal life by developing these antagonistic interests.

It is easy to condemn the capitalist system, and the increasing effort for gain which is its motive. But it is as easy to prove that, without it, civilized nations could not maintain their present numbers. Socialism would have capital without capitalists. This, however, would be capital without the ambition to use it—the objective instrument without the subjective " drive " that works it, and would be as ineffective as a locomotive without its steam. The State can do much to protect labour—and perhaps something to protect consumers—from excessive exploitation. And, by means of an Income Tax, it can enable the community as a whole to share in the capitalists' successes. This, it seems, is as far as its interference can go without blunting the ambition upon which productiveness ultimately depends. And, we must remember, that under the capitalist system, labour, with some assistance from the State, has won its way to what half a century ago would have seemed to be a condition of fantastic prosperity.

Science.—The present day is pre-eminently that of Science. Its discoveries, by enabling us to harness the mysterious forces by which we are surrounded have opened out to us a new life of movement, production and enjoyment.   As these possibilities have been perceived, increasing ingenuity has been employed to discover by experiment methods of utilizing the unknown.   But science is not, of course, wholly utilitarian.   An immense amount of research is devoted to the accumulation of new facts—in such domains as that of astronomy, natural history and anthropology—which cannot well possess any practical bearings.   There is success in discovering things, and discoveries are accordingly satisfying in themselves. They do not necessarily lead to reasoning, and they have not been used to the fullest possible extent for the formulation of laws, or the detection of clues which would connect them with laws.   Generalization has further been impeded by the " exclusiveness " of the various sciences by the view that they represent different kinds, and not merely different aspects of Nature.   Progress has consequently been halting.   Researches into the genesis and early history of mankind, for instance, would have been more fruitful had they taken into ampler account the information that is given by man's anatomy as to his essential natural requirements.

We are naturally proud of our scientific accomplishments.   But our knowledge is merely surface deep : it shows us only the material consequences of ethereal forces that altogether elude our senses and our comprehension.   Indeed, it actually seems to emphasize our ignorance.   Reviewing a life of strenuous endeavour, Lord Kelvin —perhaps the most successful man of science of our days—confessed his failure :   I know no more of electric and magnetic force, or of the relations between ether, electricity and ponderable matter, or of chemical affinity, than I knew and tried to teach to my students of natural philosophy 50 years ago in my first session as Professor." But we need not accept it as impossible to penetrate the veil which hides the real from us.   There are in all probability analogies of relationship between the perceivable and the unperceivable, which will, in time, be used as clues to a deeper understanding.

Progress.—Most of us are convinced that our civilization is " progressive "—that it is something higher and better than conditions which have preceded it.   Yet there are those who stoutly maintain that its prudent materialism is decadent ; and in India it has aroused passionate contempt.   We cannot bring its merits to a decisive test, for we are unable to dis-embarrass our minds of two contrary standards—the masculine and the feminine.   We admire romance, with its ideals of self-control, magnanimity and chivalry.   We also value prudence.   Yet romance scorns prudence, and prudence sneers at romance.

Material civilization has immensely increased the capacity for sensory pleasures. It, therefore, encourages luxury and sets a high value upon comfort. On the other hand, its deliberative mentality dulls the spirits and renders amusement a necessity. The successes at which it aims are objective—those which are realized through the behaviour of others towards us : consequently the most flagrant breaches of moral rules may be condoned if they lead to notoriety. Self-respect that rests upon comparison of self with others is hurt by any suggestions of relative inferiority. Accordingly, persuasion is preferred to command as a means of influencing others. Heresy is tolerated because under the reign of persuasion it is impossible to persecute freedom of speech. Violence is condemned, since it upsets calculations, and in defiance of experience there is an endeavour to believe that " force is no remedy ". The masculine spirit of antagonism is quelled by prudence : to " manage " an adversary, instead of directly opposing him, is a feminine characteristic, and, accordingly, women can reasonably be admitted to political privileges. A social orderliness is attained that would be impossible under romantic conditions. The mental habit of assessing oneself by comparison with others engenders a sentimental pity for those whose inferiority is exalting to ourselves. This patronizing sympathy, however unpretentious be its origin, has been of immense benefit to mankind. It ordained the abolition of slavery and the humanizing of imprisonment : it maintains hospitals : it brightens the life of slum children with playgrounds and play centres ; and it contributes very largely to such benevolent legislation as the grant of old age pensions, and the early closing of shops. It seemed to render war " unthinkable " until disillusion came in 1914.

On the other hand materialistic tendencies seriously conflict with the magnanimous virtues. For these, it is assumed, " do not pay ": they are said to be " their own reward." Modern history furnishes many large-scale illustrations of their declining influence. During the Crimean war Russia continued to pay dividends to enemy creditors—an example of chivalrous fidelity which seventy years later seemed impossibly foolish. How great is the contrast between the peace that followed Waterloo and that of Versailles ! The sacrifice of our alliance with Japan to American interests must have struck the East as the reverse of high-minded. We console ourselves with the thought that magnanimity is " quixotic "—that it is not " good business ". But, nevertheless, in our hearts we cannot help admiring its strength. In applauding the " state-craft " that is its opposite, our conscience is not at ease with itself. And it is not true that magnanimity does not pay. The spectre of revenge which still looms over Europe might have been laid by some " great-heartedness " in making peace. The class war with which we are threatened would be exorcised if capital showed more of the " sporting spirit " in its dealings with labour. There is no lesson which needs teaching to the younger generation more urgently than that prudence is to be tempered with generosity.

9 Language

" Language," it has been said, " is not a system of symbols, but a living instrument of expression." This is rhetoric not reason. For if speech were a living, not an artificial activity, it would not vary from nation to nation—almost, indeed, from village to village ; and its character would not entirely depend upon the influence of our environment during childhood. It is true that the evolution of language has proceeded from a natural source. But the forms into which it has grown are as artificial as our clothes. Its words are fabricated signals. They are, nevertheless, operated by a force that is a marvel of living activity. Between thoughts and words there is such an intimate connection as between the keys of a piano and the notes which it sounds. Far more intimate indeed. For the process of piano-playing cannot be *reversed*—the sounds cannot move the keys ; whereas speech not only expresses ideas but recalls them.

The ultimate source of language is the necessity of expressing nervous activity in movement. The urgency of relieving a nervous stress by utterances or actions is felt by everyone who is excited by anger, emulation, triumph, grief, admiration or disappointment. Darwin in his *Expressions of Emotion* contrasts the impatient wriggling and jumping of a dog when it sees its food platter with its quietude when it has settled down to its meal. We think of words as *sounds*, because it is as sounds that the words of others impress us. But in ourselves they are muscular movements of the chest, throat and mouth, which do not differ fundamentally from the cries and grimaces of infancy. If we listen critically to conversation that is passing around us we shall be struck by the large admixture of exclamations and expletives that it contains—indeed, by the number of inarticulate noises that are made, not merely to express approval or disapproval, but to warn, scold or soothe another, and are then on the same plane as the " conversation " of birds. We can, it seems, find an " instinctive " exclamatory use in the vowels. *Ah* seems naturally to express surprise : it goes up from a crowd during an exhibition of fireworks. *Ih* indicates pleasure : it is the vowel of " giggling " : *Uh* vents displeasure : it is an ejaculation of disgust. *Eh* signifies distress or doubt : it is employed as an interrogative. *Oh* calls attention. These natural meanings are overshadowed by the practical uses to which the vowels are put as, for instance, in signifying the various relationships of an idea (*strike, stroke, struck, strake, streak*). But the words *awful, cheerful* and *gloomy* appear to have an auto-suggestive effect. *Eh* seems to have made its mark upon *ache*. *Oh* is employed in the vocative.

It is, as we have seen, a law that the spontaneous evolves into the voluntary. These liberative manifestations of feeling could be made voluntarily when their use in communicating with others was appreciated. It is clear that birds and beasts use their natural cries as signals to one another. But, being bound by instinct, they can rarely initiate new utterances. Man's inventive capacities are, on the contrary, unfettered. That communication with others should be effective, it must be extended from feelings to sensations and ideas, so that, for instance, one can communicate to another, not merely a feeling of alarm, but the *cause* of the alarm. The use of utterances to express *ideas* represents, of course, a prodigious evolutionary step. But nature supplied a point of departure. Since a feeling is intimately associated with a sound, or a movement of expressive utterance, a sensation or idea could also be represented by one. For sensations and ideas are, in fact, " feelings " of a kind. If, for instance, a feeling of repletion can be indicated by a sound, why should not a sound be used to signify the food which caused the repletion ? And, indeed, the close connection between feeling and utterance would, of itself, tend to prompt an impulse to attach utterances to sensations and ideas—that is to say, to give *names* to things. We see this tendency strikingly illustrated in the nursery. Children are never content until they have named their pets and playthings.

Apart from the use of words to express relationships, the development of language is the gradual attachment of names to things. At the outset these signified particular things. But they become general names as things are generalized. If there is no natural clue to a name, it is invented. But Nature affords us a number of clues in the association of certain things with sounds and movements which can be either spontaneously or voluntarily imitated.

Sounds.—The voice can mimic sounds more or less adequately, as is illustrated by such words as *bark, whisper, rattle, shriek, cough, sneeze, thunder,* and perhaps *rain.* A sound can be used to name its cause, since it can be regarded as a quality of its cause. Hence we name a cuckoo by its note, and signify a *saw,* a *hammer* and the netal *tin* by the sounds that they produce. *Foot* (or *pad*) seems to eproduce the sounds of a footfall.

Movements.—Articulations involve movements of the lips and tongue which are, in fact, " gestures ". When once learnt in childhood they become automatic, and elude consciousness unless we force ourselves to attend to them. These movements form the consonants, as opposed to the vowels, of language. If we make them slowly and deliberately we can feel that they can, in some cases, mimic very strikingly the movements of the fingers, arms and legs. A child, learning to write, will automatically accompany the movements of its fingers with movements of its tongue. The classification of consonants as given in grammars is uninstructive because it fails to reduce their articulation to its essential elements. Our instruments for this purpose are the lips, acting one against the other, and the tongue, acting against the palate. We can articulate by (1) touching one with the other ; (2) pressing one against the other ; (3) jerking the two apart ; and (4) rubbing them together. Touchings and jerkings may be light or heavy. And, in each of these cases, the contact may be " breathed "—that is to say, may fall short of completeness. By these movements can be formed all the consonants used in European speech :

	With lips.		With fore-tongue and palate.		With hind-tongue and palate.	
	Complete.	Incomplete.	Complete.	Incomplete.	Complete.	Incomplete.
Touches—light	P	F	T	TH (*thin*)	K	C (Latin)
—heavy	P.	V	D	TH (*this*)	G	CH (*loch*)
Presses	M	FF	N	S	N (*bien*)	CH (*ich*)
Jerks—light	V	W	CH (*child*)	SH	Z	ZH (*ieu*)
—heavy			J	Y		
Rubs	—	—	L	R	LL (*ville*)	R (*rue*)

There is a fact which seems to show that this classification corresponds with intuitive feeling. The alphabetical names of ten of the above consonantal articulations are introduced by a vowel (eM) instead of being followed by one (Be). The ten include all but one of the letters classed as *presses* or *rubs*, and only one (F) that is not so classed : and this letter involves pressure if strongly pronounced.

These articulations enable us to express a good many ideas of movement by imitating in miniature the movements of our limbs. The Scandinavian and German languages have made good use of this capacity. Words such as *push, pull, pinch, run, jump, skip, stop, flap*, will be found to mimic these movements if they be pronounced slowly, and the movements of the lips and tongue be watched. When feelings are accompanied by movements they may be expressed by imitating these movements. It has been plausibly conjectured that *putrid* and *filthy* imitate expirations or expectorations of disgust while *pure* expresses their consequences. We may perhaps assign a similar origin to the words *good* and *bad :* they seem to mimic the movements of swallowing and rejection. *Rough* and *smooth* appear to imitate the impressions which these surfaces make upon our sense of touch. And articulations may be used to signify energy. Such combinations as *str* and *sw* (as in *strike* and *swim*) seem to be expressive of force.

Naming from association.—A thing for which no name suggests itself naturally may be christened after its origin or outcome. Thus *damask* was named from Damascus, and *muslin* from Mosul ; anger of a certain sort is called " indignation " because it is provoked by " unworthiness " : " lady " (*ledig*) is the title given to a woman of free birth. On the other hand, desire is called " longing " because of the tedium which follows it, and a " bit " is the consequence of a bite. Most things are, however, as inexpressible in their origins and outcomes as in themselves, and must be named purely arbitrarily, although it may be that associations which are now unsuspected may have assisted our forefathers with suggestions. May not, for instance, the *s*, which occurs so commonly in different names for the sun, be meant to represent the " whisper of the dawn " ?

Naming by invention.—These imitations and associations do not, however, carry us very far in the creation of a vocabulary. The vast majority of our ideas are named " out of the void " by random efforts. Such is the origin of children's " nursery " words, and the ever-changing vocabulary of slang. If the results are forcible, such as the American " pep " and " stunt ", they " catch on ", as it is said.   In this fashion language is growing under our eyes—as it has grown in the past—in spite of the efforts of purists to stereotype it. We may think it impossible that random effort should ever have produced the materials of a dictionary.   But at the rate of five new words a year a working language would be developed in a dozen generations.   It must be remembered that as new ideas were conceived there was a strong desire for words to express them. What a flood of strange words the science of the last half century has poured into our glossaries !

With so artificial a foundation it was only to be expected that isolated tribes should develop tongues of their own.   It is, on the other hand, surprising that, with few exceptions, all the languages of Europe—with the classical languages of Persia and India—should be traceable to the same spring of invention.   This does not necessarily imply racial affinity.   For history shows that a nation can change its language, as it can change its religion.   The large negro population of America has lost from its speech all traces of Africa. Man has a natural inclination to copy the speech of his conquerors, for, by doing so, he seems to gain superiority.   But this tendency to uniformity is met by one that acts contrary to it—the development of local peculiarities.   These may be due to the influence, upon conquering immigrants, of the peculiar articulation of the children of the soil—or *vice versa ;* or they may merely exhibit the power of localized fashion.   The changes in pronunciation that have occurred are often as great as to entirely obscure a word's kinship : there is apparently nothing in common between the Latin *filius* and its Spanish descendant *hijo.*   They tend to stereotype themselves locally, so that certain changes become characteristic of certain nations or places.   The Scandinavian tongues (including ancient Gothic) differ characteristically from the Teutonic in the use of *th, t* and *d* for *d, tz* and *t* : " the tide " (time) takes the place of " die zeit ".   Northern England pronounces " book " and " pass " as they are spelt.   Southern England defies their spelling.

The adoption of particular verbal changes to signify shades of meaning and relationships to blank ideas, must, it would seem, have been regularized by kingly or priestly influence, exercising such authority as is now conceded to the French Academy.   It is impossible otherwise to explain the uniformity that came about. This is extraordinarily rigid in the Arabic language, which, by certain changes of form, can give to any verbal root the significations of acting, acted upon, and act in the abstract.   But this unifying movement has from time to time been catastrophically reversed by

the convulsions of war.   After the fall of the Roman Empire, Latin
suffered a change which may be likened to liquifaction.   The
Romance languages are crystals that emerged from the cauldron.
There is no reason to believe that Greek or Latin could claim a more
stable ancestry.   It is only in a " patchwork " language that there
would be anomalies and irregularities of declension and conjugation.

Shifts of meaning.—Since the process of associative re-stimulation
adds to an experience suggestions of what has preceded and followed
it, words tend to exchange their original meanings for those of their
origins and outcomes.   A very curious illustration of this (already
mentioned) is given by the word *mercy*, which originally (as *merces*)
meaning a ransom, came to signify the sparing that is the consequence
of a ransom, and then (in the French *merci*) the thanks that are the
consequence of the sparing.   The word *help* is often used to express
the " escaping " that is the consequence of assistance, as in the
phrases " I could not help it ", and " not longer than I can help ".
Connection is used to signify a link which is the consequence of a
linking.   On the other hand a thing is pitiful because it excites pity.
The influence of these associative shifts on the meaning of words has
been very great, and it is surprising that so little notice is taken of it
in our dictionaries.   It compelled the French language to import
words direct from Latin to express meanings which their Roman
derivatives had lost.   *Frêle* had to be supplemented by *fragile*,
meuble by *mobile*, *sembler* by *simuler*, since the original meanings of
" breakable ", " moveable ", and " imitating " had given place to
their outcomes in " delicate ", " furniture " and " resembling ".   So
in English *innocuous* has been adopted to supply the original meaning
of *innocent*, which has come to mean the goodness which is the
cause of harmlessness.

Metaphor.—The use of a word may similarly be extended to a
thing which is connected with its original meaning by a sameness or
analogy.   Its use, then, becomes " metaphorical ".   The use of
metaphor is more general than may be supposed.   It is obvious in
our attribution to the sun of our own movements of " rising " and
" sitting ", and of our movements of " running " to rivers and trains
—similitudes which occur in various languages although expressed
by quite different words.   " Ram " is extended from the animal to
the instrument in Latin, English and French, with words that are
etymologically distinct.   In slang expressions metaphor insinuates
itself into speech in hundreds of fashions.   We use the word " do "
metaphorically when we enquire after another's health, or express
our own fatigue or the cooking of a dish : the verb " get " (go-to) in

the phrases "get beaten " and "getting well ". Metaphors are generally humorous (as when we describe ourselves as " cheap " when below par), and therefore soon gain popular acceptance. Metaphorical extension was carried to a fine art in Greek and Latin. We must marvel at the acuteness of intelligence which could perceive an analogy to *weighing* in " deliberation ", to *reassembling* in " recollection ", to the *interlinking* of things in " intelligence ". The English language is fortunate in that it has added these classical flowers of analogy to the imitative forcefulness of the Scandinavian tongue.

We owe to metaphor the uses of a great number of prepositions, adverbs and conjunctions. Prepositions of place are extended to time. *Of*—meaning " off " one thing in the direction of another—expresses derivation of any kind, as in " he did it of himself ". *By*, signifying " next in succession ", figures metaphorically in *bye-law, before, besides, because, believe* (by like), *by-the-by, bye and bye*, and a *bye* (in games). *For* (" in front " as in *therefore*) is used to express looking forward at, as in *for ever, for shame, forbear* (to be passive onwards) ; and consequently disregarding what is behind, as in *forgive, forget* and *forsake* (behaving without reference to the past). *Since* (akin to *syne*) signifies looking back at. *Ever* seems to indicate repetitive succession : hence *never* means " in no succession " ; *every*, " each in turn " ; *however*, " in the way of succession " ; *nevertheless*, " invalidated by no succession ". The same root seemingly occurs in *verus* and *very ;* the " true " is that which is reiterated ; " very beautiful " is " beautiful, beautiful, beautiful ". *If* (gif) means " given that ". *Yet* (get) is probably akin to " go to " implying a check to an obvious inference ; *still* (stop) has the same sense. *But* is " by out ", meaning " in succession from outside ", and not from the word or sentence preceding. We think much of the discoveries of modern science. But they are hardly more wonderful than the apprehension of these analogies. It has given us the " little words " which are the most durable and distinctive elements of a language, and may be likened to its nerves. The *names* for things may be borrowed from far and wide. But the particles hold their own. They prove that English is a form of Scandinavian (or Gothic) and has no immediate Saxon affinities.

Reference may be made here to an almost incredibly acute appreciation of an analogy between the process of linking one thing with another and the movements of the tongue in touching first the fore and then the hind part of the palate, as in articulating the syllables LIK or LIG. These syllables are the roots of a number of classical and English words that indicate a " connecting ". In Greek and Latin they express *gathering, reading, speaking, thinking*—all of which are connectings—and they enter into the words from which we have derived *legal, logic, analogy, recollecting* and *intelligence*. In English they figure in *link,* and also in the word *like,* with its two senses of favouring and resembling, both of which involve the establishment of a tie.

The inclusion in words of relationships.—Words are modified grammatically to signify their relationships to other words in the same sentence. But over and above these fluctuating changes, others of a permanent character are made to indicate that words bear special *relative* significations. Two words may be amalgamated as in *waist-coat.* Syllables may be prefixed or added. Thus the syllable *di* indicates a relationship of two-fold (as in divide), *dis,* one of contrariety ; *re,* a " spring back " ; *un,* or *in,* a negative. By adding certain syllables to a word the phase of its idea is indicated. Thus the suffix *tion* usually implies a condition ; that of *ment,* an instrument ; *dom* gives an idea of power ; *ty, cy, ce,* denote qualities ; *ly* (like), *y, ful, ish* and *ous,* attributives. The suffix *ness* attached to an attributive, indicates the abstract condition of possessing it—as in *faithfulness.* This expedient illustrates the ingenuity with which our forbears adapted the material to signify the abstract. For *ness* is certainly akin to " nose ", the possession of this feature being taken as analogical to the possession of a quality. Not less ingenious is the use of the suffixes *ship* and *hood* to indicate correlatives (as in *sonship* and *fatherhood*). For these words, it seems, primitively mean a basket and its cover, which not inaptly typify a correlative relationship, since one involves the other and is its contrary.

Grammatical relationships.—Coherent speech, as we have seen, *ascribes* to an individual a phase of relationship—connecting it with an active or passive condition, with a quality, an origin or outcome, with place or time, or with a condition which springs from identity with, resemblance to, or difference from something else. It uses, moreover, one of these relationships to *describe* an individual, or that which is ascribed to the individual ; and may elaborate such a description into an ascriptive form as a dependent sentence. We have already noticed the various expedients by which words are grammatically linked together so as to express these relationships. We may briefly review here what can be gathered as to the course of their evolution.

Grammar is so lifeless a science because it attempts to study a running succession piece-meal ; and, from an intelligent point of view, this is impossible.   Speech is a succession of waves—of rises and falls—of varying lengths.   The former are the important words that are stressed or accentuated—that is to say, the *ascription*, and the various *subjects* of description.   Should each wave be considered as a fall followed by a rise, or as a rise followed by a fall—as an *iambus* (∪ —) or as a *trochee* (— ∪) ?   In the former case a description will precede its subject and will be attached to it (if not an adjective) by a *post-position* or case ending as in " a blackbird's nest " ; and the ascription will be placed at the close of the sentence (a blackbird's nest have I found).   If, on the contrary, the more accentuated precedes the less accentuated, the essence of a sentence —its ascription—will be set at its commencement ; and each subject that is described will precede its description to which (if not an adjective) it will be attached by a *preposition*.   These two orders of syntax, it may be remarked, are illustrated by the two arrangements of a ceremonial procession : in one the chief follows his retinue, in the other he precedes it.   The distinction between the two is of radical importance from the grammatical point of view, and is the most fundamental of the tests that can be employed to classify languages grammatically.   It lies quite apart from their kinship in descent, evidences of which are sought in similarities between individual words.   These, it may be noted, may be misleading. For they may be merely the results of borrowing.   How large is the proportion of borrowed Latin words in English !   Moreover, original similarities may be completely disguised by colloquial changes that occur with great rapidity when languages are not stereotyped by writing.   So dialects that are closely akin may hardly have a single word that is recognizable as common to them—an anomaly that actually occurs amongst the frontier tribesmen of Assam.

The consideration of grammar from the " dynamic " point of view has not received much attention, and words are lacking to express these two contrary lines of expression.   It is not easy to name them, for they are differences between methods of linking ideas together into a chain, for which no words have been coined.   We may use the term " anatropic " for languages, such as Turkish, which by the use of post-positions or case endings lead *up* to a subject, or to an ascription, through its particulars ; and give the name of " catatropic " to those, such as Arabic, which, by the employment of prepositions, run *down* from a subject, or an ascription, to its particulars—as, for instance, in such a sentence as—" Yesterday was concluded the inquest on the bodies of the victims of the aeroplane crash at Croydon on Christmas Eve ". Thrown into an " anatropic " form this would run—" Christmas-eve-on Croydon-at aeroplane-crash-of victims-of bodies-on inquest yesterday concluded was ".

From contact between these two initial types a third has evolved which is intermediate between them. The Homeric poems are an early record of this development. Greek and Latin were originally " anatropic ", like Sanskrit, as is shown by their use of case endings. But they adopted the " catatropic " use of prepositions, and varied the position of the verb. This swing towards catatropy became very pronounced in the Romance languages that sprung from Latin : in them case endings have altogether given place to prepositions. German and English exhibit a similar catatropic trend : they generally use prepositions as connectives, but retain relics of an earlier anatropic stage in the German genitive and dative, and the English possessive case. In all these modern languages the placing of the verb has become very elastic. It normally tends towards the beginning of a sentence ; but, when a German verb includes a past participle, this is relegated to the end. We may use the term " polytropic " to describe this hybrid state, since the succession of words is continually veering from up to down and *vice versa.*

It would, of course, be beyond the scope of this summary to attempt anything of the nature of a complete classification or analysis of past and present languages. But, since the principles that have been outlined are unfamiliar, it is worth while to illustrate them in greater detail.

Archæological research has discovered a curious *liaison* between an anatropic and a catatropic language which occurred so anciently as, perhaps, 4000 B.C. In the valley of the Euphrates, the Sumerian was subverted by the Akkadian culture. The Sumerian language was anatropic, resembling Turkish ; the Akkadian was a catatropic Semitic tongue, akin to Arabic. Indeed, its vocabulary can be interpreted through its analogies with known Semitic languages ; and since its literature comprises glossaries rendering Akkadian into Sumerian, it is possible to interpret the latter. The sentences of the two languages run different ways. The ancient language of Egypt (now represented by Coptic) seems to have evolved from similar clashes between anatropic and catatropic tongues. Characters of both types are mingled in its grammar.

The existing languages of Central and Eastern Asia are of the Turkish, or anatropic, type. They use post-positions, and end their sentences with the verb. This is so with Japanese, and with the Tibeto-Burman dialects that are current over so large an area of the East. Chinese has evolved in the direction of catatropy; prepositions are used as well as post-positions, and the verb has been shifted back. Hindustani closely resembles Turkish in its syntax, having received its stamp from Turkish invaders. It is characteristically anatropic; and it is remarkable that Sanskrit, its ancient predecessor, is also a type of the anatropic style, although the Sanskrit vocabulary is akin to that of the principal European languages, and shows no trace of the Far East.

The existing type of the catatropic style is Arabic. Its sentences characteristically run from the verb downwards; the use of prepositions is universal, and post-positions (or case endings) are unknown. Of this class are the languages that are classed together as "Semitic"—Phœnician, Hebrew and Aramaic. Curiously enough, a catatropic tongue of this kind still survives in the hills of Assam. This is Khasi—a relic of widespread culture now long past—an island in a sea of Tibeto-Burman dialects.

Persian is akin to Sanskrit in its vocabulary. But, probably under Arab influence, it has changed catatropically. Post-positions have been entirely displaced by prepositions. The verb, however, remains at the end of the sentence. It approaches, therefore, the stage which we have called "polytropic"—possessing an elasticity that has earned for it the name of the "French of the East". Greek, Latin and the principal languages of modern Europe are, as we have seen, polytropic. They were, it seems, originally anatropic, like Sanskrit; post-positions (or case endings) are used, or figure in their ancestry. Their trend towards catatropy was no doubt urged by a need of greater freedom of expression. But it may be ascribed in some measure to Semitic influences. Considering how extensively the Greek and Roman worlds were pervaded by these influences—Phœnician (or Carthaginian), Hebrew, Arabic and Aramaic—it would be surprising if their languages had not been grammatically affected. It is noticeable that the Greek of the New Testament differs from that of the classical age in Semitic features—in the extended use of prepositions and the forward shifting of the verb. And it is not unlikely that Arabic influences, extending from the Universities of Spain, similarly affected the development of mediæval Latin, and the Romance languages. Such Latin as that of the *Imitatio Christi*, for example, retains but few of the peculiarities of classical phrasing.

Let us now turn to the various devices that have been employed by mankind to link ideas into connected sentences. And, first, of *ascriptive* syntax.

In Sanskrit, Greek and Latin personal endings were essential characteristics of the verb. They could take the place of separate pronouns, and were not simply used to connect a verb with the substantive that was its subject. That is to say, they were used substitutively as well as connectively. This is still the case in Italian and Spanish. In French and German they have become connectives and nothing more ; in English and other Scandinavian languages they are on the verge of disappearance. They are still used substitutively for pronouns in Turkish, Arabic and Persian. In Chinese, Japanese, and the Tibeto-Burman dialects they have never existed.

They originated, it appears, in the idea that it was more forcible to say, for instance, " hungry I " than " I hungry ". In Turkish, Arabic and Persian personal endings may be attached to any noun or adjective to express its ascription to a person—" wet I " means that " I am wet " ; " money with me ", that " I have money ".

Another essential element of the verb is the signification of present, past and future times, and of various phases of them. A number of different expedients have been adopted to denote them— separate words, interposed letters, prefixes, post-fixes and vowel changes—which probably once had *meanings* that have been effaced from memory by colloquial changes. A remarkable method of signifying the past is by re-duplication, as employed in Sanscrit, Greek and Latin : the backward repetition of a syllable symbolizes a backward repetition of the present into the past. In some cases the original meanings of tense-endings can be traced with probability. In the Romance languages the imperfect and perfect are formed by the addition of the past and present tenses of " having " to the present and past verbal stems, and the future by a similar addition to a third verbal stem—*purposive*, ordinarily called the " infinitive ". Thus " parler*ai* " means " I have to speak ". And there seems reason to believe that the *b* and *v* in *amabam*, *amavi*, and *amabo*, similarly represents the verb *habeo*.

As *auxiliary verbs*, tenses of " being " are used in Arabic, Persian, Greek and Latin, but not in Sanskrit or Turkish. The Romance languages express the past in the present, past and future by employing, as auxiliaries, tenses of " being " or " having ", according as the verb is subjective or objective. In German and English " having " is the auxiliary in both cases ; English is peculiar in the use of " being ", with a present participle, to express a continuing present. The future is expressed in Persian, and in English, by an auxiliary signifying *intention*. In German " becoming " is used to throw a participle into future time.

The variety of the shifts which man has devised to express himself is illustrated by the expedients that are employed for giving a verb a *passive* signification. In Arabic this is imparted by vowel changes. In Sanskrit, Greek and Latin peculiar personal endings were employed, which, it is surmized, were primitively *doublings*, so as to give a reflexive cast, as in the French *je m'ennui*. According to this view the passive first took shape as a subjective reflexive. It could be expressed objectively by the use of the active past participle in combination with an auxiliary verb, since a present passivity is correlative with a past activity *in its cause :* if I am being beaten some one has already begun beating me. In Hindustani tenses of " going " are used as passive auxiliaries to the past participle (I beaten go) : there is a parallel in the English " to get beaten ". Turkish introduces the letter *l* into the active verb—the characteristic letter of the verb " to become ". Persian uses tenses of " becoming " with the past participle. The Romance languages associate the past participle with tenses or participles of " being " preceded by tenses of " having " to express the perfect, or the future past. The English method is similar, using however, " shall " to signify future time. In German passive constructions are exceedingly complicated, the participle being associated with tenses and participles of " becoming " and " being ", the former being employed twice over for the future and the future past.

The most primitive method of attaching its *object* to an active verb is to include it in its meaning, so as to have, for instance, separate words for washing oneself and for washing clothes. If the object is a person, it may be attached to the verb as a pronominal postfix. This is so in Arabic and Persian—and also in Italian and Spanish when the verb is in the infinitive. The Romance languages, generally, link an accusative personal pronoun to its verb by prefixing it to the verb or the verbal participle. Pronouns apart, the object is denoted in Turkish and Hindustani by a postfix, and in Sanskrit, Greek and Latin by a case-ending. This primitively indicated *direction towards*—as in " *Romam* "—a meaning which survives in the Spanish use of the preposition *a* for objects that are persons. In Arabic, in the Romance languages other than Spanish and in English the object is marked simply by its relative position to the verb, which it follows, unless it is a connecting reference to something already mentioned. In Persian a postfix is used—an exception to the normal use of prepositions.

Other qualifications of ascriptions, such as purpose, instrument, method, place and time, when not expressed adverbially, are signified by postfixes (including case-endings), or prepositions according as the language is of the anatropic or catatropic type. In polytropic languages either method is possible. English still places its " prepositions " *after* the words which they attach, when these are adverbs of place or time (*thereupon*).

We pass to *descriptive* syntax. A subject is described as an individual or a particular by the indefinite and definite articles. These now seem to be essential features of speech. But Latin left both to be understood ; and the Greek definite article was really a personal pronoun that was used in great measure to " bracket " a noun with words that defined it. There are no articles in Sanskrit, Turkish, Hindustani or Persian : in the latter, however, a vowel may be added to a noun to signify that it is indefinite. Arabic, on the other hand, possesses a definite article which plays a very important part in its syntax. In the Romance languages the definite article is derived from the Latin demonstrative, and the indefinite from the numeral *one*, used as an indefinite pronoun. This is also the case with the articles in German and English—a similarity of evolution that is remarkable because it starts from different origins. In Danish the pronouns that are used as indefinite articles become definite if they are attached to the end of their nouns.

An adjective is placed anatropically if it precedes, catatropically if it follows its noun. The former is the case in Turkish and Hindustani, the latter in Arabic and Persian. In Greek and Latin the adjective might be separated from its noun since the two were linked together by agreements in case ending, gender and number. There are similar agreements between an adjective and its noun in the Romance languages and German. But the two cannot be separated in speech. In the Romance languages the adjective in some cases precedes, in other cases follows its noun. In German and English it always precedes.

When one noun signifies the possessor, origin or outcome of another by an anatropic post-position or case ending, the former should use its attachment by immediately preceding the latter. This is so in Turkish, Hindustani, German and English, but in Greek and Latin the two were not uncommonly divorced. In the Romance languages a preposition (*de*) has been substituted for the possessive, or genitive case ; and this construction is commonly used in Danish and English as an alternative to the use of the possessive case. In Arabic and Persian the described catatropically precedes its description, the connexion between the two being signified in Arabic by the transfer of the definite article to the description, and in Persian by a connecting vowel.

It is interesting to contrast the syntaxes of *comparison* in the languages from which we have been drawing illustrations, since the methods that are employed illustrate very strikingly the evolution of thought from sensation. " John is taller than William " may be expressed as " taller from William ", " taller as William ", or " taller to William ", according as we mentally turn our eyes from William to John, or identify the two in the quality of height (*i.e.* regard them simultaneously), or turn our eyes from John to William. The first method is apparently the more ancient : " fromness " in the standard of comparison may be indicated catatropically by a preposition (as in Arabic and Persian), anatropically either by a post-position (as in Turkish and Hindustani), or a case ending (as in Sanskrit). This construction is also followed (with a case ending) in Greek and Latin : but an alternative method was also used, in which the compared and the standard of comparison were *identified* with one another, the identification being signified by a particle meaning " as ". This is the practice in German. The Romance languages also identify the two through *que*, unless the comparison is between numbers, when they are linked catatropically by the connective *de*. The English " than " was, it seems, primitively " then ", and indicates a turning from the compared to that with which it is compared.

As a language develops there is a tendency to substitute ancillary ascriptions—that is to say dependent sentences—for descriptive words, since attributes can be defined, and timed, with more detail in a sentence, than through the agglomeration of a string of words, as in Sanskrit, or the use of participles that is so characteristic of Greek and Latin. The qualities of a subject, its possessor, origin and outcome, purpose and method, time and place are, therefore, commonly attached to it through dependent ascriptions. These are also used to express in detail an object when this is something that is felt, thought or said, as, for instance, " he thought that he had better go ". The ancillary ascription may be linked to its subject either consecutively, or through identification. The English connective " that " illustrates the former ; " as " the latter method. " He said that he would go " links his words on to his speech in sequence ; the vulgar " he said as he would go " identifies them with an indefinite *something* that is implied in *saying*. In Latin *ut* (akin to *aut*) was commonly used as an identifying connective. But there are descriptive particulars—such as those of possession and place for instance—which a dependent ascription cannot express unless its connective be itself inflected : the word *qui* (closely resembling the Turkish connective *keh*, and the Persian *kih*) was used as an inflected identifying connection, that is to say, as a *relative* pronoun or conjunction. It passed into the Romance languages. In German and English the utterance *qu* is represented by *w* or *wh* (*welcher* or *who*). But in both these languages combination in sequence is commonly preferred to identification, as the instrument for connecting the subject of a descriptive sentence with something preceding—*der* and *that* being used instead of relative pronouns.

Dependent sentences that are reasoning (*therefore* or *because*) hypothetical (*if* or *unless*) or restrictive (*but* and *although*) stand upon a different footing. They are part and parcel of the chain of ascriptive thought, and have already been reviewed in that connection.

Colloquial and literary styles.—The form in which we express thoughts in words may differ very widely from that which first presents itself. We can review various words and phrases, can make trial of them, and may reject or accept them. This faculty appears at first sight to be altogether incompatible with the view that thought progresses according to definite laws. But, in fact, it merely shows that one current of word-ideas can set up, or " induce ", other currents through familiarities of association or identities. The stream of thought follows certain laws : it is accompanied by ideas of words that have become intimately linked to the thoughts, and, if we use these words, we express ourselves colloquially. Words may, indeed, sometimes fail us, and there is a shock that stimulates an effort to hunt for them. But, generally, each thought is accompanied by the words that are its habitual associates. These words can originate a second " induced " current of words and phrases through ties either of familiarity, or of resemblance in meaning, sound or consonantal articulation. The effect of familiarity is illustrated very clearly by the " stock expressions ", or *clichés*, that occur to one when thinking of a subject : the thought of an illustration recalls the words " for instance " ; the thought of an objection suggests the deprecatory " if one may be permitted to say so " ; the sea announces itself grandiloquently as " the briny element ". Identity of meaning may present " depart " as an alternative to " go away " : identity of sound enables " fire " to recall " inspire " : identity of articulation suggests " brief " as accordant with " blessed ". Rhyme is, of course, resemblance in sound : alliteration resemblance in articulation. This induced current may provide us with a large number of alternative methods of expression, and so far it is true that we " think in words ". But in the background lies the natural procession of thoughts, each re-stimulating its successor ; and we owe our choices in expression to the similar re-stimulation of word-ideas by the word-ideas that are the habitual companions of the thoughts. The difference between the colloquial and literary, or sophisticated, language is, then, that in the former we use the words that offer themselves automatically, whereas in the latter we elaborate and polish our expressions by the use of other words and phrases that are recalled by their automatic accompaniments. There is, in fact, an evolution which illustrates the domination of spontaneity by the will.

The " induced " current of word ideas may differ very greatly indeed from the automatic, as when one thinks in his own and expresses himself in a foreign tongue. One who is acquainted with several languages has, therefore, the materials for several " induced " currents at his disposal. This is no sign of intellectual culture, for little children can often express themselves in two or three languages with facility. During the Middle Ages Latin was the European language of literary expression. But most of those who used it must have thought in their own vernacular, for which Latin was substituted by a rapid process of translation. Speech is an admirable faculty and there is therefore a tendency to elaborate and decorate it, and thus to produce an artificial, or " classical ", language, which may be very different from that of conversation. One may be well acquainted with colloquial Arabic and be quite unable to understand it in its literary form. Indeed, Arabic grammarians will insist that some of the most useful—and ancient—words in ordinary use *cannot* be written. There is a similar contrast between modern Greek as spoken and as used in journalism. This desire to obtain " preciosity " by refinement, assisted by a gush of patriotic sentiment, has led to the resuscitation of languages, such as Czech, and Erse, which were almost as dead as Cornish.

The impressive effect of a language (as of all forms of Art) depends greatly upon its spontaneity, and literature loses its vitality if it severs itself altogether from the speech of ordinary emotional life. We can then understand how a movement has come about, notably in America, to abandon literary form, and invigorate composition, not merely by phrasing it colloquially but by borrowing the " slang " that gives force to speech by stripping it of all polish. But it is still generally accepted that literature, to be an art, should involve skill in expression—that its phrasing, while of the same order as that of speech, should be more stylish—that is to say, more artificial. Its style is in some measure determined by the fashion of the day. But it is also influenced by profounder considerations—by appreciations of harmony in signification, sound and rhythm, which are the fruits of cultured sensibility. It is harmonious to use dignified words to express exalted thoughts, and, in phrasing sentences, to place words of leading importance where they will command attention. Rhyme and alliteration are harmonious. We think of them as the special instruments of the poet. But if we scrutinize mellifluous passages of prose, we shall be surprised to find how much use is made of them; Rhythm—that is to say, a regularly cadenced accentuation—is harmonious. We give effect to it, and are affected by it, in " well-balanced " sentences.

So far we have been referring to *technical* features of style. But there are also features of *sentimental* value which contribute immensely to its attractiveness. Ideas may stimulate *feelings*, and a writer can take advantage of this, not merely by direct appeals to emotion, but by the use of words which in themselves may possess no emotional power, but can, through associations and analogies, provoke little stirs of sentiment that pass across the current of thought like sunshine and shadow on a stream. So the lecturer's pointer becomes an enchanter's wand which charms while it teaches. This sentimental allusiveness is admirably illustrated by the *Essays of Elia.*

The development of writing and of the alphabet.—The use of marks to signify vocal and articulated sounds was a discovery far more difficult than the use of sounds to express ideas. It appears to have been unknown to the Greeks of Homer's days, although it was then already long established in Egypt and Mesopotamia. There are many peoples of the present day—far removed from savagery—who owe their first acquaintance with writing to missionary influences of quite modern date. The letters that have been used in Europe from the earliest days to the present—even the *runes* of Scandinavia —were borrowed from Semitic peoples—Phœnicians, Hebrews or Arabs—who had settled on the shores of the Mediterranean. Indeed the word " alphabet " is of Semitic origin. Writing is so striking and useful an accomplishment that a conquering nation has not hesitated to learn from those whom it has humiliated. The Sumerians—a people of apparently Turkish affinities who inhabited Mesopotamia as far back as history can take us—used the characters known as " cuneiform ". They were conquered by an Arab race who adopted the Sumerian characters for the writing of their own language. Some five millenia later, the Turks, on conquering the

Arabs, adopted the Arabic characters for the writing of Turkish. How curiously this illustrates the flux and reflux of history !

The simplest method of writing a word is to make a picture of the idea which it represents. The hieroglyphics of Egypt, the cuneiform of Mesopotamia, and the ideographs of China can be traced to this " pictographic " origin. Outlines, as we have seen, can be imitated, or " followed ", by movements of the arm and fingers : such imitations are largely used by the deaf and dumb in communicating with one another. It could easily have been discovered by accident or in play, that imitative movements could trace themselves upon a surface—as that of sand, for instance— and, when things were once pictured, the usefulness of the designs would be realized. The drawings could soon be abbreviated into signs, each of which would be associated with a word. But, until words were analyzed into syllables and letters, it would be necessary to have a separate sign for each word in the language.

This analysis came about through the accumulating consequences of a mental process—that of isolation through comparison—which has already been described in Section III. To give a fanciful illustration : The syllable *ti* can be isolated from *tiger* because it also occurs in the different word *tidy*, and the *t* can be isolated from *ti* because it also occurs in the different syllable *to*. The letters would be named from striking words that commenced with them. We get the word " alphabet " from the Semitic names for an ox (*alif*) and a tent (*beth*). But they would represent sounds, not ideas, and writing became phonographic instead of pictographic.

When words had thus been broken up into their component sounds, a phonographic system of writing could be invented directly, and without reference to pictographic signs. For there is an analogy between an utterance and a mark, in the both are the *consequences of movement*. In very ancient days marks were used to particularize the ownership, or makership, of things, to signify numbers and as *aide-memoires*. In this form they had no connection with *sounds*. But the process of marking, once invented, could be used to symbolize vocal articulations if the resemblance between movement and articulation was apprehended. Resting upon analogies of movement, marks could not be used for vowels, and it is a curious fact that in some languages—Arabic, for instance—the vowel signs are outside the written alphabet. The *Ogam* inscriptions that occur on memorial stones in Southern Ireland (and in Kent), use dots and dashes to signify sounds, as does the Morse code of signals. They are generally attributed to Irish invention, but are more probably

Scandinavian. Ireland was extensively colonized by Scandinavian immigrants. The invention of Ogam is, however, more likely to have followed than to have preceded the adoption of the early Runic characters of Scandinavia. These were apparently derived from Mediterranean sources—the outcome of the ancient connection between Scandinavia and the Ægean through the amber trade, and through the southward migration of Northmen to obtain profitable service. It was, indeed, to a body-guard of Scandinavians that the Byzantine emperors owed their safety during several centuries.

PART V

EXPERIENCE AND EDUCATION

The fruits of experience are commonly held to be knowledge, and the dexterities of action and utterance that are our " accomplishments ". But in reality they are much more than this. For it is through experience that the highest of our faculties grow into existence—our powers of thinking and willing, our varied tastes, and our emotional appreciations such as admiration and faith. Experience is, then, creative as well as associative. And in its associative phase it extends further than may appear. For we owe to it, not merely our muscular and mental associations—our habits, manners, morals and knowledge—but the sentimental associations between certain persons, things or ideas and particular feelings—the attachments and repugnances that are of far more importance than knowledge or skill in orientating our lives. We are born into life ; but we are nurtured into humanity. Our foster-mother is experience.

We gain experience indirectly as well as directly. Education is indirect experience. When we learn from another we imitatively " borrow " his experience and apply it to ourselves. So a child learns that fire burns, without actually suffering the pain of being burnt. Experience, may, accordingly, be defined as the effects of life in the development of faculties and the construction of memorial and sentimental associations—effects which may come about either directly or through imitative borrowing from others.

1 Evolution through Experience

The growth of an animal from its birth to maturity is obviously affected by its experience, since its development is checked or marred if its food or environment is unsuitable. So far, experience is involved in the material evolution of all living organisms but the very simplest. But, amongst the humbler animals, its influence upon the evolution of motives and capacities is inconsiderable. They come into the world equipped with faculties that are efficient from the hour of birth, and with ready-made memorial concatenations which regulate their lives with machine-like precision. These may have ultimately sprung from the effects of ancestral experience, slowly operating through the course of ages, possibly under the nervous shock of cataclysmic changes of climatic and other conditions which stimulated abnormal energy. But, once acquired, they were stamped upon the organism hereditarily, so that it is practically enslaved by them. As we ascend the animal kingdom, there is a gain of freedom. A bird can learn infinitely more than a reptile. But all animals except man are obsessed by hereditary instincts that limit their capacities of learning. A young cuckoo, although nurtured by hedge-sparrows, develops the habits and utterances of its kind. Man is, however, born almost free. A baby can be taught any language, any manners, any religion that you please. And since its accomplishments are not opposed by any innate promptings, it feels the pride of success in acquiring them, and will voluntarily practise them of itself. There are, then, before it almost unlimited possibilities of development.

There is nothing more wonderful in Nature than the development of man from primitive savagery to civilization. It is a peculiar " artificial " phase of evolution. The evolution of species has been accompanied by changes in their physical organization. The civilization of man is attended by no such changes. Between the primitive savage and the highest representative of modern culture there do not seem to be any *specific* differences of body or mind. Yet the gulf that separates them is even wider than is commonly realized. For current theories as to man's most primitive condition underrate the simplicity from which he has sprung. It is vaguely surmised, for instance, that his original home was Egypt or Mesopotamia. But such suppositions are absolutely contradicted by indisputable inferences that can be drawn from his bodily constitution. The character of his teeth, and the inordinate length of his intestine, demonstrate that he is naturally a vegetarian, living on fruits and soft roots. His " Garden of Eden " must, therefore, have been situated in a locality where these are in season all the year round. His skin is unprotected against changes of temperature. His original home must, accordingly, have enjoyed a warm equable climate. He could hardly have learnt the use of fire except through accidental experiences of the effect of hot lava streams ; and his acquaintance with navigation must, it seems, have been forced upon him by changes in sea level which compelled him to cross the water in order to keep in touch with his food, or his friends. It follows that his birthplace was a volcanic region in the tropical seas—such as Polynesia or the Malay archipelago. In the latter have been discovered the fossil remains of the ape which most resembles man ; and there still exists, in the ourang-utang, the nearest of man's brute relations. Amongst the present inhabitants of Polynesia there are types, such as the Maori, which are physically on a par with the European. And there are arguments to show that Polynesian civilization, such as it is, goes back to immense antiquity. Polynesia is, it appears, the home of three most peculiar customs— that of tattooing, circumcision and the " couvade ", under which on the birth of a child its father takes to his bed and is fed like an infant. In Polynesia, savage decorative art has attained its highest development : the carved ornamentation of canoes, for example, shows a finished intricacy of design which can hardly be surpassed by the skill of modern Europe. And Polynesia is a centre from which America as well as Asia could have been colonized.

It is owing to his extraordinary adaptability that man has been able to wander and settle over most of the globe—that he inhabits the interior of Africa and the Arctic circle. And it is clear that his ubiquity is at least as ancient as the glacial epoch of geology. For the palæolithic remains of the Ice-age are plainly those of the Eskimos of the day—of wanderers from more favoured centres of population. They tell as no more of the civilization that had been attained in more hospitable regions than we could learn in present-day Greenland of the culture of Italy.

Man's vagrant propensities have probably been the cause of the variations that have differentiated the human species into " races of mankind ". There are reasons to infer that, over a long course of years, differences in soil, temperature, climate, and other factors of unknown nature, produce racial changes both in appearance and character. For, in spite of the complications that are caused by immigration and inter-breeding, the inhabitants of particular regions exhibit a generally prevalent uniformity of type. Tallness of stature, lightness of hair and complexion, and energy of willed control are, for instance, associated with the Baltic ; shortness, dark hair and complexion, and emotional excitability with the Mediterranean countries of Europe ; the Negro type with Central Africa, the Mongolian with Central Asia. A similar localization of type is to be observed amongst animals and birds. There are in India three kinds of hare, and two kinds of florican, each confined to a definite region of its own : the Burmese peacock differs in its colouring from that of India. The influence of environment operates very slowly—so slowly as hardly to be detected during historical times. But it is illustrated very clearly by the changes that occur in sheep that have been introduced from England into Australia and South America ; and, amongst mankind, by the very marked difference of type between Australians and New Zealanders. In Europe the effect of migration has been obscured by inter-breeding. There has been a constant flow of population from the North to the South. The ruling classes of the ancient Greeks and Romans are believed to have been Northerners who descended upon the Mediterranean, as did the Normans of later days. Amidst Mediterranean surroundings both streams of immigrants lost their northern characteristics. The Goths, who appeared on the Danube shortly after the commencement of our era, were a Scandinavian people, as is shown by the Gothic translation of the Bible that was made in the fourth century by the missionary Ulfilas. They conquered and colonized Italy and Spain. But, although traces of Scandinavian character may still be found in the inhabitants of these countries, the type has practically disappeared. It is, however, impossible to determine how far these changes can be attributed to environment, since they assuredly resulted largely from inter-marriage. For, although, under the law discovered by Mendel, a type may occasionally assert itself in purity amongst the offspring of mixed parentage, racial characters become submerged by cross-breeding. The Scandinavian characteristics are, for instance, far less prominent on the east coast of Denmark than upon the west, owing to the effect in race-mixture of the maritime trade of Copenhagen. In London they have been diluted almost out of existence. But we must not deny that locality and climate affect the human body and character because their influence is obscured by the inter-action of another cause.

Judging from their capacity for inter-breeding it is probable that all the races of mankind have evolved from a single source, which gave rise to two well-marked stocks—the one straight-haired and thin-lipped, the other crinkly-haired and thick-lipped. It is noticeable that both these stocks are represented in the South Sea Islands,

2 Self-acquired and Imitative Experience

Could experience only be acquired directly, man's advance would be limited by the possibilities of a single life period. But the poverty of his innate endowments is made up to him by his extraordinary imitative powers. We learn by imitation. We acquire dexterities by copying another's movements, as when one watches a professional at golf. We gain knowledge from another by connecting ideas together as they are connected by his words—spoken or written. We contract prejudices by associating with certain ideas likes and dislikes that are aroused in us by another's words. These imitations in thought and feeling are, of course, involuntary, or spontaneous. We have seen that imitation may be spontaneous as well as deliberate. Children involuntarily " pick up " the manners and accents of those around them. But this spontaneous mimicry develops into deliberate, or effortful, imitation, under the law to which we have so often referred. Learning, when deliberate, involves effort. This may be re-stimulated, as an optimistic ambition, by an idea of success ; but, generally, it is stimulated by a discord—the fear of reproach, humiliation or punishment, or the apprehension of failure. For those who do not associate success with learning the more unpleasant of these discords is alone effective. " *La crainte est le commencement de la sagesse* ".

We habitually under-rate the educational effect of our imitative faculties—and traduce our birth-right of freedom—by attributing to "instinct " the promptings which are, in fact, those of acquired habit. We think that our habits of body and mind are inborn because we forget the process of their acquirement. Our earliest memories rarely carry us back beyond the age of four, and by this time a child has become engrained with most of the habits that distinguish man from the brute. It has learnt to eat and to speak : it has become accustomed to wear clothes, and has acquired the manners of civilized behaviour and notions of decency. There are two facts which demonstrate the poverty of man's inherited endowments—firstly, that children that are brought up in bestial surroundings are practically inhuman ; and, secondly, that mankind may be thrown back from civilization into barbarism by such a catastrophe as the fall of the Roman Empire. This, it may be remarked, was no isolated reversion. The researches of archæology have brought to light a succession of civilizations of high order, most of which have passed into obliteration. What is left of the Sumerian, Hittite and Babylonian civilizations—of the culture of Knossos and Mycenæ? During more than three centuries Roman civilization had a footing in England. Hardly a trace of it remains. These reversions are very disconcerting to those who would believe in the continuity of human progress. But they are the natural results of man's innate freedom. The strings by which he is controlled are mostly of his own making. He can, therefore, break them.

Education is, then, the transmitting force upon which the artificial evolution of man depends for its continuity : and, until writing was invented, the progress of the past was lost if a generation was left untaught. Civilization may, in fact, be compared to a chain of cameos, of increasing complexity of design, each of which is attached to its predecessor by a link. The cameos represent the accumulated attainments of each generation : the links represent the educational influences through which each generation takes over the attainments of its forefathers. If a link is broken, the cameos that precede it are lost. Or we may liken the civilizations of the past to a succession of forest-clearings which were cultivated for a time and then relapsed into jungle—owing to the destructiveness of war, to catastrophes of Nature, to plagues, or to a loss of energy that resulted from spiritual decadence.

3 Creative Experience

We give this name to experience when it has the effect, not merely of forming muscular, mental or sentimental associations, but of bringing *faculties* into existence. It is a surprising reflection that the most " human " of our capacities are not inborn but acquired— amongst them the *will*, which is commonly considered the most exalted of our endowments. To develop this conclusion some recapitulation will be necessary. We must briefly review the capacities that are undoubtedly inborn in us, endeavouring to distinguish them according as they originate from the feminine or the masculine elements in our nature, or from inter-actions between the two.

Both elements, being nervous energies, possess, we may feel assured, the faculty of receiving impressions : indeed, the masculine germ in its free condition exhibits activities which could only be directed by sensory susceptibilities of some sort. Our analysis of the conditions under which conscious perception comes into being, seems to show that susceptibility to environal stimuli through the sense-organs is a feminine characteristic, whereas it is through masculine emotion that sense-impressions become transformed into conscious sensations. It follows that in the process of objective perception the masculine horizon is limited by the feminine—that the masculine is susceptible, not to external stimuli directly, but to their effects upon the feminine. When, for instance, we are affected by music, it would be the feminine that receives vibrations, and the masculine that transforms them into sounds. Subjective conditions, on the other hand, generate conscious ideas through the inter-action of the feminine. We may assume that, as nervous energies, both elements possess the faculty of repeating past experiences under the re-stimulating influence of conditions that have previously accompanied these experiences—the faculty that is the source of memory, habit, muscular dexterity and of intelligence. Both elements certainly possess the capacity of producing muscular movements. Those of the feminine are the purposeful, or practical, movements of approach and recoil, to which we owe the instinctive detachment of outside impressions from ourselves and their externalization by being attached to their causes. Those of the masculine are efforts, and expressions of emotion, which are primitively purposeless. Movements may also be instinctively imitative. In this case they are prompted by the process of associative re-stimulation : the sensation of a movement prompts the movement. If, as we have conjectured, external sensation is a feminine capacity, imitative movements originate from the feminine side. This conclusion is borne out by their unemotional character. A like peculiarity marks *habit* as a feminine product. It is passionlessly practical—the very antithesis of emotion. Within the body there dwell, then, two " familiar spirits " which urge it in different directions. Or, changing the metaphor, we are as marionettes, with strings that are pulled by two different operators—redeemed, however, from mechanical subservience by the fact that we may be taught by education and experience to respond to one more sensitively than to the other.

The feminine element is specially characterized by the two conditions of attractedness and repelledness—the conditions of which we are conscious as likes and dislikes, or inclinations. The stimuli which *innately* rouse them are comparatively few and simple— the things which satisfy such appetitive cravings as hunger, thirst and lust, the harmonious and the familiar, the discordant and the strange, and a few poignant sensory experiences. But their range is capable of indefinite extension through a feminine capacity of vast importance—that of forming new inclinations under the masculine influence of pleasure and displeasure. A thing which gives pleasure or displeasure becomes a stimulus of like or dislike. We owe to this elastic susceptibility the multitude of acquired tastes that differentiates civilization from savagery.

The masculine element asserts itself in the two-phased (expansive or contractive) energy of emotion, of which we are conscious as pleasure and displeasure, exhilaration and depression. Pleasure and displeasure are masculine reactions to the effects of passing sensory impressions. Exhilaration and depression are conditions of a more enduring nature—phases of a standing " head " of emotional energy to which we owe the *activity* of our lives. It is acutely affected by the pleasure or displeasure that is generated by sensory impressions, and, when strongly excited, it has a remarkable effect upon the course of thought, throwing it into an imaginative phase, in which individuals are created out of qualities.

Other innate endowments arise from antagonistic reactions between the two elements. From contrariness in their conditions springs the irritation of anger, the forcefulness of spontaneous courage and desire, the intensifications of emotion experienced in the joy of success, the sorrow of failure and the pleasure of amusement, and, most notable of all, the muscular manifestation of energy in effort. From the *union* of the two elements may proceed the mysterious faculty of consciousness—that condition which obscures by its unity the duality of our nature—which stands apart from both feminine and masculine, and can, therefore, observe the action of both. In the form of a vague awareness of pleasure and pain this may exist before ideas give it a reflective turn. A baby shows consciousness of comfort and discomfort before it can have acquired any definite ideas. In this vague condition, consciousness may be possessed by animals of low organization.

Upon these innate foundations experience builds up a number of artificial structures. The most elaborate of them is the edifice of our ideas. These, it has been shown, are all ultimately derived from impressions that we receive through the senses or by self-conscious apprehension. Apart from experience, the mind is idealess—that is to say, the mind can hardly be said to exist at all. Without ideas there can be no thought. Accordingly, we owe to experience not only our capacity for rational (or practical) thought, but the current of emotional changes which are re-stimulated by thoughts and give our reflections a sentimental, as opposed to a practical, complexion.

Another remarkable artificiality is the changeable variety of our tastes, whether in food, dress or amusements. These arise from refinements of sensibility that are developed by practice or from associations that are brought about by trial, imagination or accident. They are primarily subjective pleasures, which are externalized by being attached to their causes. This is an instinctive process. But the tastes themselves are generated by experience.

It is innate in us to suffer nervous discord, for this is the inevitable consequence of duality. The effects of discord in intensifying emotion and energizing effort can then be traced to a susceptibility that is inborn. It is an emotional, or masculine, characteristic, to respond to a shock by a muscular effort. This is the ultimate origin of the will. Until thought has come into existence, effort is merely a struggle, although it may be guided by associations between sensory impressions and muscles that have been formed by successful experiences. With the formation of ideas a new kind of discord comes into being—that between an *idea* and a nervous condition of feeling. An *idea* of an inclination is formed, and until the idea is realized there is the mental discord of discontent. This is the origin of effortful *desire*. But a further complication must come about before this one-idea'd impulse passes into the broader and more comprehensive effort that is involved in willing. The effort must be led by ideas of success or failure, which give its vision a wider scope. These ideas can, however, only arise from experience. There can be no notions of success or failure until they have actually been achieved or suffered. Volition is, then, the offspring of experience : and we can understand why it sets itself against spontaneity and gradually overcomes it. In its origin it is masculine. But it readily submits itself to the influence of feminine inclinations. So it develops into prudence and the faculty of deliberate deceit.

Fostered by the very regularity of life which it produces, prudence has entirely changed man's character. It has domesticated him by bridling his emotions. But, if it raises him in one way, it lowers him in another. It dulls his noblest aspirations : it sets before him an inferior set of values ; and it appears actually to be diminishing his reproductive powers. It is paradoxical, but seems to be true, that mankind becomes emasculated by an undue predominance of feminine influence.

Our emotional susceptibilities—our feelings of admiration, respect, faith, pity and contempt—are also the creations of experience. For they arise from our associating with certain qualities feelings of " ex-revulsive ", or spiritual, pleasure or displeasure which, under the influence of the feminine element, dispose us towards, or away from, their possessors. But these " ex-revulsive " feelings are, in fact, re-stimulations of emotional *crises* that follow success and failure, and these *crises* could not be experienced unless we had actually won or lost. Nor could the all-powerful notions of superiority and inferiority come into existence until we had enjoyed the one or suffered the other. These notions are not, then, ingrained in our nature, but acquired by experience, and we have an explanation of the remarkable fact that their influence upon man varies with the stage of his culture. The resentment of inferiority, which we call individual, class or national " self-consciousness ", is far more apparent in our time than in the more submissive, less critical, days of the past, when men accepted authority—and even slavery— with an unquestioning resignation that to us seems pathetic.

4 Associative Experience

We do not recognize the extent to which memory—the automatic re-stimulation of past experiences—enters into our lives. It is through memory, we all admit, that a string of words is repeated " by heart ", and we cannot deny that the rapid movements of a pianist's fingers are memorial when he is playing " from memory ". But it is less easy to realize that habits are, in fact, memories, that it is memory that holds us to conventional manners and morals, that we follow the usages of society because we " remember " them just as we work hard because we have acquired industrious habits. And it is still more difficult to understand that our beliefs and prejudices —even such important matters as nationality and religion—actually rest upon a memorial basis. Yet it is evident that we possess all these associations because they have been instilled into us, and that, although their acquisition may involve effort, their retention becomes automatic. And we know that they can be lost altogether through a sudden catastrophic " lapse of memory ".

These associations that become engrained in us by experience may be distinguished as muscular, moral, inclinational or emotional, and mental. Of the first class are all our actions and utterances but the simplest and crudest ; and it is, indeed, by no means clear that man's erect attitude is not *acquired*. It is through the association of muscular experiences with sight that our eyes give us impressions of distance and solidity. The learning of these accomplishments may be no easy matter, and may involve strenuous repetition, as will be appreciated by watching the tentative efforts of a baby. For they rest upon accuracy of co-ordinated re-stimulation in a number of different sets of nerves : in playing tennis, for instance, the visual perspective of a moving ball must re-stimulate movements of the body and hand that are precisely the same in direction, timing and strength as those which have succeeded on a previous occasion with a ball in like condition. Men vary in their capacity for co-ordinated restimulation. The difference between skill and clumsiness is, then, in fact that between good and bad memorial powers of a particular kind. And since skill is acquired by effort, and successful effort gives the exhilaration of pride, dexterity of any kind re-stimulates admiration—that is to say, is naturally attractive.

Moral associations include all manners and customs which are conventional, and are not the " heart-felt " products of admiration or idealism. They are, so to speak, " habits of body ". Such of them as are merely expressive may be " picked up ". But most of them involve some measure of self-control, and need an effort for their acquirement, although they soon pass into the automatic stage. Discipline begins with the repression of physical inclinations that are inopportune : it grows as it is practised, and becomes a habit that can fight down fear, and even repress anger from showing itself. Submission to the law comes to us through being inculcated : it becomes so habitual that the most tempting theft, the most excusable violence, are put aside as " not done ". Industry and punctuality must be *learnt*. When habitual they may become so insistent as to be eccentric obsessions.

By inclinational and emotional associations are meant " habits of mind "—the beliefs that underlie our attachments, affections, and convictions. We recognize their artificiality in calling them " bents of mind ". They arise from the association of like or dislike (which may be practical or emotional) with particular objects—a connection that may be formed by the words of a teacher as well as by actual experience. They originate, therefore, not from effort, but from feeling. But they are conserved by the force of habit. Such are our loyalties and prejudices—perhaps the most influential of all our motives. It is through memorial association that our faith remains constant in religion, king and country, as well as in our private attachments. And it is, of course, purely through memorial association that certain symbols affect us emotionally—the national anthem and flag for example.

It is easy to acquire habits of body and mind—that is to say, manners and beliefs. Children pick up with great facility the behaviour and opinions of those around them. But when these associations have once been formed, it is exceedingly difficult to modify or reconstruct them. Having become familiar, they oppose themselves to change almost as obstinately as inherited instincts. It is a curious paradox that the consequences of experience resist any experience that would disconcert them, and also any reasoning that is based upon experience—or " common sense ", as we call it. They will give way to it only upon conditions—that it hold out offers of sensory gratification, material advantage, or social distinction. Hence, amongst peoples of simple tastes, who believe that distinction comes rather from inherited position or personal character than from wealth or display, manners and beliefs may remain unaltered during centuries. On the other hand, in a society which has developed tastes for luxury and amusement, and is permeated with the profit-seeking spirit, old-fashioned customs and prejudices dissolve very rapidly indeed. During the last two generations the life and mentality of Europe have undergone more change than in the five centuries preceding. Quite recent history has given us a striking illustration of the dissolving effect of profit upon prejudice. Whilst France and England were, generally, bitter against Germany, merchants of both countries were endeavouring to trade with her.

Habits of body and mind will, however, also yield to idealistic enthusiasm. They go down before the gusts of emotional feeling which convert individuals and revolutionize societies, and breathe a dramatic spirit into conventional life. So the Arabs became changed by the doctrines of Muhammed, the English by Puritanism, the French by the self-assertive iconoclasm of the 18th century. Similarly, if truth be idealized, it can prevail against prejudice even when it is unaided by material considerations. But truth is not generally an object of enthusiastic admiration.

Mental associations constitute " knowledge ". For this is a tissue of potential *liaisons* that connect a vast number of subjects with attributes of quality or condition, origin or outcome, purpose, method, place, time, identity, resemblance, difference or quantity. They have all originated as ascriptions that have been made under the influence of direct observation or of another's words. But, once constituted, they persist as potentialities of being re-stimulated through association or analogies.

T

5 Education

It is an obvious reflection that, since the evolution of human culture depends upon education for its continuity, it is possible through education to control its course. We need not passively accept the trend of environal influences. The ideas from which sprung, for instance, the disciplined self-control of the Spartans and the Puritans deflected the course of history. But they were idealistic discoveries that lay off the track of man's ordinary life, and gained ground because they were systematically impressed upon the young. The effect of these idealistic cross-currents has by no means been always beneficial. But the mere fact that they run counter to evolution is not of itself against them. For evolution may run backwards as well as forwards—towards parasitic degeneracy as well as towards increasing energetic efficiency. The obsessing influence of prudential motives is, for example, the natural evolutionary consequence of material civilization. Prudence has its advantages. Few, however, will deny that it involves a loss of " value " in life—a step on the down-hill path to decadence. What can a nation do that is more *prudent*—or more dangerous—than to employ foreign mercenaries to fight its battles for it ? Prudence is enfeebling in that it stifles emotion. It must be infused with idealism ; and it is only through education that we can hope so to leaven it.

Education, of course, includes much more than the instruction that is received at school or college. The most enduring of educational influences are those of the home. We are haunted throughout life by the impressions of childhood. Thanks to its mother, a child of six is already quite " civilized ". Were it not indeed for the instructive solicitude of maternal love, man would never have raised himself much above the ape. There is, moreover, an " atmosphere " in home life that infects us, quite apart from the ideas, language and manners with which we are instilled. It may breathe into us religious sentiments that are rarely stifled by after-experiences, and certain attitudes towards life and society that are as persistent. An Oriental, however Europeanized at school and college, can rarely assimilate the European respect for women. One who has been brought up in Puritan discipline is harassed through life by qualms of conscience. He may defy them—clergymen's sons are not the most moral of men—but he never achieves the light-hearted irresponsibility of the true hedonist. In a commercial atmosphere one absorbs the spirit of profit-getting. There is nothing in the Jewish character that is *instinctively* directed towards money-making, and large classes of the Jewish sect are quite uncommercial in their sympathies. But to " spoil the Egyptians " has been the natural ambition of men who have been despised and ostracized, and hence the atmosphere of Jewish families has been very generally that of usury. There is a precisely parallel case in India, where one caste has for centuries been so closely identified with close-fisted commerce that it is customary to speak of its " instinct " for money-making. As civilization becomes more and more material a *bourgeois* atmosphere spreads into the most aristocratic families and into the highest political circles. On the other hand, in families whose tone is artistic or idealistic, children retain their primitive sensibilities, and throughout life cannot be sobered into the disposition that is called " matter of fact ".

It is true that some children react against their home influences in a spirit of antagonism. But, speaking generally, we can hardly escape from the effects of these first associations. They are the foundations of the Temple of Life. We build upon them with materials that are drawn from our educational experiences in the narrower sense of the term—from the lessons that we learn at school and college. In reviewing these we may conveniently maintain the distinction that has been drawn between creative and assertive experiences.

The creative effects of education.—The processes of combination, comparison and deduction, by which ideas are formed, can be impelled by ascriptions that are expressed by other persons. Our conception of " distance ", for example, is *evolved* by comparing a number of pairs of objects that are separated from one another, and isolating the quality of " apartness ". It is *taught* by ascribing distance as the condition which keeps two objects apart. In this fashion teaching and reading rapidly impart to us ideas which it cost our forefathers much time and trouble to conceive.

Of purely sensory tastes, such as those for delicacies of the table, luxuries and comforts, the less acquired during youth the better. For they are clogs upon the spirit of adventure in which one should enter upon life's campaign. But it is all to the good that a liking for bodily exercise should be cultivated. And those who can contract an interest in natural history insure themselves against dullness in after life.

Whatever be the defects of the boarding-school system, there can be no doubt that it strengthens power of will. It is a tremendous experience for a boy to be suddenly transplanted from the secure familiarity of home life into a strange and alien environment where the exercise of determination and self-control is necessary for self-protection. According to my own very considerable experience of young men, some educated at public schools, others with a less definite break with home life, the former can be more generally depended upon for discipline and determination, although they may yield to the latter in intelligence and initiative.

It is often claimed for education that it improves the faculties of memory and intelligence. But this pretension cannot be accepted off-hand. For memory seems to be strongest during childhood, and gradually to weaken with advancing years. Are not the novels that delighted us in youth better remembered than those which relieve the boredom of middle age ? Devices for improving the memory act by substituting analogies for purely memorial associations—that is to say, by enlisting the aid of intelligence. This, we may repeat is the appreciation of samenesses—of analogies—between two different things which assimilate them, and may render them amenable to the same law—such as the analogy, for instance, which enables one to comprehend the causes of day and night by turning an orange round a candle. But men who have had no school education not infrequently possess very great intelligence. It is true, however, that some analogies are more difficult to grasp than others, and quickness in apprehending them can, it seems, be developed by practice. Mathematical identities and contrarieties, for instance, which to some minds are self-apparent, are very puzzling to others until they have become familiarized by study.

It is in the development of *emotional appreciations* that the creative power of education is most notable. These are of immense importance to our lives since they establish the " values " that we attach to particular qualities—that is to say, determine the qualities that will stimulate our admiration. They may strike us æsthetically or idealistically. Æsthetic appreciation is less spontaneous, more sophisticated, than idealistic, since it is swayed by the habit of fashion : it is also greatly affected by skill in technique, and this, being a voluntary accomplishment, takes many phases. Æsthetic judgment may, therefore, vary with the period and the locality. Music or painting that appeals to a Chinaman may, to a European, seem merely grotesque. Æsthetic appreciations are, then, so far artificial that they must be cultivated. It is none the less true that they add immensely to the happiness and resourcefulness of life.

Admiration is one of the most blissful of feelings, and Art provides charms for stimulating it. Education is very incomplete if it makes no attempt to introduce its pupils into a Garden of Delights which, however artificial in its origin, is very real in its effects upon us. This has now come to be generally recognized.

Idealistic appreciations are far less affected by the fashion of the day. For the qualities that arouse them are natural and spontaneous, not deliberate and artificial. Our appreciation of them is therefore an inborn faculty and, in developing it, education is creative only by accentuating points of excellence that would otherwise escape notice. Some of them, courage and justice for example, are obviously admirable. The strength of others, as of generosity and mercy, may not be so apparent. Education focusses our eyes upon it.

If these admirable qualities are associated with personalities, our admiration extends to their possessors. So we love God and honour the King. But, as ideals, they are admirable in themselves and possess the outstanding merit of being untarnishable by disillusionment. Our admiration for a person may be quenched by further acquaintance with him. But our admiration for a quality cannot be prejudiced by our experience of other qualities that conflict with it. We do not appreciate courage the less because we have unfortunate experiences of cowardice.

It is exhilarating to admire, and ideals, therefore, afford great happiness to those who are inspired by them. And, since admiration generates sympathetic feeling, idealism invigorates one with an energy that is stronger than will power, and can withstand the growing influence of the deliberate faculties. It is a remedy for the decadence that follows an over-development of prudence.

Some ideals are strongly emphasized in school life. Courage, emulation, and patriotism are vigorously instilled. They are useful to the State. The liberty of independence is extolled. It is the most effective argument for the democratic system of government. These ideals are all *strong*. But history shows that, when followed with blind enthusiasm, they bring countless miseries upon mankind. No such charge can be brought against the Christian ideals of harmony in loving-kindness, justice and gratitude, of self-control in honesty, purity, sincerity and humility, and of magnanimity in mercy, forgiveness, tolerance and generosity. They are harmless to others, if not actually beneficent. Yet they have only to be understood to be admired. What is more excellent than harmony, more powerful than self-restraint, more noble than self-restraint that is exercised for others ? Nevertheless, with the exception of honesty, they are relegated, so to speak, to a corner of the school curriculum—are treated as " Sunday " subjects and so lose " work-a-day " significance. Honesty is insisted upon, for it is essential for industrial life. But the other Christian virtues are presented rather as pious sentiments than as commanding principles of action, and for this reason do not take their place as ruling motives of life.

It may well be that they have suffered from their association with religion. For it is not conducive to the development of our noblest feelings that they should be ascribed to mysterious causes and not be recognized as our own ; or that their cult should be associated with the morality of the Old Testament, much of which breathes a spirit that contradicts them. And religious opinion is indisposed to admit the dramatic hyperbolism of such injunctions as " take no thought for the morrow ", which, if accepted as they stand, imply that idealism is irreconcilable with prudence and cannot be used, in Christ's own words, to " leaven " it. Religious authority cannot, then, be expected to promote the *rational* teaching of Christian morality. Yet it is only through its spread that our civilization can hope to escape the moral and material dangers that threaten it. Feelings of sympathy, self-abnegation and magnanimity can counteract the sterilizing effect of egotistical prudence, and are (as is now generally admitted) the only antidote against the bitterness that inevitably antagonizes employers and work-people when each regards the other as material to be exploited. There are, then, sound economic reasons for pressing them upon the admiration of both classes during the impressionable years of school life. These reasons are, however, by the way. For morality ceases to be idealistic when it looks for profit. But it may be profitable, nevertheless. Had the Peace of Versailles been tempered with magnanimity, Europe would not have been so long disorganized by apprehensions of revenge.

It may be objected that ideals cannot reliably contribute to the foundations of civilization inasmuch as they tend to fade away. It is true that admiration cannot maintain itself indefinitely at white heat, and that beauties which once transported us may lose all but " sentimental " interest. But idealism so far resembles prudence in that it can produce an enduring " habit of mind ", that will maintain its effect upon us even when enthusiasm has waned. That is to say, idealistic teaching affects us associatively as well as creatively.

The associative effects of education.—These arise from the action of education in putting on a *memorial* basis activities of body and mind that have originated through imitation, effort or emotion—that is to say, in converting activities into " aptitudes " by rendering them habitual. Thus a movement that can repeat itself accurately becomes a dexterity, behaviour becomes automatic as a habit, affections and beliefs are engrained as " bents of mind ", strings of thoughts and words present themselves without effort.

Most of the gifts that are necessary for success in life's work—whether in an art, a craft, a business or a profession—are actually dexterities of action or speech. They are acquired through technical, or vocational, training, which is as distinct from general education as labour is from life. In ancient days they were learnt in apprenticeships, and it is probable that this is a more efficient means of special training than courses of instruction in school or college. Dexterities also include the accomplishments of playing instruments, singing and painting, as well as skill at games. The associations, on which the *morals* and *manners* of life so greatly depend, are originally the products, either of a prudent regard for social well-being, of a desire for distinction, or of the idealistic admiration of some quality of mankind. But they are inculcated as undeniable obligations that need no arguments. The respect for vested interests in social position or property, that gives stability to civilization, maintains itself because it is impressed as a habit. Industry and discipline must have become habitual if they are to be enduring. Self-control can be cultivated by little acts of self-repression that in themselves are ridiculous. Prudence, of course, becomes habitual; and considering the facility with which it is picked up in our present-day atmosphere, unnecessary pains are taken to instil it into the young. Fortunately, the effect of such maxims as " Safety First " are counteracted in some measure by the influences of the cinema.

In addition to the conduct ordinarily called " moral ", school morality enjoins observances of " good form " which are even more imperative. Amongst them are the obligations to obey one's chief, or " captain ", and to subordinate oneself to the interests of the fellowship—the vital element in *esprit de corps*, so essential to " team-work ". This is a most admirable quality for the service of democratic government. For a party-leader is at ease if his followers are good " party-men " : his grossest errors will pass uncensured.

To acquire muscular aptitudes, morals and manners, some effort is ordinarily needed. Habits of mind, on the other hand, grow independently of the will. Respect for the king, consideration for one's family and friends, belief in one's religion are not " learnt " :

they are emotionally " imbibed " through admiration that is aroused by the suggestion of the teacher. They rapidly become habitual. Our reverence for Queen Elizabeth, Bacon, and Shakespeare is rather a habit of mind than an active emotion. These conventional beliefs are most useful instruments for giving solidarity to a nation or a class. People are not united unless in some measure they feel alike. They are unified if they admire the same national celebrities ; and, from the political point of view, biographers have good reason to conceal the shortcomings of their heroes. They are also unified by what is called the " social sense ". For this is the habitual acceptance of the approval or disapproval of one's fellows as the criterion of what is good or bad, and is to be considered as success or failure.

To impart the *mental associations* which constitute " knowledge " is the chief function of education as popularly understood. Knowledge may be appreciated from three points of view—the technical, the rational and the emotional (or " sentimental "). It is *technically* fruitful if it fits us for our special calling in life ; *rationally* fruitful if it enables us to interpret correctly the present, the past or the future ; *emotionally* if it intrigues, entertains, exalts or inspires us. In the first two cases it must be *true :* in the second case its truth is of little importance, since fiction may be as interesting, as amusing, or as inspiring, as actuality.

It is noticeable that the subjects of language and mathematics that occupy so large a share of school *curricula* are primarily *instruments* for acquiring knowledge. They become objects in themselves under the law which has so frequently been mentioned. Both being admirable attainments, are admiringly elaborated. Language becomes an art in itself, quite apart from its meaning ; and, as a succession of harmonies in voicing, pronouncing and spacing, develops into a kind of music. And mathematics, from being a simple instrument for measurement and calculation, grow into processes which possess the mysterious profundity of metaphysics, and seem to afford us magical glimpses of the real nature of things. But, in reality, its capacities are severely limited by the truth of the assumptions of fact upon which its comparisons are based. If these are incorrect, mathematical deductions from them must be incorrect also. Accordingly, since our acquaintance with the strength and endurance of materials is uncertain, engineers and architects must multiply their calculated quantities four or five times in order to provide for the " factor of safety " ; and we can understand how the Romans could have built so enduringly by " rule of thumb ", and how architecture that was almost innocent of arithmetic, could have achieved the triumph of a Gothic cathedral. Aviation, perhaps the most novel discovery of our own times, could obtain no assistance from mathematics until facts had been collected by actual experiences of flying. Its pioneers—the brothers Wright—have declared that " having set out with absolute faith in existing scientific *data*, we were driven to doubt one thing after another, until finally we cast it all aside, and decided to rely entirely upon our own investigations ". On the other hand, the success of mathematics in deducing from experience a series of complicated future happenings, does not of itself prove that its ultimate theories are correct. During centuries, astronomical calculations, which started from the delusion that the sun went round the earth, could nevertheless, predict eclipses accurately.

Languages and mathematics apart, the various branches of knowledge trespass upon one another's provinces so as to be hardly amenable to rigid classification. They may be divided into two groups according as the studies from which they proceed are concerned with man's faculties and attainments, or with his physical environment, including his bodily self—distinctions which roughly correspond to those between " the humanities " and " physics ". Of the first kind are theology, philosophy, psychology, logic, political economy, politics and history, of the second, the biological, electrical, chemical and mechanical sciences.

The value of " the humanities " is almost wholly emotional or sentimental. They are of little " practical " utility, since in their development generalizations which dignify human nature have been far more influential than the lessons of experience. Systems of theology vary from nation to nation—each being convinced that its own is true—and have been continually changing their dogmas. The conclusions of philosophy and psychology have always been discredited by irreconcilable differences of opinion between their various schools, and the frequency with which their doctrines change. Logic has hardly ventured to claim that it can improve the reasoning faculties. It is generally realized that political economy cannot be trusted in practical affairs : it consented to the blunders of the Peace of Versailles, and cannot judge for us authoritatively between protection and free trade. Political theories transport us only so long as they are in the air : put into harness, they are sadly halting. History, which might be the most useful of all the sciences, is generally directed to entertain, to flatter, or to vindicate the historian's prejudices. It is dramatic rather than scientific, and is seldom content to trace events to their causes by dispassionate analysis.   Much of it is consequently quite misleading. The character and behaviour of its personalities are rarely drawn to life, for the historian very naturally shrinks from besmirching the reputation of the dead, and from belittling those who are regarded as national heroes.

The physical sciences are rational so far as they classify facts, and draw inferences from them that are warranted by laws of experience or by incontrovertible analogies.   But when so limited to " matters of fact ", they lack " sentimental " interest, and do not afford a very wide field for mathematical treatment.   Men of science are consequently tempted to dignify or enlarge their subjects by generalizations that are imperfectly warranted by their experiments.   Scientific theories have, therefore, been constantly changing.   The doctrine of the Conservation of Energy, which a few years ago was unassailable, is now trembling to its fall.   Unless facts are sharply distinguished from theories, and the validity of the latter is appraised by strictly comparing them with the observations and laws from which they are deduced, the study of science is not more effective than that of theology in stimulating the reasoning faculty.

This brings us to the momentous question : Should boys be taught to *think ?*   Most schoolmasters would reply unhesitatingly in the affirmative.   But in practice they hardly act upon this opinion. For one thing, it is not easy to give reasons for all that their pupils are expected to believe ; and intelligent questions add greatly to the labour of teaching.   And there must always be an uncomfortable suspicion that intelligence is a dangerous possession.   It will refuse respect to those who are not really efficient : it is apt to judge men by their deeds instead of by their words : it shakes accepted beliefs by burrowing into their foundations, and imperils the reputation of acknowledged authorities : it will not even accept without question such popular ideals as those of liberty and democracy.   It consequently seems to threaten social stability by judging of things independently of class or national feelings.   On the other hand, we must remember that it is to individual originality that mankind owes whatever progress it has achieved—to intelligence that has been able to apprehend connecting analogies and to argue from them as to causes and consequences.   Faith, however useful as a buttress, cannot advance one inch on the past.   If, then, education is to lead and not merely maintain, it must give some play to the intelligence. The conclusions of science must be referred to the experiences upon which they are based and not merely taught as dogmas.   Their acceptance will then be intelligent. History should include a description of the authorities from which it is taken, with some discussion of their credibility. And if dogmatic religion withers under so critical an examination, its place can be taken by Christian idealism, for this rests upon foundations which reason cannot undermine, and possesses excellencies which reason must admit.

It is because education does not involve thought that its results have generally been disappointing. Not a few teachers will admit that youths, on leaving school, are less *intelligent* than when they entered it. Schooling has been compulsory in England for over half a century. Yet there is little to be perceived of a general rise of intelligence, or of more discrimination as to the journalistic and political food which the people enjoy. The curious paradox is explained that many of the most inventive, most artistic and wisest of mankind have had no school education worth the name. The conclusion seems inevitable that reasoning, while owing its materials to the teaching of experience, is not improved—may indeed be impaired—by the experience of being taught at school.

INDEX

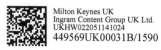